Physics for Surgeons

An Aid to the MRCS OSCE

Physical Examination for Surgeons

An Aid to the MRCS OSCE

Edited by

Petrut Gogalniceanu
Specialist Registrar in General Surgery, London Postgraduate School of Surgery, and Honorary
Clinical Lecturer, University College London, London, UK

James Pegrum
Specialist Registrar in Trauma and Orthopaedic Surgery, Oxford Deanery, Oxford, and Honorary
Clinical Lecturer, Queen Mary University of London Sports and Exercise Department, London, UK

William Lynn
Specialist Registrar in General Surgery, London Postgraduate School of Surgery, London, UK

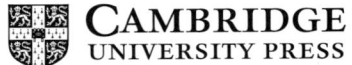

CAMBRIDGE
UNIVERSITY PRESS

University Printing House, Cambridge CB2 8BS, United Kingdom

Cambridge University Press is part of the University of Cambridge.

It furthers the University's mission by disseminating knowledge in the pursuit of education, learning and research at the highest international levels of excellence.

www.cambridge.org
Information on this title: www.cambridge.org/9781107625549

© Cambridge University Press 2015

This publication is in copyright. Subject to statutory exception and to the provisions of relevant collective licensing agreements, no reproduction of any part may take place without the written permission of Cambridge University Press.

First published 2015

Printed in the United Kingdom by TJ International Ltd. Padstow Cornwall

A catalogue record for this publication is available from the British Library

Library of Congress Cataloging-in-Publication Data
Physical examination for surgeons : an aid to the MRCS OSCE / [edited by] Petrut Gogalniceanu, James Pegrum, William Lynn.
   p. ; cm.
ISBN 978-1-107-62554-9 (Paperback)
I. Gogalniceanu, Petrut, editor. II. Pegrum, James, editor. III. Lynn, William, 1982-, editor.
[DNLM: 1. General Surgery–methods–Case Reports. 2. General Surgery–methods–Problems and Exercises. 3. Physical Examination–methods–Case Reports. 4. Physical Examination–methods–Problems and Exercises. 5. Signs and Symptoms–Case Reports. 6. Signs and Symptoms–Problems and Exercises. WO 18.2]
RD33.55
617.0754076–dc23   2014039487

ISBN 978-1-107-62554-9 Paperback

Cambridge University Press has no responsibility for the persistence or accuracy of URLs for external or third-party internet websites referred to in this publication, and does not guarantee that any content on such websites is, or will remain, accurate or appropriate.

....

Every effort has been made in preparing this book to provide accurate and up-to-date information which is in accord with accepted standards and practice at the time of publication. Although case histories are drawn from actual cases, every effort has been made to disguise the identities of the individuals involved.

Nevertheless, the authors, editors and publishers can make no warranties that the information contained herein is totally free from error, not least because clinical standards are constantly changing through research and regulation. The authors, editors and publishers therefore disclaim all liability for direct or consequential damages resulting from the use of material contained in this book. Readers are strongly advised to pay careful attention to information provided by the manufacturer of any drugs or equipment that they plan to use.

To my grandfather, Petru Cretescu, and my parents,
Calina and Dan Gogalniceanu
PG

Thank you for the continued support shown by Madeleine,
John, Julia and William
JP

To Emma – for her love and support
WL

To Catherine, Alistair, my mother and father
Hardi Madani

To my mother Azhar and father Hilal Sheena
Yezen Sheena

Contents

List of contributors xii
Introduction xv
Acknowledgments xvi
List of abbreviations xvii

Section 1. Principles of surgery

1 **Principles of surgical practice** 1
Petrut Gogalniceanu, James Pegrum, William Lynn and Vijay M. Gadhvi

2 **Surgical history and documentation** 16
Petrut Gogalniceanu

Section 2. General surgery

3 **Examination of peripheral stigmata of disease in general surgery** 27
Petrut Gogalniceanu, William Lynn and Andrew T. Raftery

4 **Examination of the abdomen** 34
Petrut Gogalniceanu, William Lynn and Andrew T. Raftery

5 **Examination of abdominal scars** 61
Petrut Gogalniceanu, Parveen Jayia and Andrew T. Raftery

6 **Examination of the groin** 69
Petrut Gogalniceanu, William Lynn and Andrew T. Raftery

7 **Examination of a stoma** 80
William Lynn, Petrut Gogalniceanu and Andrew T. Raftery

8 **Renal access and transplant examination** 84
Petrut Gogalniceanu and Andrew T. Raftery

Section 3. Breast surgery

9 **Examination of the breast** 89
Petrut Gogalniceanu, Yezen Sheena and Michael Douek

Section 4. Pelvis and perineum

10 **Examination of the anus** 99
Petrut Gogalniceanu, William Lynn and Andrew T. Raftery

11 **Examination of the pudendum and vagina** 102
Maria Memtsa and Wai Yoong

12 **Examination of the penis** 109
Paul Erotocritou, Vassilios Memtsas, Petrut Gogalniceanu and Justin Vale

13 **Examination of the scrotum** 112
Paul Erotocritou, Vassilios Memtsas, Petrut Gogalniceanu and Justin Vale

Section 5. Orthopaedic surgery

14 **Generic joint examination** 121
James Pegrum, Petrut Gogalniceanu and Chris Lavy

15 **Examination of gait** 128
James Pegrum and Chris Lavy

16 **Examination of the cervical and thoracic spine** 130
James Pegrum and Chris Lavy

17 **Cervical spine injury: assessment in trauma** 138
James Pegrum and Chris Lavy

18 **Examination of the shoulder** 140
James Pegrum, Petrut Gogalniceanu and Chris Lavy

19 **Examination of the elbow** 152
James Pegrum and Chris Lavy

20 **Examination of the lumbar spine and sacroiliac joint** 154
James Pegrum and Chris Lavy

21 **Examination of the hip** 162
James Pegrum, Petrut Gogalniceanu and Chris Lavy

22 **Examination of the knee** 175
James Pegrum, Petrut Gogalniceanu and Chris Lavy

23 **Examination of the ankle** 190
James Pegrum and Chris Lavy

Section 6. Vascular surgery

24 **Examination of the carotid artery** 203
Petrut Gogalniceanu and Vijay M. Gadhvi

25 **Examination of an abdominal aortic aneurysm** 208
Petrut Gogalniceanu and Vijay M. Gadhvi

26 **Arterial examination of the upper limbs** 212
Petrut Gogalniceanu and Vijay M. Gadhvi

27 **Arterial examination of the lower limbs** 223
Petrut Gogalniceanu and Vijay M. Gadhvi

28 **Examination of the lower limb venous system** 237
Petrut Gogalniceanu, William Lynn and Vijay M. Gadhvi

29 **Examination of ulcers** 247
Petrut Gogalniceanu, William Lynn and Vijay M. Gadhvi

Section 7. Heart and thorax

30 **Examination of the thorax and lungs** 255
Martin T. Yates, Petrut Gogalniceanu and Ian Hunt

31 **Examination of the heart and great vessels** 264
Martin T. Yates, Petrut Gogalniceanu and Ian Hunt

Section 8. Head and neck surgery

32 **Examination of the ear** 271
Rajeev Mathew, S. Alam Hannan and Parag M. Patel

33 **Examination of the nose** 281
Rajeev Mathew, S. Alam Hannan and Parag M. Patel

34 **Examination of the throat** 288
Rajeev Mathew, S. Alam Hannan and Parag M. Patel

35 **Oral and maxillofacial examination** 292
David C. McAnerney, Petrut Gogalniceanu, Rajeev Mathew and Dan Gogalniceanu

36 **Examination of the neck and thyroid** 307
William Lynn, Petrut Gogalniceanu and John Lynn

Section 9. Neurosurgery

37 **Global neurological examination** 319
Harry Bulstrode, Yezen Sheena and Diederik O. Bulters

38 **Focal neurological examination** 332
Harry Bulstrode, Yezen Sheena and Diederik O. Bulters

Section 10. Plastic surgery

39 **Examination of skin lesions and lumps** 353
Edmund Fitzgerald O'Connor, Yezen Sheena, Petrut Gogalniceanu and Henk Giele

40 **Examination of scars** 359
Edmund Fitzgerald O'Connor, Yezen Sheena and Henk Giele

41 **Examination of flaps and grafts** 362
Edmund Fitzgerald O'Connor, Yezen Sheena and Henk Giele

42 **Examination of burns** 367
Yezen Sheena, Edmund Fitzgerald O'Connor, Petrut Gogalniceanu and Henk Giele

43 **Examination of the hands** 371
Yezen Sheena, Edmund Fitzgerald O'Connor, Petrut Gogalniceanu and Henk Giele

Section 11. Surgical radiology

44 **Principles of plain film** 383
Hardi Madani, Petrut Gogalniceanu, James Pegrum, John Curtis and Helen Marmery

45 **Chest x-ray** 386
Hardi Madani, Petrut Gogalniceanu, John Curtis and Helen Marmery

46 **Abdominal x-ray** 396
Hardi Madani, Petrut Gogalniceanu, John Curtis and Helen Marmery

47 **Mammogram** 404
Hardi Madani, Helen Marmery and Trupti Kulkarni

48 **Facial x-ray** 409
Hardi Madani, John Curtis and Helen Marmery

49 **Cervical spine x-ray** 414
Hardi Madani, John Curtis and Helen Marmery

50 **Shoulder x-ray** 418
Hardi Madani, John Curtis and Helen Marmery

51 **Elbow x-ray** 424
Hardi Madani, John Curtis and Helen Marmery

52 **Wrist and distal forearm x-ray** 426
Hardi Madani, John Curtis and Helen Marmery

53 **Pelvis and hip x-ray** 433
Hardi Madani, John Curtis and Helen Marmery

54 **Knee x-ray** 437
Hardi Madani, John Curtis and Helen Marmery

55 **Foot and ankle x-ray** 444
Hardi Madani, John Curtis and Helen Marmery

56 **Principles of CT** 449
Hardi Madani, John Curtis and Helen Marmery

57 **Head CT** 451
Hardi Madani, John Curtis and Helen Marmery

58 **Chest CT** 455
Hardi Madani, John Curtis and Helen Marmery

59 **Abdomen CT** 457
Hardi Madani, John Curtis and Helen Marmery

60 **Aorta CT** 463
Hardi Madani, John Curtis and Helen Marmery

61 **Kidneys, ureter and bladder CT** 469
Hardi Madani, John Curtis and Helen Marmery

62 **Lower limb CT angiogram** 471
Hardi Madani, John Curtis and Helen Marmery

Section 12. Airway, trauma and critical care

63 **Examination of the trauma patient** 473
Petrut Gogalniceanu and Vijay M. Gadhvi

64 **Examination of the critically ill surgical patient** 485
Petrut Gogalniceanu, Julia Niewiarowski and Vijay M. Gadhvi

65 **Assessment of the airway for intubation** 491
Julia Niewiarowski, Rajeev Mathew and Vijay M. Gadhvi

66 **Assessment of the compromised airway** 494
Julia Niewiarowski, Rajeev Mathew and Vijay M. Gadhvi

67 **Examination of a tracheostomy** 497
Julia Niewiarowski, Rajeev Mathew and Vijay M. Gadhvi

Index 499

Contributors

Harry Bulstrode BMBCh MA Cantab MRCS
Specialist Registrar, Neurosurgery, Wessex Neurological Centre, Southampton, and Wellcome Research Training Fellow, University College London, London, UK

Paul Erotocritou MBBS BSc MRCS FRCS(Urol)
Specialist Registrar, Urology, London Deanery, London, UK

Petrut Gogalniceanu BSc MEd MRCS(Eng)
Specialist Registrar, General Surgery, London Postgraduate School of Surgery, London, UK

Parveen Jayia MBBS MRPharmS MRCS
Specialist Registrar, General Surgery, London Postgraduate School of Surgery, London, UK

William Lynn BSc MRCS(Eng)
Specialist Registrar, General Surgery, London Deanery, London, UK

Hardi Madani BPharm(Hons) MPhil MBBS MRCS(Eng)
Specialist Registrar, Clinical Radiology, Royal Free Hospital, London Deanery, London, UK

Rajeev Mathew MA MBBS MRCS DOHNS
Specialist Registrar, ENT Surgery, St Georges University Hospital, London, UK

Maria Memtsa MBBS BSc
Specialist Registrar, Obstetrics and Gynaecology, London Deanery, London, UK

Vassilios Memtsas MD
Ninewells Hospital, Dundee, UK

David C. McAnerney BSc(Hons) BDS(Hons) MBBS MFDS(Eng) MRCS(Eng)
Specialist Registrar, Oral and Maxillofacial Surgery, Norfolk and Norwich University Hospital, Norfolk, UK

Julia Niewiarowski MBBS BSc FRCA
Specialist Registrar, Anaesthetics, Oxford Deanery, Oxford, UK

Edmund Fitzgerald O'Connor BSc MBBS MRCS PgCert MedEd FHEA
Plastic Surgery Registrar – Pan Thames, St Andrew's Centre for Plastic Surgery and Burns, Chelmsford, UK

James Pegrum BSc MSc(SEM) MRCS(Eng) Dip Mtn Med UIAA
Specialist Registrar, Trauma and Orthopaedic Surgery, Oxford Deanery, Oxford, and Honorary Clinical Lecturer, Queen Mary University of London Sports & Exercise Department, London, UK

Yezen Sheena MRCS MBBS BSc(Hons)
Specialist Registrar, Plastic Surgery, Health Education East of England, Cambridge, UK

Martin T. Yates MBChB MRCS
Specialist Registrar, Cardiothoracic Surgery, St George's Hospital, London, UK

Senior authors

Diederik O. Bulters BSc MBChB FRCS(SN)
Consultant Neurosurgeon and Honorary Senior Clinical Lecturer, Wessex Neurological Centre, Southampton, UK

John Curtis FRCP DMRD FRCR
Consultant Radiologist, University Hospital Aintree, Liverpool, UK

Michael Douek MD FRCS(Eng) FRCS(Gen)
Reader in Surgery and Consultant Breast Surgeon, King's College London, London, UK

Vijay M. Gadhvi BSc(Hons) MSc (DIC) MBBS(Hons) MRCS(Eng Gl) FRCS
Consultant Vascular, Endovascular and General Surgeon, Basildon and Thurrock University Hospital, Basildon, UK

Henk Giele MBBS MS FRACS FRCS AFRACMA
Consultant Plastic Reconstructive and Hand Surgeon, Oxford University Hospitals, Oxford, UK

Dan Gogalniceanu MD PhD FDS
Professor of Oral and Maxillofacial Surgery and former Chief of Service, Department of Oral and Maxillofacial Surgery, Sf. Spiridon University Hospital and Gr. T. Popa University of Medicine and Pharmacy, Iasi, Romania

S. Alam Hannan BSc MBBS AKC MRCS DLORCS FRCS(ORL-HNS)
Consultant Otorhinolaryngologist – Head and Neck Surgeon, Royal National Throat, Nose and Ear Hospital, London, UK

Ian Hunt FRCS(CTh)
Consultant Thoracic Surgeon, St George's Hospital, London, UK

Trupti Kulkarni MBBS MS MRCS FRCR
Consultant Radiologist, Aintree University Hospital, Liverpool, and Breast Screening Radiologist, Wirral Breast Unit, Clatterbridge, UK

Chris Lavy OBE MD MCh FCS FRCS
Consultant Orthopaedic Surgeon, Nuffield Department of

Orthopaedics, Rheumatology and Musculoskeletal Science, University of Oxford, Oxford, UK

John Lynn MS FRCS
Consultant Endocrine Surgeon, The Cromwell Hospital, London, UK

Helen Marmery FRCR MRCS MBChB
Consultant Musculoskeletal Radiologist, Royal Free Hampstead NHS Trust, London, UK

Parag M. Patel FRCS (ORL-HNS) MSc
Consultant in Otolaryngology and Skull Base Surgery, St George's Hospital, London, UK

Andrew T. Raftery BSc MBChB (Hons) MD FRCS(Eng) FRCS(Ed)
Former Consultant Surgeon, Sheffield Kidney Institute, Sheffield Teaching Hospitals NHS Foundation Trust, Northern General Hospital; Member (formerly Chairman), Court of Examiners, Royal College of Surgeons of England; Member of Panel of Examiners, Intercollegiate Speciality Board in General Surgery; Member of Council, Royal College of Surgeons of England; Honorary Clinical Senior Lecturer in Surgery, University of Sheffield, Sheffield, UK

Justin Vale MD
Consultant Urological Surgeon, Imperial College Healthcare Trust, and Adjunct Professor of Urology, Imperial College London, London, UK

Wai Yoong MD FRCOG
Consultant in Obstetrics and Gynaecology, North Middlesex Hospital, London, UK

Introduction

The Intercollegiate Membership of the Royal College of Surgeons (MRCS) examination aims to assess a junior doctor's competence to enter surgical training. This is based on the candidate's understanding of core clinical and professional principles needed to diagnose and treat surgical disease. The exam is the first step in a process that transforms a doctor into a surgeon and provides a common foundation of practice for all surgeons in the UK, irrespective of their subspecialty.

Focused, systematic and diagnostic physical examination skills are a key aspect of surgical practice. Their purpose is to assess anatomical form and test physiological function in order to allow a professional opinion to be formulated.

The book provides one method of performing physical examination from a surgeon's perspective, addressing key topics in the objective structured clinical examination (OSCE) part of the assessment. It also addresses related diagnostic skills, such as history taking, communication, critical care assessment and interpretation of surgical radiology images.

It aims to be a practical manual, being neither exhaustive nor specific to a single syllabus. It includes chapters on topics such as gynaecology and neurosurgery, which, although not tested in the MRCS exam, may be relevant to the practice of general surgery.

We recommend the consultation of reference manuals for the acquisition of finer details and clinical knowledge. Updated details of the MRCS examination format, syllabus and requirements must be obtained from the relevant examining bodies.

Each chapter contains the following key elements:

1. At-a-glance **checklists** on how to perform any physical examination routine.
2. **Examination notes**, including focused questions and answers.
3. Mind maps of **differential diagnoses**, to facilitate the easy formulation and recall of diagnoses.
4. Tips, mnemonics and examples.

We hope this book will be of use in caring for your patients.

PG, JP and WL
London, 2015

Acknowledgments

We would like to thank Joanna Chamberlin of Cambridge University Press for her role in commissioning and guiding the creation of this book, and Hugh Brazier for his expert review, advice and support during the copy-editing process.

We would like to thank the following specialists:

General surgery

Dr Parminderjit Jayia and Dr Teresa Jacobs

Surgical radiology

Dr N Mir, Consultant Radiologist, Royal Free Hospital
Dr D Yu, Consultant Interventional Radiologist, Royal Free Hospital
Dr N Woodward, Consultant Interventional Radiologist and Programme Director, Royal Free Hospital
Dr A Malhotra, Consultant Breast Radiologist, Royal Free Hospital
Dr A Wigham, Interventional Radiology Fellow, Royal Free Hospital
Dr F Ingham, Consultant Radiologist, Barnet Hospital
Dr J Berger, Consultant Radiologist, Barnet Hospital
Dr A Marcus, Consultant Interventional Radiologist, Barnet Hospital

We are also grateful to the PACS teams at the Royal Free and Barnet Hospitals, especially Mr James Lovell, whose help with the radiology chapter was invaluable.

Abbreviations

AAA abdominal aortic aneurysm
ABG arterial blood gas
ABPI ankle–brachial pressure index
ACJ acromioclavicular joint
ACL anterior cruciate ligament
ADM acellular dermal matrix
A&E accident and emergency
AF atrial fibrillation
AFX atypical fibroxanthoma
AIN anterior interosseous nerve
ALS Advanced Life Support
ALT alanine transaminase
ALT anterolateral thigh (flap)
AMTS Abbreviated Mental Test Score
ANC axillary node clearance
AP anteroposterior
APTT activated partial thromboplastin time
ARDS acute respiratory distress syndrome
ASD atrial septal defect
ASIS anterior superior iliac spine
ATA anterior tibial artery
ATFL anterior talofibular ligament
ATLS Advanced Trauma Life Support
AVF arteriovenous fistula
AVM arteriovenous malformation
AVN avascular necrosis
AXR abdominal x-ray
BCC basal cell carcinoma
BCT brachiocephalic trunk
bHCG beta human chorionic gonadotropin
BiPAP bi-level positive airway pressure
BNO bowels not opened
BNP brain natriuretic peptide
BPH benign prostatic hypertrophy
BPPV benign paroxysmal positional vertigo
BS bowel sounds
CA carcinoma
CABG coronary artery bypass graft
CCA common carotid artery
CCF congestive cardiac failure
CCrISP care of the critically ill surgical patient
CEA carotid endarterectomy
CES cauda equina syndrome
CFA common femoral artery
CHL conductive hearing loss
CIA common iliac artery
CMC carpometacarpal (joint)
CNS central nervous system
COPD chronic obstructive pulmonary disease
CP chest pain
CPAP continuous positive airway pressure
CPEX cardiopulmonary exercise
CRP C-reactive protein
CRT capillary refill time
CSF cerebrospinal fluid
CT computed tomography
CTA CT angiogram
CVA cerebrovascular accident
CXR chest x-ray
DH drug history
DIEP deep inferior epigastric perforator (flap)
DIP distal interphalangeal (joint)
DKA diabetic ketoacidosis
DM diabetes mellitus
DNA did not attend
DP dorsalis pedis

DP dorsoplantar
DPL diagnostic peritoneal lavage
DRE digital rectal examination
DSA digital subtraction angiogram
DVT deep venous thrombosis
ECA external carotid artery
ECG electrocardiogram
EDH extradural haematoma
eGFR estimated glomerular filtration rate
EIA external iliac artery
EMSB Emergency Management of Severe Burns
ERCP endoscopic retrograde cholangiopancreatography
ERPC evacuation of retained products of conception
ET endotracheal
EVAR endovascular (abdominal aortic) aneurysm repair
FAST focused assessment with sonography in trauma
FBC full blood count
FDP flexor digitorum profundus (tendon or muscle)
FDS flexor digitorum superficialis (tendon or muscle)
FEVAR fenestrated endovascular aneurysm repair
FFP fresh frozen plasma
FH family history
FNA fine-needle aspiration (biopsy)
FPL flexor pollicis longus (tendon or muscle)
FTSG full-thickness skin graft
GCS Glasgow Coma Scale
GI gastrointestinal
GMC General Medical Council
HAS human albumin solution
Hb haemoglobin
HIV human immunodeficiency virus
HPC history of presenting complaint
IBD inflammatory bowel disease
ICA internal carotid artery
ICP intracranial pressure
ICS intercostal space
IIA internal iliac artery
IM intramuscular
IMA inferior mesenteric artery
IMF inframammary fold
INR international normalised ratio
IP interphalangeal
ITU intensive therapy unit
IV intravenous
IVC inferior vena cava
IVU intravenous urogram
JVP jugular venous pressure
KUB kidneys, ureters and bladder
LAT lateral
LBO large bowel obstruction
LCL lateral collateral ligament
LD latissimus dorsi (flap)
LFT liver function test
LIF left iliac fossa
LMP last menstrual period
LRTI lower respiratory tract infection
LSA left subclavian artery
LSV long saphenous vein
LUQ left upper quadrant
LVF left ventricular failure
M, C & S microscopy, culture and sensitivity
MAP mean arterial pressure
MCP metacarpophalangeal (joint)
MDT multidisciplinary team
MI myocardial infarct
MM malignant melanoma
MMSE Mini-Mental State Examination
MRA magnetic resonance angiogram

MRC Medical Research Council
MRCP magnetic resonance cholangiopancreatography
MRI magnetic resonance imaging
MRSA Methicillin-resistant *Staphylococcus aureus*
MT metatarsal
NAI non-accidental injury
NG nasogastric
NIV non-invasive ventilation
NKDA no known drug allergies
OA osteoarthritis
OGD oesophagogastroduodenoscopy
OPG orthopantomogram
ORIF open reduction internal fixation
PA peroneal artery
PC presenting complaint
PCL posterior cruciate ligament
PD peritoneal dialysis
PE pulmonary embolism
PEVAR percutaneous endovascular aneurysm repair
PFA profunda femoris artery
PID pelvic inflammatory disease
PIP proximal interphalangeal (joint)
PMH past medical history
PR per rectum
PSH past surgical history
PTA posterior tibial artery
PTFL posterior talofibular ligament
PUJ pelviureteric junction
PV per vaginam
RA rheumatoid arthritis
RBC red blood cells
RCS Royal College of Surgeons
RFF radial forearm flap
RIF right iliac fossa
ROM range of movement
RSA right sublclavian artery
RSTL relaxed skin tension lines

RTA road traffic accident
RUQ right upper quadrant
SAH subarachnoid haemorrhage
SBO small bowel obstruction
SCC squamous cell carcinoma
SCM sternocleidomastoid muscle
SDH subdural haematoma
SFA superficial femoral artery
SFJ saphenofemoral junction
SH social history
SIJ sacroiliac joint
SIRS systemic inflammatory response syndrome
SLAP superior labrum anterior to posterior (tear)
SLE systemic lupus erythematosus
SLNB sentinel lymph-node biopsy
SMA superior mesenteric artery
SNHL sensorineural hearing loss
SOB shortness of breath
SPJ saphenopopliteal junction
SSV short saphenous vein
STSG split-thickness skin graft
SUFE slipped upper femoral epiphysis
SVC superior vena cava
TAA thoracic aortic aneurysm
TAP thoracodorsal artery perforator (flap)
TB tuberculosis
TBPI toe–brachial pressure index
TBSA total body surface area
TEVAR thoracic endovascular aneurysm repair
TFT thyroid function test
TIPPS transjugular intrahepatic portosystemic shunt
TM tympanic membrane
TMJ temporomandibular joint
TOP termination of pregnancy
TOS thoracic outlet syndrome
TP tibioperoneal (trunk)

TPN total parenteral nutrition
TRAM transverse rectus abdominis myocutaneous (flap)
TWOC trial without catheter
UC ulcerative colitis
UO urine output
US ultrasound
VATS video-assisted thorascopic/thoracic surgery
VTE venous thromboembolism
WBC white blood cells
WHO World Health Organization

Section editors: Petrut Gogalniceanu, James Pegrum, William Lynn
Senior author: Vijay M. Gadhvi

Section 1 Principles of surgery

Chapter 1

Principles of surgical practice

Petrut Gogalniceanu, James Pegrum,
William Lynn and Vijay M. Gadhvi

- The purpose of medicine in general is to improve physical, intellectual and emotional health.
- Surgery aims to achieve this through the scientific manipulation of human anatomy and physiology, aiming to restore form and function and alleviate pain, whilst reducing the number of complications that can arise during the process.
- The surgeon's role is twofold:
  1. to identify the problem (diagnosis)
  2. to provide a solution (design and implement a management plan)
- The surgeon needs to establish a relationship of trust with the patient, based on honesty, competence and good communication, in order to address complex aspects of diagnosis and treatment.
- The management of patients should be done in a professional, timely and efficient manner, with the goal of treatment being positive outcomes rather than good intentions.
- Surgical intervention should result in either an increase in the patient's length of life or an improvement of their quality of life in a timely, ethical and patient-centred manner.
- Ethics can be defined as the respect for human life and its autonomy.

Physical Examination for Surgeons, ed. Petrut Gogalniceanu, James Pegrum and William Lynn. Published by Cambridge University Press. © Cambridge University Press 2015.

Section 1: Principles of surgery

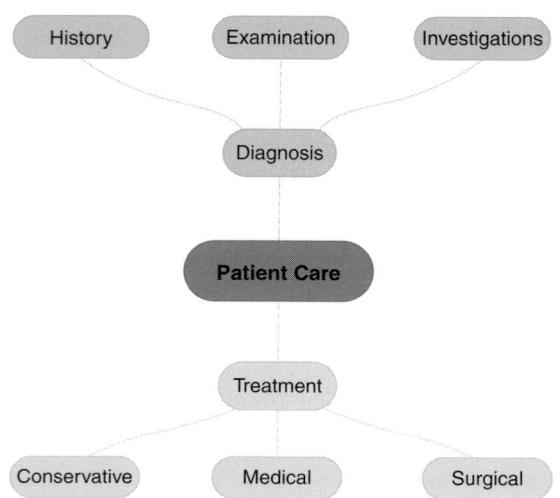

Principles of diagnosis

How is a diagnosis reached?

Three steps:

1. History taking
2. Physical examination
3. Investigations

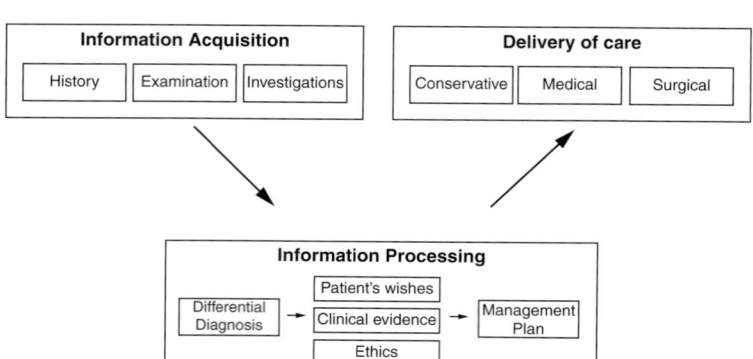

Differential diagnoses

How can a differential diagnosis be made?

A logical differential diagnosis can be formulated by applying a list of pathological processes to any organ in an anatomical area. The surgical sieve used in this book is **C-MIT**:

- **C**ongenital
- **M**echanical: extrinsic, mural, intraluminal
- **I**nfective or **I**nflammatory: autoimmune, bacterial, viral, fungal, protozoal
- **I**schaemic or haemorrhagic (vascular): stenosis, embolism, thrombosis, haemorrhage, dissection, aneurysmal change, vasospasm
- **T**umour: primary, secondary (metastases), lymphoproliferative
- **T**rauma: penetrating, blunt, chemical, electrical, thermal

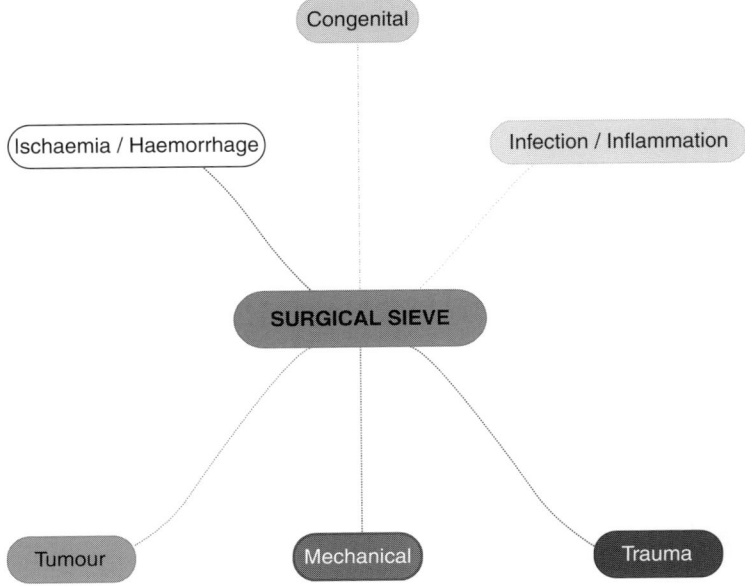

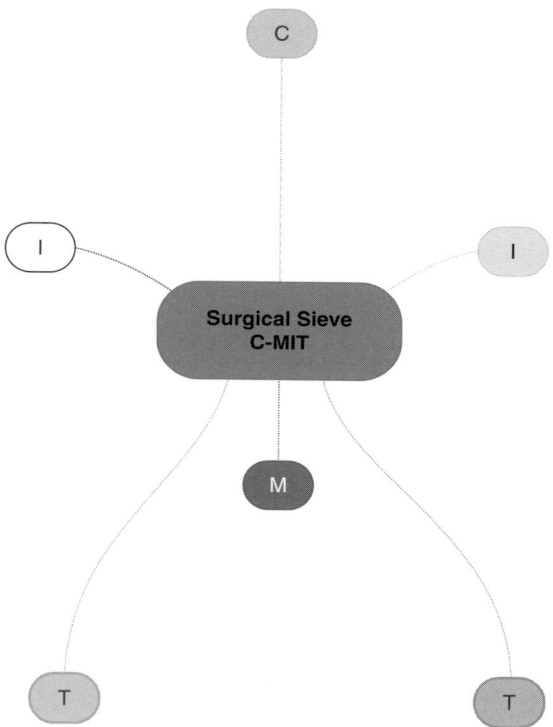

All the differential diagnoses in the book are conveyed in the same diagrammatic manner, based on the pathological processes mentioned above.

Principles of examination

What checks must be made prior to beginning the physical examination?

- The surgeon must prepare for the examination.
- Check physiological parameters (vital signs) and fluid balance from the observations chart.
- Examine patient's bedside or environment.
- General examination of the patient from the end of the bed.

How should the examining surgeon prepare before commencing an examination?

> **Mnemonic**
>
> **WIPER**

- **W**ash hands, remove all jewellery and watches and expose arms above elbows.
- **I**ntroduce yourself.
- **P**urpose and **P**ermission: explain purpose and gain verbal consent (permission) to proceed with the examination.
- **E**xpose the patient appropriately for the examination you are about to perform.
- **R**ecline: position the patient appropriately.

> **Example**
>
> *'Good morning, Mrs Taylor. My name is Mr Smith. I am a surgical registrar working for Mr Johnson. I understand you have pain in your calf. I would like to examine you to find out the cause. Would that be OK?'*
>
> Find a chaperone.
> Expose the patient's legs, removing shoes and socks. Cover the inguinal area and perineum with a sheet.
> Place the patient flat with one pillow on an examination couch.

What physiological parameters should be checked in every examination?

The first part of the physical examination is to inspect the patient's observation chart for physiological parameters (vital signs). If the observation chart contains inaccurate, incomplete or old vital signs it is the examiner's responsibility to assess and measure these at the time of examination.

The vital signs or physiological parameters are grouped in the following manner and must always be documented:

- Cardiac: heart rate and rhythm (HR) and blood pressure (BP)
- Respiratory: respiratory rate (RR) and oxygen saturation (Sats)
- Temperature (degrees Celsius)
- Glasgow Coma Scale (GCS) score
- Blood sugar levels (if available)
- Fluid balance (positive or negative), including urine output (ml/h in the last 3 hours), drain, NG and stoma output, as well as oral intake

> **Example**
>
> HR 95 SR[1]　　　RR 18　　　T 37.2 °C　　　Glucose 3.9
>
> BP 135/82　　　Sats 98% RA[2]　　　GCS 15/15
>
> Urine: 20 – 32 – 35 ml/hour
> Drain: 50 ml in 24 hours
> Fluid balance 340 ml +ve in 24 hours

What 'bedside' observations should be made?

Look for any signs in the patient's immediate environment that would hint at the patient's health:

- Evidence of acute illness: attachment to cardiac monitors, defibrillators or infusion pumps
- Floor: purulent discharge, bleeding, incontinence, vomitus
- Surgical appliances: drains, catheters, vacuum suction devices, blood transfusions, parenteral feeding bags
- Orthopaedic appliances: prostheses, walking aids, external fixation devices

> **Tip**
>
> Inspect the bedside for clues, **'MD'**:
>
>   **3 Ms**: monitors, mobility aids, medical equipment (e.g. ventilators, dialysis machines)
>   **3 Ds**: drips, drains, drug infusions

How is the general examination performed from the end of the bed?

The surgeon stands at the end of the bed keeping her/his hands in a neutral position (e.g. behind the back) so as to emphasise the lack of patient

---

[1] SR describes a sinus rhythm pulse. Other pulse rhythms notations may include AF (atrial fibrillation), irreg irreg (irregularly irregular), VF (ventricular fibrillation) or VT (ventricular tachycardia). The last two can only be assessed if the patient is attached to a cardiac monitor.

[2] RA or 21% O_2 signifies normal 'room air' concentration of oxygen. Saturations should always be reported with the concentration of oxygen that the patient is breathing.

contact and focus on the global observation of the patient. Only once this is completed can the examiner move to the right-hand side of the patient's bed (for right-handed examiners) and proceed with the organ-system-based assessment. Also assess the patient's general appearance and behaviour:
- Pain
- Lethargy, confusion or agitation
- Malnutrition, obesity

How can the peripheral stigmata of disease be remembered?

Airway – stridor, anaphylaxis

Breathing – dyspnoea, cyanosis, use of accessory muscles, patient position to facilitate breathing

Circulation – external bleeding

Deficit of neurology – consciousness, comfort (pain), cognition (**3Cs**)

Dermatology – jaundice, rashes, pallor

Emaciation – cachexia, malnourishment, evidence of catabolism

Fluid status – dehydrated, overloaded/oedematous

Facies – syndromes

Foul smell – foetor, melaena, urine/faecal incontinence, infected tissue/pus, alcohol

---

Mnemonic

JACCOL is a quick method of remembering the peripheral stigmata of systemic disease from the end of the bed:

Jaundice, **A**naemia, **C**lubbing, **C**yanosis, **O**edema, **L**ymphadenopathy

---

Tips

Always terminate the examination if the patient is in discomfort or in danger, or if there is a sudden deterioration in the patient's status. Resuscitate the patient as described in the ALS or CCrISP guidelines.

Inspection: always ask patient to show where the problem is found.

Palpation: always ask the patient if he/she has any pain before palpating or asking them to move a body part.

Principles of investigation

How are surgical investigations classified?
- Laboratory-based
- Physiological tests
- Imaging
- Invasive diagnostic tests

What laboratory tests can be performed?
- Blood tests: full blood count, urea and creatinine, electrolytes, liver function tests, C-reactive protein, immunology assays
- Blood bank: group, save and crossmatch blood and blood products
- Microbiology: microscopy, culture and sensitivity (any fluid or tissues)
- Histopathology: microscopic analysis of tissues

What basic physiological tests can be performed at the bedside?
- ECG
- Spirometry/peak flow
- ABPI

What imaging tests can be performed?
- Simple imaging: plain x-rays (abdomen, chest or limbs) and ultrasonography
- Complex imaging: computed tomography (CT) scanning or magnetic resonance imaging (MRI)

What are the invasive diagnostic tests available?
- Endoscopy: OGD, colonoscopy, ERCP, endoscopic ultrasound, cystoscopy
- Biopsy: fine-needle aspiration (FNA), true-cut biopsy, excision biopsy
- Percutaneous angiography

Chapter 1: Principles of surgical practice

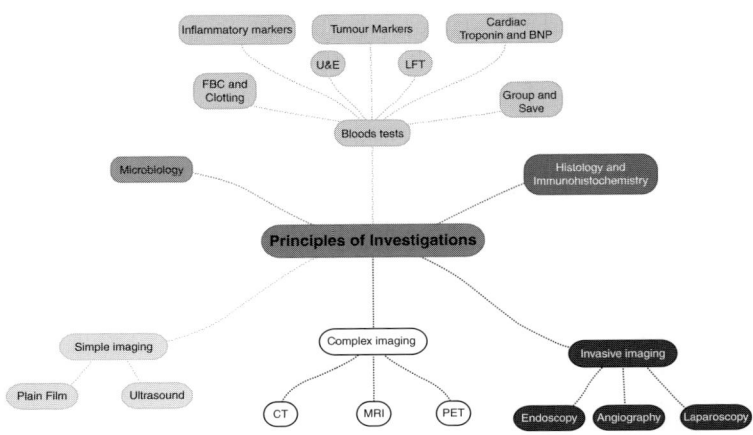

How to examine anything...

Tip

What are the features of surgical disease in any organ?

1.	Abnormal anatomy: increase or decrease in size	e.g. palpable gallbladder
2.	Abnormal physiology: loss of function	e.g. jaundice
3.	Pain	e.g. positive Murphy's sign

General examination
- Bedside
- JACCOL
- WIPER
- Physiological parameters

Inspection
Skin:
- Skin lesions: masses, ulcers, fistulas
- Scars: well healed, tethering, hypertrophic, keloid
- Lacerations: clean, irregular, flaps, contamination

- Colour changes: rashes, erythema, jaundice, pallor, ecchymosis, cyanosis, necrosis or gangrene[3]

Soft tissues:[4]

- Swellings: hypertrophy, abscesses, tumours, aneurysms, haematomas, fractures, hernias.
- Tissue loss: excision, atrophy, aplasia, necrosis

Bone:

- Deformities
- Amputations

Palpation

Skin:

- Temperature: cold or hot
- Hydration: normal, dry, moist
- Sensitivity: pain-free, tender, anaesthesia, paraesthesia

Soft tissues:

- Swelling or fluctuance
- Tissue loss
- Crepitus (surgical emphysema or infection)

Viscera:

- Tenderness
- Organomegaly/distension
- Atrophy
- Pulsations or movement

Vascular:

- Presence or absence of pulses
- Capillary refill time
- Evidence of haemorrhage

Neurology:

- Sensation
- Movement
- (Reflexes)

---

[3] Mnemonic for skin colour changes: **REJPECT**: **R**ashes, **E**rythema, **J**aundice, **P**allor, **E**cchymoses, **C**yanosis, **T**errifying changes (necrosis and gangrene).

[4] Remember there can be only two types of soft tissue changes: too much or too little.

Bones:
- Site of pain
- Abnormal mobility/crepitus
- Steps

Percussion
- Dull
- Resonant

Ausculation
- Normal physiological sounds
- Bruits or pathological sounds

Principles of treatment

Any patient that is acutely compromised must be managed according to established national guidelines:

- **Trauma patients**: Advanced Trauma Life Support (ATLS)
- **Critically ill patients**: Care of the Critically Ill Surgical Patient (CCrISP; Royal College of Surgeons) or Advanced Life Support (ALS; UK Resuscitation Council)

All critically ill patients require multidisciplinary input from critical care or acute medicine physicians, and their care must be escalated to the responsible senior surgeon (consultant).

What are the methods of managing stable surgical patients?

1. Conservative management
    a. screening
    b. surveillance and monitoring ('watch and wait')
    c. rehabilitation
    d. postoperative care

2. **Medical management** (pharmacological and physiological)
    a. prophylactic
    b. therapeutic
    c. symptomatic

3. Surgical management (anatomical)
    a. endoscopic
    b. percutaneous
    c. endovascular

d. laparoscopic
e. open

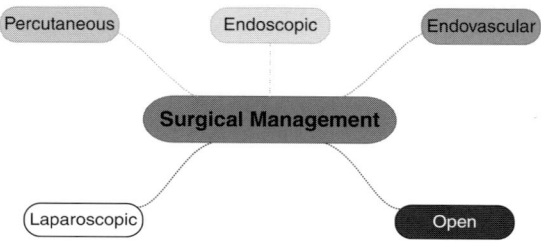

What are the initial steps in managing a surgical patient?

4 × 3 *(as required; not all are necessary, but each must be considered as a checklist)*

3 letters	3 As	3 tubes	3 fluids
Airway	Analgesia	IV access	IV fluids
Breathing	Antiemetics	NG tube	Blood tests
Circulation	Antibiotics	Foley catheter	Urine tests

How do you manage any fracture?

4 Rs:

- **Resuscitate**: assume any fracture occurred as a result of high-energy trauma and carry out ATLS if this is the case.
- **Reduce**: any misaligned joint or limb needs to be straightened. Assess neurovascular status before and after reduction.
- **Restrict**: after straightening the limb immobilise it in a plaster cast or for femoral fractures skin traction. This is followed by formal management with either on-going plaster or surgical fixation.
- **Rehabilitation**: Following removal of cast or surgical fixation appropriate physiotherapy input is required.

How can any operation be structured?

3 Ps: **P**rocedure planning, **P**osition patient, **P**erioperative WHO checklist.
3 Ps: **P**ostoperative management plan, **P**ain control, **P**roblem checks (complications).

What are the WHO perioperative checks?

Before induction of anaesthesia	Before skin incision	Before patient leaves operating room
Patient identity	Identity of patient, procedure and site	Name of procedure performed
Procedure name	Team members introduced	Instrument, sponge/swabs and needle count correct
Consent signed	Unexpected anticipated surgical, anaesthetic or nursing steps	Labelling of specimens
Site of surgery	Estimated operation time	Equipment problems identified
Anaesthesia and monitoring equipment applied and working	Estimated blood loss	
Allergies	Antibiotic prophylaxis	Recovery and postoperative management concerns
Risk of aspiration	Imaging displayed	
Risk of > 500 ml blood loss		

Postoperative assessment

	Checks
A	**Assess vital signs/Analgesia/Antiemetics** What are the observations? Is the patient in pain? Is the patient nauseated?
B	**Breathing** Is there shortness of breath (LRTI, PE, pulmonary oedema) or sputum production?

(cont.)

	Checks
C	**Cardiovascular** Is the patient in shock? Does the patient have chest pain?
D	**Is there a neurological Deficit?** Is there **DVT** prophylaxis in place? Is **diabetes**/blood sugar controlled?
E	**Evaluate surgical site** Is there bleeding? Is there infection? Is the wound intact? Is the operated organ's function intact?
F	**Fluid balance** Is the patient in urinary retention? Fluid output 24 hours? Fluid input 24 hours? What is the fluid balance?
G	**Gastrointestinal** Is the patient eating and drinking? Has the patient passed flatus? Has the patient passed stool?
H	**Haemoglobin** What is the postoperative Hb?
I	**Infection** Is there evidence of fever, rigors or sweating? What are the WBC and CRP? Are antibiotics prescribed? Microbiology results?
K	**Potassium (K), sodium, urea, creatinine** What is the renal function?
L	**Lines** What IV access is present?
M	**Medication review** What drugs can be stopped? What drugs must be started?

(cont.)

	Checks
O	**Occupational therapy**
P	**Physiotherapy**
S	**Social issues**
	What personal problems are present?
Concerns × 3	Any patient/family concerns?
	Any nurse concerns?
	Any doctor concerns?

What bedside documents need to be checked each time a patient is reviewed?

- Drug chart:
    - thromboprophylaxis
    - analgesia
    - oxygen
    - fluid prescription
- Fluid balance chart
- Physiological parameters/observations chart (including stool chart and blood glucose checks)
- Recent laboratory results

Section 1: Principles of surgery

Chapter 2: Surgical history and documentation
Petrut Gogalniceanu

Surgical history

Introduction

Age

Occupation

Presenting complaint (PC)
- Symptom 1 duration
- Symptom 2 duration
- Symptom 3 duration

History of presenting complaint (HPC)
- Quality: what, where and how
- Quantity: how much and impact on life
- Time line: duration, onset, progression, offset
- Associated features, risk factors and complications

Past medical history (PMH)
- Similar problems in the past
- Medical history: MJTHREADS (**M**I, **j**aundice, **T**B, **h**ypertension, **r**heumatoid, **e**pilepsy, **a**sthma/COPD, **d**iabetes, **s**urgery or **s**trokes)
- Anaesthetic history
- General risk factors: stroke, ischaemic heart disease, angina, shortness of breath, COPD, renal failure, diabetes, change in bowel habit, DVT, PE
- Women: last menstrual period (LMP), vaginal bleeding or discharge, pregnancies, deliveries

Past surgical history (PSH)
- Open surgery
- Laparoscopy

Physical Examination for Surgeons, ed. Petrut Gogalniceanu, James Pegrum and William Lynn. Published by Cambridge University Press. © Cambridge University Press 2015.

- Endoscopy/endovascular procedures
- Ultrasound/CT/MRI imaging
- Surgical fitness assessment: mobility, able to climb one flight of stairs, ability to lie flat, maximal exercise distance
- Bleeding risk: bleeding disorders

Drug history (DH)

- Allergies
- Regular medications
- Medications taken since symptoms have started
- Anticoagulant or antiplatelet agents: warfarin, heparin, aspirin, clopidogrel
- Recreational drugs

Social history (SH)

- Smoking
- Alcohol
- Home + 3 others (work, social, personal)

Family history (FH)

- Relevant hereditary conditions
- Exposure to any risk factors of acquired disease

Systems review (SR)

- Systems review if not already undertaken

Summary of findings and confirmation that they are correct

Any questions? Any concerns?

Inform patient of future plans

Proceed to examination

Examination notes

What is the purpose of the history?

- The primary aim of the history is to establish a list of differential diagnoses based on the patient's history of presenting complaint and risk factors.
- The second aim is to determine the patient's medical, social and functional background, which would guide further therapy and management.

What are the four cardinal presentations of surgical disease?
- **P**ain
- **I**nfection
- Abnormal **A**natomy (morphology/shape)
- Abnormal **F**unction (physiology)

> **Mnemonic**
>
> **PIAF**:
>   Pain, Infection, Anatomy, Function

What are the principal orthopaedic presenting complaints?
- Pain
- Reduced range of movement
- Reduced function
- Deformity

> **Example 1.** Vascular
>
> - Calf pain on walking 15 metres (pain)
> - Cold limb with reduced sensation in the toes (abnormal function)
> - Ulcers on toes (abnormal anatomy)
> - Redness and purulent discharge from toenails (infection)
>
> **Diagnosis**: short-distance claudication associated with infected toe ulcers: critical ischaemia of the lower limb

> **Example 2.** Bowel
>
> - Abdominal pain (pain)
> - Bowels opening 8 times per day (abnormal function)
> - Abdominal distension (abnormal anatomy)
> - Fresh blood and mucus in stool; recently ate burger at a music festival (infection)
>
> **Diagnosis**: infective colitis/gastroenteritis; consider neoplasia in middle-aged or elderly patient

What are the main pathological processes causing surgical disease?

- Congenital disorders
- Mechanical: intraluminal, mural, extraluminal
- Infection and inflammation: bacterial, viral, protozoal, autoimmune
- Ischaemia and haemorrhage (vascular): bleeding, thrombosis, embolism, stenosis, occlusion, aneurysmal change, ischaemia
- Tumours: primary and secondary; benign or malignant
- Trauma: physical (blunt or penetrating), thermal (burns), chemical and electric

Mnemonic

C-MIT

How should a presenting complaint be assessed?

The use of mnemonics (e.g. SOCRATES[5]) provides reassurance to the doctor but does not aid logical and systematic symptom assessment or fluid presentation of findings. Instead, four universal factors can be used to describe any symptom: quality, quantity, timing and associated risk factors/context.

- **Quality** of symptom: the site, nature and character of the presenting complaint need to be determined. Establish the presence of the four cardinal presentations: pain, abnormal function, abnormal shape and evidence of local or systemic infection.
- **Quantity**: establish the magnitude or proportion of the symptom and impact on patient – e.g. How bad is the pain (score out of 10)? How many times per day does it occur? What was the volume of blood lost? How big is the lump?
- **Timing**:
    - onset of symptom: gradual, sudden or exacerbated by specific factors
    - progression: constant or intermittent; getting worse, getting better or staying the same
    - duration
    - offset: sudden, gradual, alleviated by specific factors
- **Associated risk factors** and context.

---

[5] Site, Onset, Character, Radiation, Associated factors, Timing, Exacerbating and alleviating factors, Severity.

Presenting Complaint

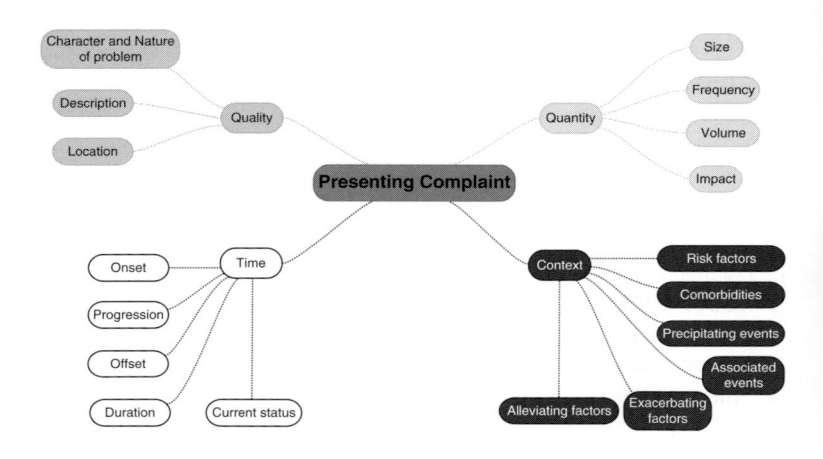

- **Quality**
  - Character and Nature of problem
  - Description
  - Location
- **Quantity**
  - Size
  - Frequency
  - Volume
  - Impact
- **Time**
  - Onset
  - Progression
  - Offset
  - Duration
  - Current status
- **Context**
  - Risk factors
  - Comorbidities
  - Precipitating events
  - Associated events
  - Exacerbating factors
  - Alleviating factors

How can the past medical history aid diagnosis?

- Recent surgery or endoscopy needs to raise awareness regarding iatrogenic injuries to surrounding anatomical structures (e.g. bleeding or perforation).
- Recent traumatic injury may predispose to undiagnosed blunt visceral injuries, e.g. blunt aortic injury, ruptured spleen, perihepatic haematomas, diaphragmatic hernias, vertebral fractures.
- Any previous operation in the abdomen predisposes to adhesional bowel obstruction and herniation.
- Insertion of prosthetic material, such as meshes in hernia repairs or orthopaedic metal work, can result in infection of the foreign materials.
- Any previous endoluminal stenting can lead to stent obstruction or migration:
  - Blockage of biliary stents can lead to ascending cholangitis.
  - Blockage of colonic stents used for palliation in bowel cancer can cause bowel obstruction.
  - Migration of aortic stents used in EVAR can cause endoleaks or acute ischaemia.
- Previous surgery for cancer may indicate tumour recurrence.
- A history of inflammatory diseases or immunosuppression can be a predictor of abscess formation and associated complications:
  - Crohn's disease: perianal fistulas or inflammatory strictures.
  - diverticulitis: bowel perforation or diverticular abscess formation.

How is fitness for surgery assessed during the history-taking process?

A surgical diagnosis implies a potential operative intervention. It is the surgeon's duty to decide whether the patient is a candidate for an operation. Furthermore, the surgeon needs to consider if the patient is able to survive not just the intervention, but also any potential complications of surgery. The correct operation in the wrong patient is as dangerous as an incorrect operation in the right candidate. This is determined according to four main criteria:

Bleeding and VTE risk
- Hereditary or acquired bleeding disorders (e.g. haemophilia) or thrombophilias.
- Anticoagulant (warfarin and heparin) and antiplatelet medication (aspirin and clopidogrel).
- Steroid use.
- Platelet deficiencies.
- Chronic renal disease: uraemia impairs platelet function.
- Chronic liver disease: abnormal clotting factor synthesis.
- Operations with high risk of bleeding will need group and save and crossmatching of blood, as well as intraoperative blood or red cell salvage equipment for autologous transfusion.

Anaesthetic risk
- Any cardiac or respiratory disease can increase anaesthetic morbidity.
- Recent myocardial infarcts, COPD, asthma and poor exercise tolerance need to be ascertained and further assessed using echocardiography, lung function testing or cardiopulmonary exercise (CPEX) studies.
- Surrogate measures of cardiorespiratory fitness include ability to climb stairs, maximum walking distance on a flat surface and ability to sleep lying flat.

Surgical risk
- Previous surgery, radiotherapy or localised infections (e.g. peritonitis) can create anatomically hostile operating fields.
- Chemotherapy, poor nutrition, steroid use or immunosuppression may lead to poor wound healing and risk of surgical site infections.
- High-risk operations will require liaison with ITU specialists regarding high dependency care postoperatively.
- Previous deep-vein thromboses, cancers, pregnancy, dehydration and immobility may predispose to future venous thromboembolisms.

- Patients who are unable to lie flat for any reason may not be candidates for certain procedures.
- Patients with terminal surgical or medical conditions (e.g. metastatic cancer, end-stage respiratory disease) may only be candidates for palliative surgery or conservative management.

Medical risk

The management of a wide range of medical problems requires adjustment in the perioperative period:

- Diabetes sufferers may need insulin sliding scales, and may need to be operated on first on the list.
- Patients with chronic renal impairment may need dialysis just before and after an operation.
- Patients with adrenal insufficiency may require conversion from oral to intravenous steroids.
- Patients with pacemakers may need pacemaker checks pre- and postoperatively, as well as the use of bipolar rather than monopolar diathermy intraoperatively.
- Patients who are carriers or actively infected with certain organisms (e.g. MRSA, HIV) may require special prophylactic and intraoperative interventions.
- Antibiotic or latex allergies need to be identified early in the preoperative assessment, to ensure patient safety during anaesthesia.
- Patients with significant comorbidities and anaesthetic risk may not be candidates for surgery. They may instead require conservative management or further preoperative assessment by an anaesthetist.

Written communication of a surgical consultation

Model
Name, hospital number, date of birth
Age
Occupation
Context of consultation: outpatient clinic/ward referral/letter to GP and responsible consultant
Presenting complaint
Background:
• PSH
• PMH

- DH
- SH
- FH

Current status
Examination findings
Investigations
Management to date
Current problems
Plan

Example

24/07/2015

Mr J. Smith, dob 01/04/1950, Hospital Number: 123456

Dear Dr Thomas,

Thank you for referring Mr Smith to Miss Jones's vascular outpatient clinic.

Presenting complaint: Right calf pain for 6 months

Background:

Type II diabetes on metformin

Smokes 20 cigarettes/day for 35 years

On 75 mg aspirin and 40 mg simvastatin

Allergic to PENICILLIN (rash)

Currently:

Mr Smith complains of pain in the right calf on walking 50 yards in the last 6 months. This is brought on by exercise and relieved by rest. He has no rest pain or history of ulcers, gangrene or soft tissue infections. He does not complain of back pain, sciatica or knee pain. There is no history of calf pain or swelling.

On examination:

Blood pressure 130/90 mmHg. Heart rate 85, regular.

The right foot is cooler than the left. There is no evidence of cellulitis, ulcers or gangrene in either leg. The aorta is not palpable. The femoral and popliteal pulses are present bilaterally. The DP and TP pulses are present in the left foot but absent in the right. Capillary refill time is 4–5 seconds on the right and 3 seconds on the left. Buerger's test is negative bilaterally.

ABPI is 0.5 on the right and 0.85 on the left.

Doppler signals on the right side: monophasic dorsalis pedis; absent tibialis posterior; biphasic femoral.

No evidence of venous or lymphatic disease in either leg.

Impression/diagnosis:

I feel Mr Smith has short-distance claudication in his right leg secondary to peripheral arterial disease. This may be affecting the right SFA.

Plan:

I have organised a CT angiogram of his lower limbs (creatinine 75, eGFR > 60) with oral rehydration.

I have encouraged him to give up smoking, control his blood sugar levels and exercise for at least 20 minutes each day. He is already on best medical therapy with aspirin and a statin.

I will see him in 2 weeks' time once the CT angiogram has been discussed in the vascular MDT. If he develops any aggravation of his symptoms in the meantime I have advised him to attend A&E.

Many thanks.

Yours sincerely,

Mr A. Johnson

Vascular SpR to Miss Jones

Bleep 1234

Surgical consent

Patient: name, date of birth, hospital number

Procedure:

Responsible clinician:

Benefits:

Complications:

- Local:
  - bleeding
  - infection
  - scarring/herniation
  - damage to surrounding structures (viscera, arteries, veins, nerves)
  - failure of procedure

- General:
  - loss of life
  - cardiopulmonary complications (myocardial infarcts, chest infections)
  - deep vein thrombosis and pulmonary embolism
  - pain and neuropathy

Type of anaesthesia:
- local
- regional
- general

Other procedures:

Blood transfusion:

Patient: name, signature, date

Surgeon: name, signature, date

Examination notes

What are the variable, operation-specific, local complications?

- Damage to surrounding structures – depending on procedure, this involves iatrogenic damage to surrounding arteries, veins, nerves or viscera:
  - any abdominal laparoscopy: bowel, bladder or vascular injury
  - any endoscopy: viscus perforation and bleeding (especially if biopsies are performed) requiring surgery
  - laparoscopic cholecystectomy: bile duct injury
  - inguinal hernia repair: chronic groin pain due to ilioinguinal nerve entrapment, ischaemic orchitis in men
  - carotid endarterectomy: hypoglossal and vagus nerve injuries, stroke

- Failure of procedure – this involves either disease recurrence in the future or inability to perform the intended procedure:
  - any laparoscopic surgery: conversion to open
  - laparoscopic cholecystectomy: stone retention in the common bile duct and need for ERCP
  - hernia repair: hernia recurrence
  - cancer surgery: incomplete resection margin, tumour recurrence

Information giving

- Introduction: name and position
- Ascertain who you are talking to (patient, relative or friend)
- Outline purpose of discussion
- Establish rapport (verbal and non-verbal communication)
- Ascertain knowledge of events so far
- Identify any concerns or expectation
- Explain circumstances/indications (prepare ground)
- Deliver information in small increments

- Allow time for patient to reflect
- Observe patient's reactions
- Any questions?
- Reiterate key points
- Outline a plan for the future
- Check patient's understanding and any further questions
- Give patient targeted objective until next meeting
- Provide information for further understanding (e.g. brochure or websites)
- Provide contact details if any future concerns (secretary, nurse specialist)
- Thank patient and end consultation

Explaining a procedure

- Introduction: name and position
- Ascertain who you are talking to (patient, relative or friend)
- Outline purpose of discussion
- Establish rapport (verbal and non-verbal communication)
- Ascertain knowledge of events so far
- Explain indication for procedure
- Explain procedure:
    - name and what it means
    - what it involves
    - duration
    - setting: inpatient or outpatient
    - local, regional or general anaesthesia
    - pain levels expected
    - recovery period
- Benefits of procedure
- Complications of procedure (and relative risks of these occurring)
- Alternative procedures
- Allow time for reflection
- Any questions?
- Check patient's understanding and any further questions
- Give patient targeted objective until next meeting/procedure
- Provide information for further understanding (e.g. brochure or websites)
- Provide contact details if any future concerns (secretary, nurse specialist)
- Thank patient and end consultation

Section editor: Petrut Gogalniceanu
Senior author: Andrew T. Raftery

Section 2: General surgery

Chapter 3: Examination of peripheral stigmata of disease in general surgery

Petrut Gogalniceanu, William Lynn and Andrew T. Raftery

Checklist

WIPER
- Patient supine, exposed from nipples to knee. Genitals covered.
- Groins need to be accessible but only uncovered when examined. Chaperone as required.

Physiological parameters

Bedside
- Catheters, drains, central lines
- Position in bed: restless (colic) vs. immobile (peritonitis)
- Thigh flexion: psoas sign

Peripheral stigmata of gastrointestinal disease
- Malnourishment, weight loss, cachexia
- Jaundice
- Pyoderma gangrenosum/erythema nodosum (Crohn's disease)

Hands
- Nails: clubbing, splinter haemorrhages, koilonychia, leukonychia
- Palms: palmar erythema, Dupuytren's contracture, liver flap tremor
- Radial pulse: rate, rhythm
- Blood pressure

Physical Examination for Surgeons, ed. Petrut Gogalniceanu, James Pegrum and William Lynn. Published by Cambridge University Press. © Cambridge University Press 2015.

Eyes
- Anaemia (pale conjunctiva)
- Jaundice (sclera)
- Xanthelasmas

Lips
- Perioral telangiectasias (Peutz–Jeghers disease)
- Aphthous stomatitis

Tongue
- Glossitis
- Icteric frenulum

Neck
- Left supraclavicular lymphadenopathy (Virchow's node, Troisier's sign)

Chest
- Spider naevi/angiomas
- Gynaecomastia
- Scratch marks (pruritus)
- Axillary hair loss

Examination notes

What are the signs of metastatic cancer?
- Cachexia
- Jaundice
- Ascites
- Bone pain
- Shortness of breath (lung metastasis, pleural effusions, pulmonary emboli)
- Scars from previous surgery
- Radiotherapy skin changes
- Tunnelled lines for long-term chemotherapy or nutrition
- Symptoms related to paraneoplastic syndromes

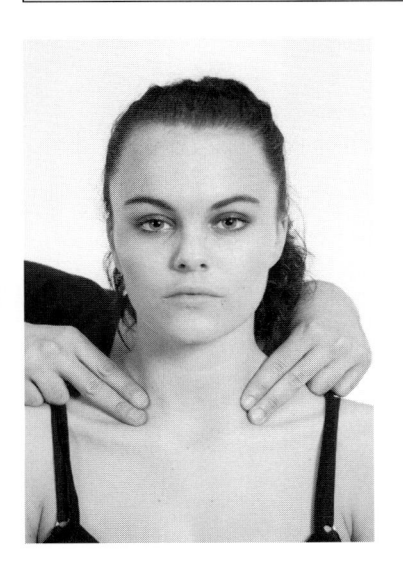

Palpation of the supraclavicular lymph nodes as part of the abdominal examination. This should also include palpation of the axillary and inguinal lymph nodes.

What are the signs of chronic liver disease?

Chronic liver disease leads to impaired hepatic synthetic function and portal hypertension. These lead to:

Mechanism	Signs
Coagulopathy	Ecchymosis and petecchiae
Impaired bilirubin metabolism	Jaundice Pruritus and scratch marks
Increased levels of serum oestrogen	Loss of secondary hair Palmar erythema Gynaecomastia Testicular atrophy Telangiectasia/spider naevi
Low albumin	Ascites Ankle and sacral oedema Cachexia
Portal hypertension	Splenomegaly

(cont.)

Mechanism	Signs
Portosystemic shunts	Gastro-oesophageal varices Retroperitoneal varices Anorectal varices Periumbilical varices (caput medusae)

What do the following peripheral stigmata of surgical disease signify?

Peripheral signs	Clinical findings	Relevance
Skin		
Jaundice	Yellow discolouration of the skin, sclera and lingual frenulum associated with dark brown urine	Impaired bilirubin metabolism; prehepatic, hepatic or posthepatic
Pyoderma gangrenosum	Ulcerative cutaneous lesion usually found on the skin of the legs and associated with systemic diseases	Associated with inflammatory bowel disease, and more rarely with primary biliary cirrhosis and hepatitis
Erythema nodosum	Tender nodular erythema affecting the skin on the anterior aspect of the lower limbs (hypersensitivity reaction)	Associated with inflammatory bowel disease, lymphoma, sarcoidosis, TB and streptococcal infections
Spider naevi (naevi aranei)	Small, blanching vascular lesion with a central arteriole surrounded by radially placed thin capillaries resembling a spider; usually found above the nipples	Chronic liver disease, thyrotoxicosis, oestrogen therapy

(cont.)

Peripheral signs	Clinical findings	Relevance
Hands		
Clubbing	Loss of Lovibond's angle (angle between distal phalanx and nail bed); Schamroth's sign (loss of diamond-shaped space between two opposed fingernails); bulbous or drumstick appearance of terminal parts of the fingers	See *Differential diagnoses*
Splinter haemorrhages	Longitudinal extravasation of blood in the nail bed	Bacterial endocarditis, mitral stenosis
Koilonychia	Spoon-shaped nails	Iron deficiency anaemia
Leukonychia	White discolouration or spots of the nails	Hypoalbuminaemia (chronic liver or renal disease), lymphoma
Palmar erythema	Red palms secondary to increased levels of oestrogen and angiogenic factors	Chronic liver disease, metastatic cancer, oestrogen therapy, pregnancy, thyrotoxicosis, polycythaemia, idiopathic
Beau lines	Arrested nail growth causing transverse nail depression	Severe systemic disease, sepsis or malnutrition
Asterixis	Coarse tremor of the wrists at rest ('liver flap')	Decompensated chronic liver disease/ encephalopathy
Eyes		
Xanthelasma	Yellow plaques on the inner canthus of the upper eyelid	Hyperlipidaemia
Xanthoma	Cutaneous lipid plaques (called xanthelasmas if found in the periorbital region)	Hyperlipidaemia

(cont.)

Peripheral signs	Clinical findings	Relevance
Corneal arcus	White rim of opacity around the border of the cornea; in the elderly it's known as arcus senilis and may be idiopathic	Abnormal lipid metabolism, e.g. hypercholesterolaemia
Mouth		
Perioral telangiectasia	Perioral melanin deposits causing pigmentation	Peutz–Jeghers syndrome: associated with multiple hamartomatous polyps in the GI tract; increased risk of GI cancer; cutaneous melanin deposits also seen at other sites
Angular stomatitis	Cracked mouth corners	Iron deficiency anaemia
Glossitis	Inflamed, smooth and erythematous tongue due to depapillation	Iron deficiency anaemia, vitamin B deficiencies, infections

Differential diagnoses

What causes finger clubbing?

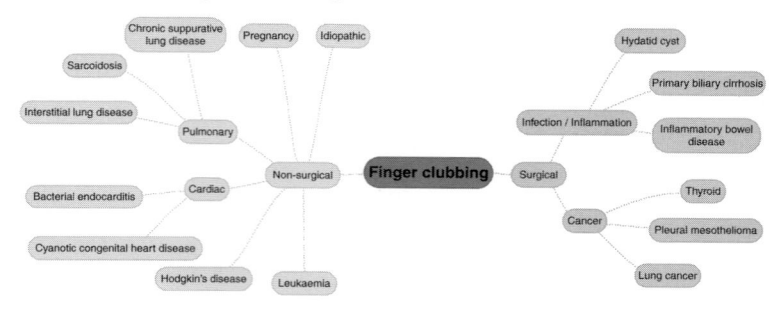

Finger clubbing

- Non-surgical
  - Pulmonary
    - Chronic suppurative lung disease
    - Pregnancy
    - Idiopathic
    - Sarcoidosis
    - Interstitial lung disease
  - Cardiac
    - Bacterial endocarditis
    - Cyanotic congenital heart disease
  - Hodgkin's disease
  - Leukaemia
- Surgical
  - Infection / Inflammation
    - Hydatid cyst
    - Primary biliary cirrhosis
    - Inflammatory bowel disease
  - Cancer
    - Thyroid
    - Pleural mesothelioma
    - Lung cancer

What are the causes of jaundice?

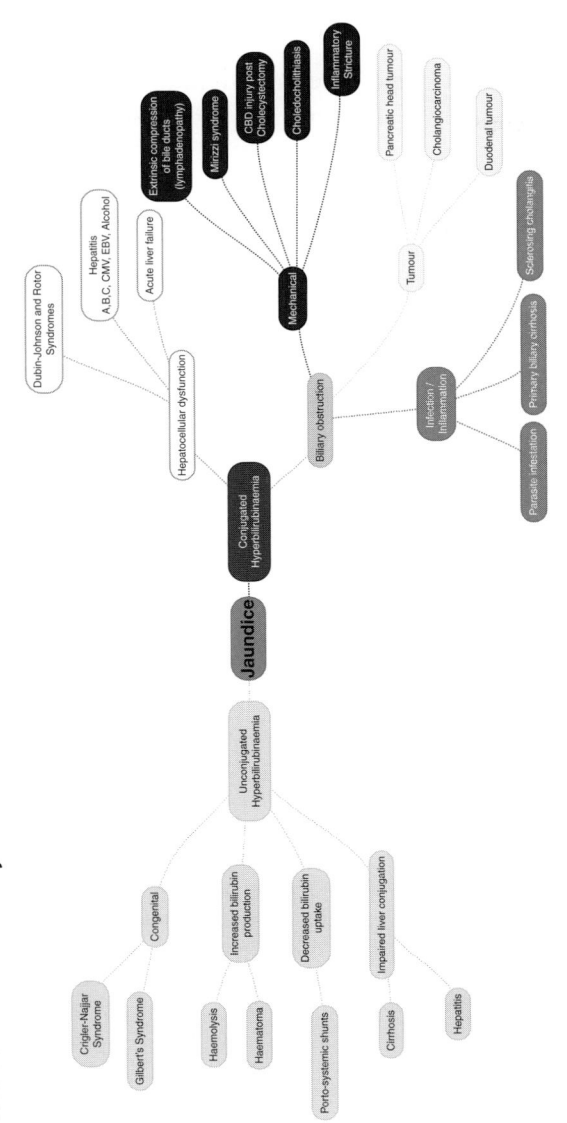

Jaundice

Unconjugated Hyperbilirubinaemia

- **Congenital**
  - Crigler-Najjar Syndrome
  - Gilbert's Syndrome
- **Increased bilirubin production**
  - Haemolysis
  - Haematoma
- **Decreased bilirubin uptake**
  - Porto-systemic shunts
- **Impaired liver conjugation**
  - Cirrhosis
  - Hepatitis

Conjugated Hyperbilirubinaemia

- Dubin-Johnson and Rotor Syndromes
- **Hepatocellular dysfunction**
  - Hepatitis A, B, C, CMV, EBV, Alcohol
  - Acute liver failure
- **Biliary obstruction**
  - **Mechanical**
    - Extrinsic compression of bile ducts (lymphadenopathy)
    - Mirizzi syndrome
    - CBD injury post Cholecystectomy
    - Choledocholithiasis
    - Inflammatory Stricture
  - **Tumour**
    - Pancreatic head tumour
    - Cholangiocarcinoma
    - Duodenal tumour
  - **Infection / Inflammation**
    - Sclerosing cholangitis
    - Primary biliary cirrhosis
    - Parasite infestation

33

Section 2: General surgery

Chapter 4

Examination of the abdomen

Petrut Gogalniceanu, William Lynn and Andrew T. Raftery

Checklist

WIPER

Physiological parameters
- Check peripheries for stigmata of abdominal disease.

Inspection
- **Skin**: scars, stomas, sinuses/fistulas, distended veins, drains

  Ask patient to cough. Observe for pain, peritoneal irritation, hernias or musculoskeletal pain.

- **Abdominal wall**: hernias (cough + head-up + heels off bed): inspect ventral abdominal wall, umbilicus, groins and scars
- **Abdominal cavity**: distension, pulsations, masses, visible peristalsis
- **Flanks**: scars, flank bulges

  Ask patient to lean forward. Inspect for hernias as patient strains.

- **Back**: scars, sacral oedema, pressure ulceration
- **Ankles**: peripheral oedema, calf swelling

Palpation

Kneel and look at patient's face to identify discomfort during palpation.

- Light palpation, four quadrants: identify peritonitis, distension, musculoskeletal pain (use four fingers of one hand).
- Deep palpation, nine regions: identify masses, organomegaly, rebound tenderness, guarding (use two hands).

Physical Examination for Surgeons, ed. Petrut Gogalniceanu, James Pegrum and William Lynn. Published by Cambridge University Press. © Cambridge University Press 2015.

- Liver, gallbladder and spleen → on inspiration
- Kidneys → ballot with two hands
- Aorta → lateral to medial palpation with two hands
- Scars: incisional hernias → cough
- Groins: inguinal and femoral hernias, inguinal lymph nodes → cough
- Scrotum
- Lower ribs and pelvis
- Specific abdominal signs (see table on pages 49–50)

Percussion
- Percussion tenderness: peritoneal irritation
- Ascites: dullness in flanks, shifting dullness, fluid thrill
- Liver size, spleen size
- Palpable bladder

Auscultation
- Bowel sounds
- Abdominal aortic aneurysm bruit
- Renal artery stenosis bruit
- Liver/splenic bruits

To complete the examination...
- Digital rectal examination
- External genitalia
- Urine dipstick

Examination notes

The examination of the abdomen is a broad screening examination that may lead to a focused assessment of other systems. It remains the trademark examination of the general surgeon. A systematic anatomical approach is needed to provide an authoritative opinion.

The examination of the abdomen can be structured around three anatomical layers: skin, abdominal wall and abdominal content.

> **Tip**
>
> **'Gift box' analogy:**
> - Wrapping paper – skin
> - Box – abdominal wall
> - Content – abdominal cavity

Section 2: General surgery

The abdomen is then further divided into nine anatomical regions (3 × 3) or four surgical quadrants.

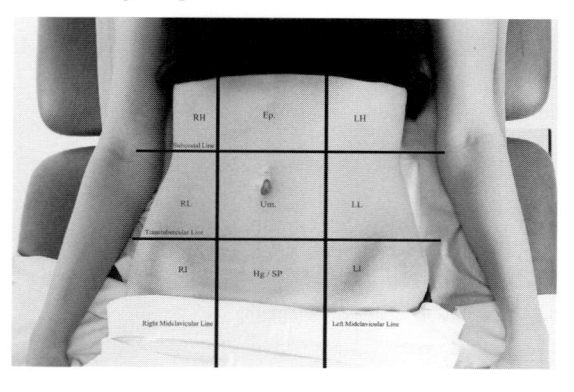

Division of the abdomen into nine regions. RH, right hypochondrium; Ep, epigastric area; LH, left hypochondrium; RL, right lumbar area; Um, umbilical or periumbilical area; LL, left lumbar area; RI, right iliac fossa / right inguinal area; Hg/SP, hypogastric or suprapubic area; LI, left iliac fossa / left inguinal area.

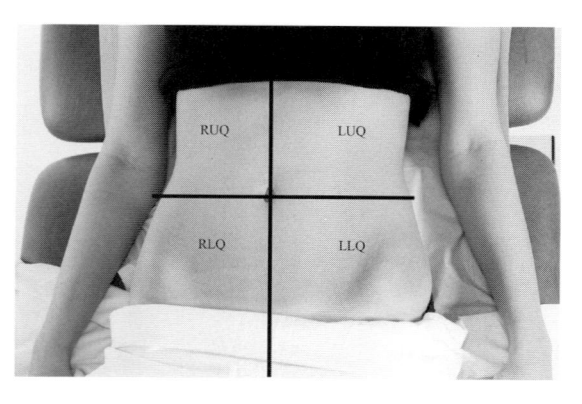

Division of the abdomen into four quadrants. RUQ, right upper quadrant; LUQ, left upper quadrant; RLQ, right lower quadrant; LLQ, left lower quadrant.

What organs can be palpated in each abdominal area?

	RUQ	Epigastrium	LUQ	
	Liver Gallbladder Hepatic flexure of colon	Stomach Pancreas Transverse colon	Spleen Splenic flexure of colon	
R renal angle Renal mass/ tenderness	**R flank** Ascending colon Kidney	**Periumbilical** Aorta Small bowel	**L flank** Descending colon Kidney	**L renal angle** Renal mass/ tenderness
	R iliac fossa Caecum Appendix R iliac artery R ovary	**Suprapubic area** Bladder Uterus	**L iliac fossa** Sigmoid colon L iliac artery L ovary	
	R groin Inguinal hernia Femoral hernia Lymphadenopathy	**Genitals** Vagina Penis & scrotum DRE	**L groin** Inguinal hernia Femoral hernia Lymphadenopathy	

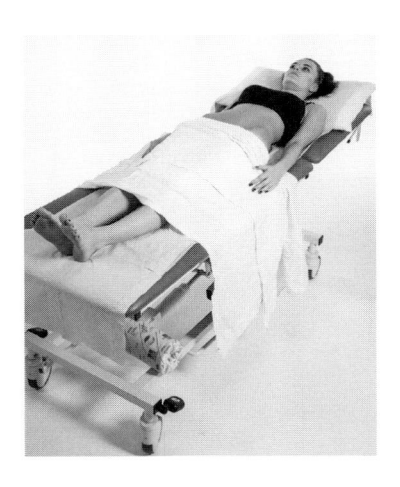

Position and exposure of the patient for abdominal examination. The patient must lie flat with a pillow under the head. Note that the legs and back must be exposed, in addition to the abdomen. The abdomen must be exposed from the lower chest (below the breasts) to the pubis, with access to the groins for examination of the inguinal areas, genitalia and femoral pulses.

Section 2: General surgery

When examining the abdomen, the surgeon must ask three questions:
1. Is there any surgical disease or process involving the skin (layer 1)?
2. Is there any abdominal wall pathology (layer 2)?
3. Is there any pathology arising from the abdominal cavity (layer 3)?

Layer 1: What skin changes should be identified?
- Scars (previous surgery), stomas, sinuses, fistulas, lacerations
- Trauma: haematomas or ecchymosis
- Infective: erythema, cellulitis, abscesses
- Tumours: benign or malignant growths

Layer 2: What abdominal wall changes should be identified?
- Hernias
- Soft tissue masses

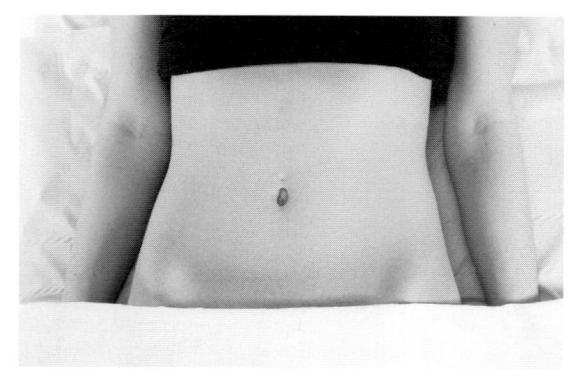

Inspection of the abdomen. This should be done from the right side of the bed, inspecting from above, but also from the side of the abdomen to look for changes in abdominal contour (distension, peristalsis, pulastions). The back and flanks must also be visualised as part of the abdominal inspection.

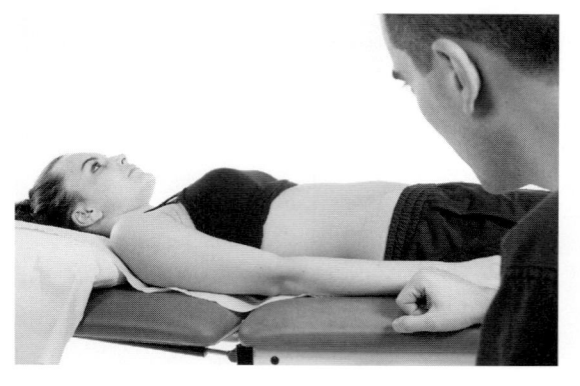

(cont.)

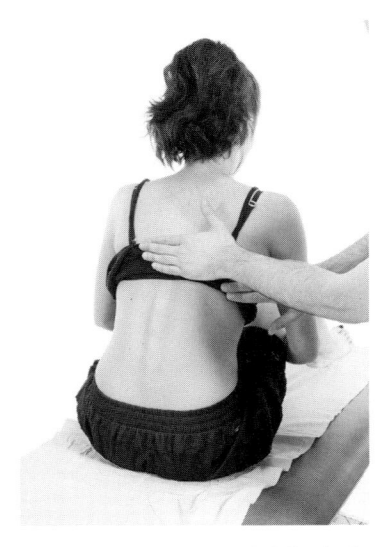

Layer 3: What markers of abdominal cavity pathology should be identified?
- Pain or peritoneal irritation
- Distension
- Masses

Where should hernias be identified?
- A hernia is 'an abnormal protrusion of an organ or tissue through the wall of the cavity in which it is contained'. Hernias must be actively sought out and excluded through inspection and palpation in the following areas:
    - inguinal canal
    - femoral canal
    - obturator canal
    - peri- or intraumbilical area
    - pararectal space (Spigelian hernia)
    - midline of the abdomen (epigastrium)
    - deep to scars (incisional)
- Patients can be asked to cough or lift their head or feet off the bed in order to raise intra-abdominal pressure and make hernias apparent.
- Any abdominal, flank or groin incision needs to be examined to rule out incisional herniation.
- Midline ventral hernias (midline fascial defects) must be differentiated from divarication of the recti (lateral displacement of abdominal recti muscles with stretching of the underlying connective tissues but absence of a fascial defect).

- Desmoid tumours are rare causes of pain originating in the abdominal wall. They are fibrous tumours originating in muscular or aponeurotic tissue. Although rare, these are usually found in scar tissue, at the site of previous trauma or in the rectus abdominis muscle. On examination, they are fixed to abdominal wall structures and have normal overlying skin. They occur in Gardner's syndrome (familial polyposis coli, desmoid tumours, osteomas of the mandible and multiple sebaceous cysts).

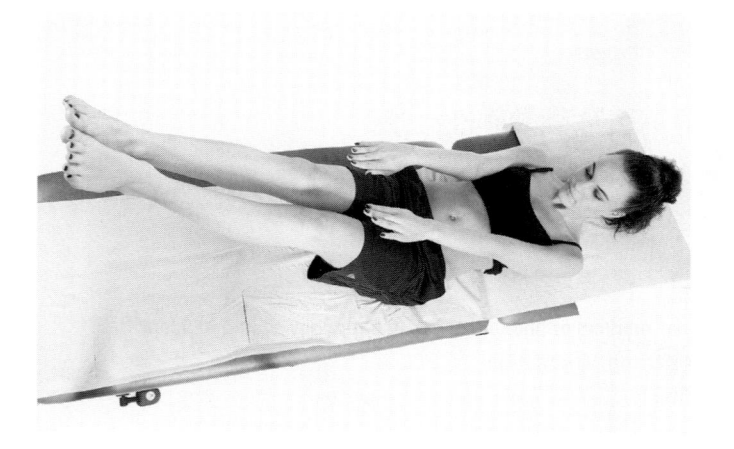

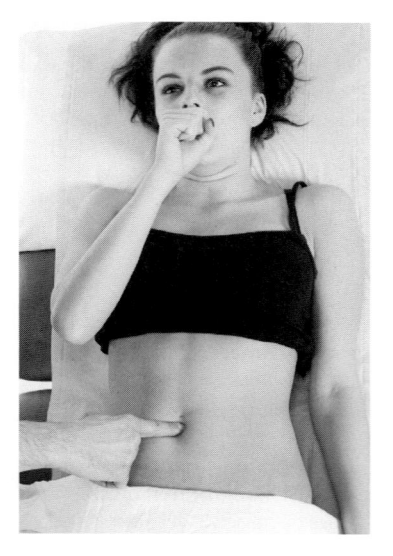

Testing the abdominal wall for hernias: (A) ventral hernias and (B) umbilical or paraumbilical hernias. Hernias are more apparent with increased intra-abdominal pressure. The patient should be asked to cough, and to lift the legs off the bed, and should finally be examined standing.

Chapter 4: Examination of the abdomen | 41

What is the purpose of light palpation?
Light palpation aims to determine whether there is:
- Peritoneal irritation: generalised or localised pain, rigidity or rebound guarding
- Distension: 5 Fs (see below)

What is the purpose of deep palpation?
Deep palpation investigates tenderness or changes in individual organs in the nine abdominal regions.

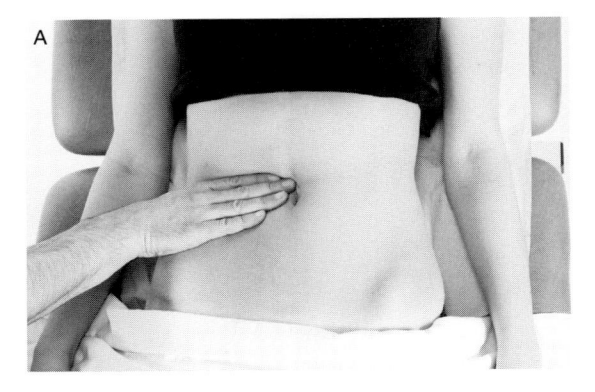

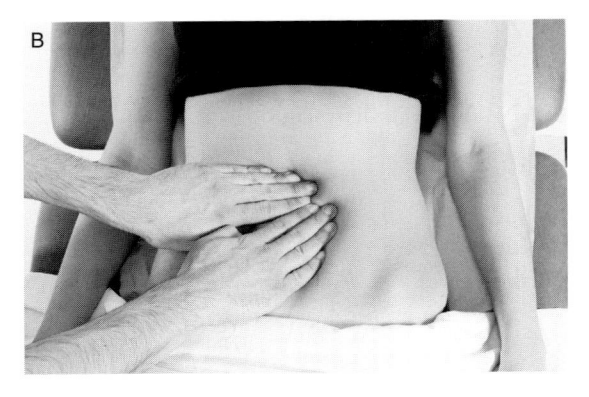

Palpation of (A) liver and (B) spleen is done in inspiration, in both cases starting in (C) the right iliac fossa and moving towards the right and left upper quadrants, respectively. Palpation of the appendix starts away from the area of pain and ends in the right lower quadrant (C), where rebound tenderness is tested. (D) The kidney is balloted with two hands.

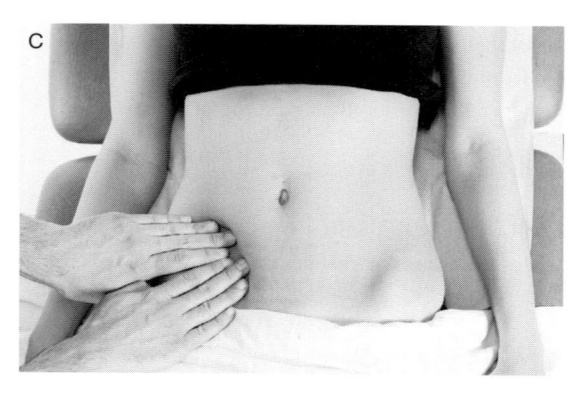

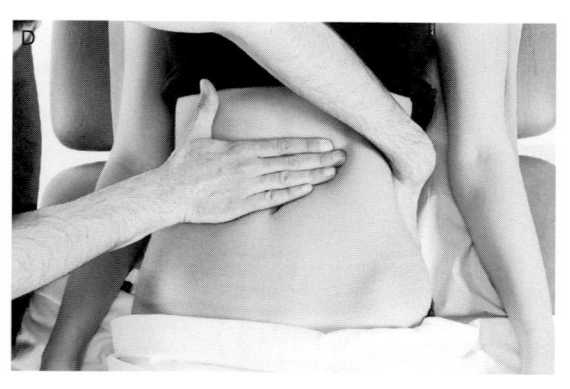

What are the causes of abdominal distension?

The 5 Fs:

- Fat
- Faeces (constipation)
- Flatus (gas, i.e. obstruction)
- Fluid (ascites, haemorrhage)
- Fetus (pregnancy; also note other gynaecological causes of distension such as fibroids or large ovarian cysts)

Where can the small and large bowel be palpated?

Large and small bowel can be palpated in any part of the abdomen, as they are mobile, partially fixed structures. In the context of bowel obstruction, the abdomen will be distended and resonant on percussion due to gas-filled bowel loops. Alternatively, the abdomen may be dull on percussion if the bowel loops are filled with intestinal fluid or blood.

How is visceral abdominal pain explained from an embryological perspective?

- Epigastric pain: viscera arising from the foregut give rise to midline dull epigastric pain
- Periumbilical pain: viscera arising from the midgut give rise to midline dull periumbilical pain
- Suprapubic pain: viscera arising from the hindgut give rise to midline dull suprapubic pain

What are the anatomical origins of abdominal pain?

In craniocaudal order:

- Psychological
- Neurological (spinal or intercostal nerve irritation)
- Chest
- Skin (shingles)
- Abdominal wall
- Intraperitoneal organs
- Retroperitoneal organs
- Pelvis

> **Tip**
>
> A common error is to include only gastrointestinal or hepatobiliary causes of abdominal pain (abdominal causes) in the differential diagnosis, whilst ignoring other anatomical sources e.g. thoracic (e.g. lower lobe pneumonia, MI) or neurological (herpes zoster).

What is the purpose of the cough sign?

- Peritonitis: in the presence of localised inflammation (peritonitis), coughing produces localised pain which the patient involuntarily identifies (Dunphy's sign).

- Hernias: coughing increases intra-abdominal pressure and makes any hernias more prominent.
- Musculoskeletal pain: coughing strains the abdominal wall and causes pain at the site of soft tissue pathology.

What are the features of peritonitis?
- Rebound tenderness: on palpation of the abdomen, the pain is worse on suddenly lifting the hand off the abdomen than it was on initially palpating it. This is explained by the contact between the peritoneum and the inflamed structures below it on applying pressure (this causes tenderness only), and sudden peritoneal irritation experienced when the hand is quickly withdrawn. Ensure this is done gently and not repeated, in order not to cause unnecessary discomfort.
- In patients with severe peritonitis, asking them to cough or even lightly percussing the abdomen can lead to symptoms of peritonitis (percussion tenderness).
- Pelvic peritonitis can also be established through a rectal examination, where the tip of the finger in the anus can elicit a powerful intraperitoneal response. Free fluid from perforated viscera or intra-abdominal pus collects in the dependent parts of the pelvis (rectovesical or rectouterine pouch), which can be examined through a digital rectal examination.

How can peritonitis be classified?
- Peritonitis can be either generalised or localised. Generalised peritonitis causes tenderness on palpation of any part of the abdomen, with a typical 'board-like rigidity' of the abdomen. Localised peritonitis is characterised by rebound guarding, pain on percussion or coughing in one isolated area. Localised peritonitis can lead to generalised peritonitis.
- Peritonitis can be primary or secondary. Primary peritonitis can occur spontaneously (spontaneous bacterial peritonitis) in patients with chronic liver disease. Secondary bacterial peritonitis arises secondary to a source of intra-abdominal infection (e.g. perforated bowel).

Why does gastric, duodenal or gallbladder inflammation or perforation present with right iliac fossa pain?
Inflammatory fluid from upper abdominal viscera can drain through the right paracolic gutter and pool in the iliac fossae and pelvis to cause lower abdominal pain.

Why can appendicitis cause RUQ pain?
A high caecum or long appendix (retrocolic) with an inflamed tip may cause RUQ pain. Similarly, pus from a perforated appendix may form an abscess in the subhepatic space.

How should the aorta be palpated?
The aorta divides into the left and right common iliac arteries at the L4 level, which roughly corresponds to the umbilicus in thin patients. The aorta should therefore be palpated bimanually above the umbilicus. The four fingers of the hands move lateral to medial to isolate the aorta between them. The hands are moved deeper with each of the patient's expiratory movements, thereby overcoming voluntary guarding. Never press vigorously on a tender or obvious aneurysm, because of the risk of rupture.

> **Tip**
>
> AAA cannot be excluded just on clinical examination. Ultrasound scanning is the first-line screening and diagnostic imaging modality in patients at risk.

Is there any purpose in palpating below the umbilicus in a patient with AAA?
Yes, but in the right and left iliac fossae to identify any iliac extension of the aneurysmal disease.

Why should the ribs and pelvis be palpated as part of the abdominal exam?
- Fractured ribs can cause liver or splenic lacerations.
- Pain from fractured ribs or pelvic bones may be interpreted as intra-abdominal pain.
- Pelvic fractures may be associated with iliac vascular or renal tract injuries.

How should the spleen be palpated?
Start in the right iliac fossa and move superolaterally towards the left upper quadrant. The patient may be rotated towards the right side, to allow the spleen to displace medially from beneath the left costal margin.

What are the differences between splenomegaly and a left renal mass?

	Splenomegaly	**Renal mass**
Displacement	Towards RIF	Inferiorly
Edge	Palpable anteromedial notch	Smooth
Palpation	Non-ballotable	Ballotable
Palpation	Cannot get above spleen	Can palpate above kidney
Percussion	Dull	Resonant (overlying bowel gas)
Auscultation	Friction rub	No friction rub

What are the causes of lymphadenopathy?
See Chapter 36, *Examination of the neck and thyroid*.

What urine tests should be performed in patients with abdominal pain?
- Urine dipstick:
  - blood (renal calculi, urinary tract infections or urogenital tract trauma, menstruation)
  - leukocytes and nitrites (urinary tract infections)
  - ketones and glucose (diabetic ketoacidosis causing abdominal pain)
- Microscopy, culture and sensitivity (M, C & S), if there is any evidence of urinary tract infection
- Pregnancy testing in all women of child-bearing age irrespective of reported sexual activity. Ambiguous results or those not in keeping with clinical findings require blood serum testing for bHCG. This is essential in any woman:
  - undergoing imaging requiring radiation exposure
  - with abdominal pain where an ectopic pregnancy must be excluded
  - undergoing surgery or anaesthesia, as these can be technically and physiologically complicated by pregnancy, and fetal viability may be compromised

What are the basic imaging tests that can be requested?
Erect chest x-ray, abdominal x-ray and a transabdominal ultrasound scan

What is the purpose of a chest x-ray in the abdominal examination?
- To rule out free air under the diaphragm from perforation of a hollow viscus (erect chest radiograph)
- To rule out consolidation of the lower lobes of the lungs causing pain radiating to the abdomen
- To diagnose hiatal hernias
- To identify pulmonary metastases from abdominal viscera

What is the purpose of an abdominal x-ray in the abdominal examination?
- To rule out large or small bowel obstruction
- Other signs that could be identified are:
    - abnormal calcifications: chronic pancreatitis, abdominal aortic aneurysm, renal or gallbladder calculi, appendicoliths
    - loss of peritoneal shadow lines/psoas shadows in retroperitoneal pathology
    - pneumobilia: air in the biliary system
    - Rigler's sign
    - evidence of bowel volvulus
    - gallstone ileus (small bowel obstruction, air in the biliary tree)

What is the purpose of the transbadominal ultrasonography in the abdominal examination?
- Identify free fluid or abscesses
- Solid organ assessment:
    - abdominal aortic aneurysms
    - liver: tumours, fatty infiltration, cirrhotic changes
    - gallbladder: gallstone disease, cholecystitis, intrahepatic or common bile duct dilatation
    - pancreas: swelling or oedema consistent with pancreatitis
    - kidneys, ureters and bladder: tumours, hydronephrosis or hydroureter
    - spleen: splenomegaly, metastatic deposits or rupture (poor sensitivity)
    - ovaries: tumours or cysts

What advanced imaging investigations may be requested following an abdominal examination?
- Computed tomography (CT) or magnetic resonance imaging (MRI) of the abdomen
- MRI is preferred in imaging pelvic structures (first-line modality) and the pancreas and biliary tract (MRCP – second-line modality following US)

What bedside investigations should be performed in all patients with fresh rectal bleeding?
- Anoscopy/proctoscopy
- Rigid sigmoidoscopy

What causes bulging of the flanks?
- Ascites
- Abdominal muscular paralysis secondary to transverse lateral flank or upper quadrant incisions which transect the motor fibres of the intercostal nerves
- Incisional hernias
- Renal haematoma or abscess (rarely)

What are the signs of lymphoproliferative diseases?
- Widespread lymphadenopathy
- Splenomegaly +/– hepatomegaly
- Signs of sepsis or opportunistic infections

What is a Sister Mary Joseph nodule?
Sister Mary Joseph nodule is an umbilical metastatic deposit caused by ovarian, gastric, hepatic or pancreatic peritoneal carcinomatosis.

What is Virchow's node?
Virchow's node is an abnormal, palpable left supraclavicular lymph node. This was initially associated with lymphatic metastasis from gastric cancer, but subsequently used as an indicator of upper abdominal visceral cancer metastasis (Troisier's sign). Virchow's node is found on the left where the thoracic duct (main truncal lymphatic vessel) drains lymph into the confluence of the left subclavian and left internal jugular veins.

What are the specific surgical eponymous signs?

Sign	Clinical features	Diagnosis
Spleen		
Kehr's sign	Left shoulder tip pain due to splenic rupture	Splenic rupture
Liver		
Murphy's sign	Palpation of the RUQ on inspiration. In the presence of acute cholecystitis, the patient suddenly stops breathing when the gallbladder comes in contact with the examiner's hand. It is negative in patients with renal or bile-duct-related RUQ pain	Acute cholecystitis
Boas' sign	Hyperaesthesia inferior to the right scapula	Acute cholecystitis
Gastrointestinal		
Rovsing's sign	Pressure in the LIF causes pain in the RIF with appendicitis	Appendicitis
Abdominal wall and peritoneum		
Obturator sign	Ipsilateral hip and knee are flexed; internal rotation of the hip (heel moves outwards) stretches obturator internus, which causes pain if in contact with an inflamed appendix	Peritonitis (usually in appendicitis)
Psoas sign	Inflammatory processes in the retroperitoneum irritate the psoas muscle, causing ipsilateral hip flexion. Straightening the leg causes further pain	Peritonitis (usually in retrocolic appendicitis)
Howship–Romberg sign	Medial thigh pain; hip is internally rotated	Obturator canal hernia

(cont.)

Sign	Clinical features	Diagnosis
Cullen's sign	Periumbilical ecchymosis	Retroperitoneal bleed: acute pancreatitis, ruptured AAA
Grey Turner's sign	Bilateral flank ecchymosis	Retroperitoneal bleed: acute pancreatitis, ruptured AAA

Differential diagnoses

What are the causes of abdominal wall ecchymosis?
- Blunt trauma to the abdominal wall
- Recent surgery
- Retroperitoneal bleed (Grey Turner's sign: bilateral flank ecchymosis; Cullen's sign: periumbilical ecchymosis) – e.g. acute haemorrhagic pancreatitis, ruptured abdominal aortic aneurysm or kidney
- Subcutaneous low-molecular-weight heparin injections for VTE prophylaxis
- Underlying bleeding diathesis/coagulopathy: e.g. thrombocytopenia, warfarin therapy

What are the causes of renal angle tenderness?
- Renal colic
- Hydronephrosis
- Pyelonephritis
- Perinephric abscess
- Lower lobe pneumonia
- Inflamed retrocaecal appendix (right side)

What causes abdominal bruits?
A bruit is caused by turbulent (abnormal) blood flow within a vessel. Bruits are rare and have a poor sensitivity.
- RUQ/flank:
    - hepatoma
    - hepatic cancer
    - renal artery stenosis

- LUQ/flank:
  - dilated or tortuous splenic artery (splenomegaly)
  - renal artery stenosis
- Epigastrium:
  - abdominal aortic aneurysm
  - mesenteric ischaemia/coeliac artery compression syndrome
  - pancreatic cancer
- Arteriovenous malformation or fistula (in any organ)

What are the surgical causes of abdominal pain?

Surgical Causes of Abdominal Pain

- **Congenital**

- **Infective / inflammatory**
  - Ascending cholangitis
  - Acute Cholecystitis
  - Acute pancreatitis
  - Acute appendicitis
  - Diverticulitis +/− Abscess
  - Liver abscess
  - Colitis
    - Infective
    - Indeterminate
    - IBD
  - Peptic ulcer Disease
  - Perinephric abscess

- **Trauma**
  - Blunt
  - Penetrating
  - Visceral damage
    - Bile, blood or faecal Peritonitis

- **Mechanical**
  - HPB
    - Choledocholithiasis
    - Biliary Colic
  - Urinary
    - Hydronephrosis / hydroureter
    - Renal / Ureteric Colic
    - Urinary retention
  - Hollow viscus obstruction
    - Incarcerated / strangulated Hernia
    - Bowel obstruction
  - Gastric
    - Gastric volvulus
    - Hiatus hernia

- **Tumour**
  - Peritoneal Metastasis

- **Ischaemic / Haemorrhagic**
  - Mesenteric angina
  - IVC thrombosis
  - Ischaemic bowel
    - Mesenteric embolism / thrombosis
    - Ischaemic colitis
  - Aortic dissection
  - Aortic aneurysm
    - Rupture
    - Acute aortic syndrome
  - Splenic or Hepatic Infarction

52

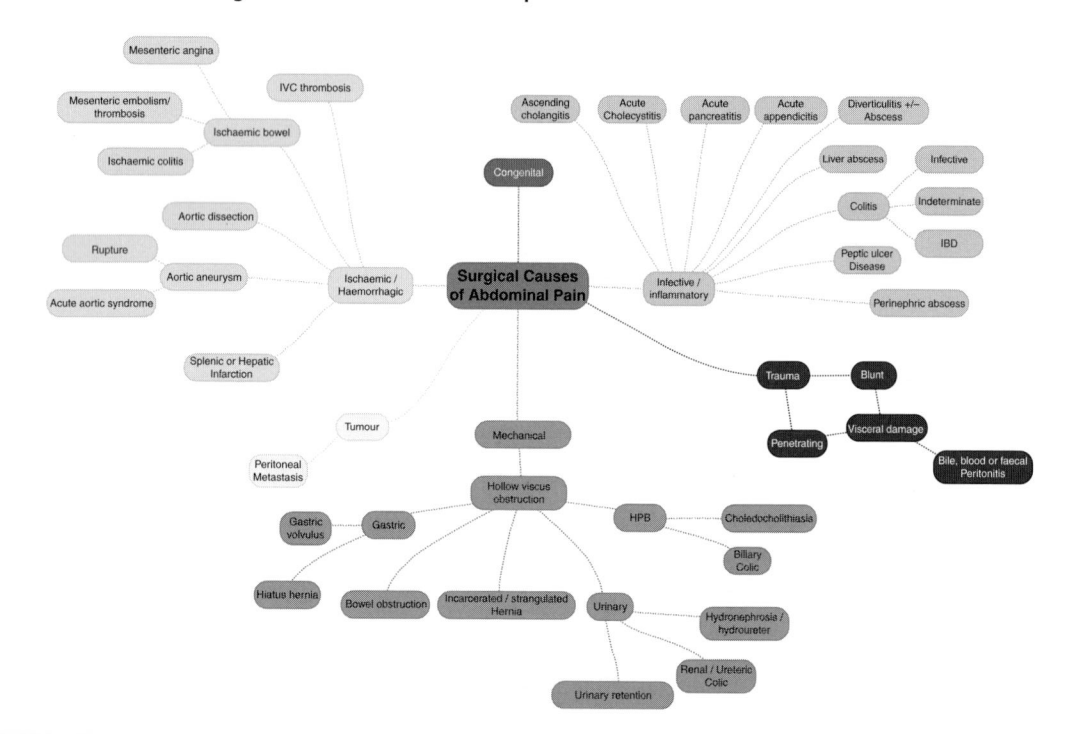

What are the gynaecological causes of abdominal pain?

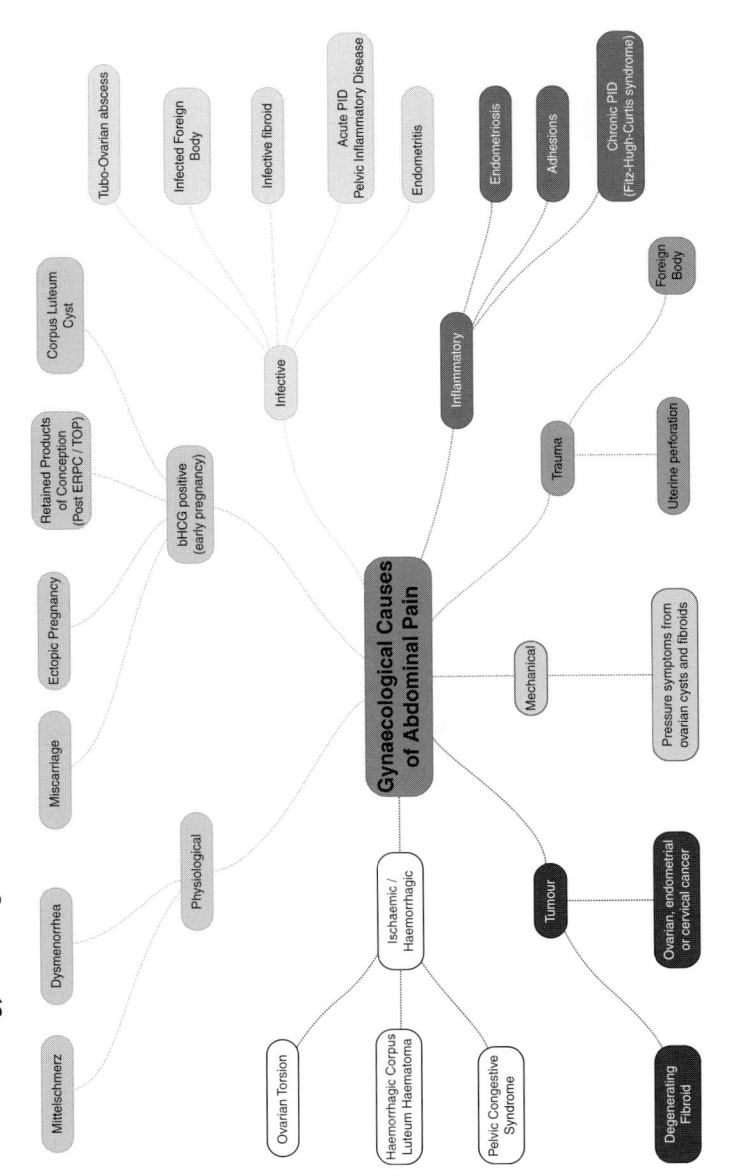

- **Gynaecological Causes of Abdominal Pain**
  - **Physiological**
    - Mittelschmerz
    - Dysmenorrhoea
  - **bHCG positive (early pregnancy)**
    - Miscarriage
    - Ectopic Pregnancy
    - Retained Products of Conception (Post ERPC / TOP)
    - Corpus Luteum Cyst
  - **Infective**
    - Tubo-Ovarian abscess
    - Infected Foreign Body
    - Infective fibroid
    - Acute PID Pelvic Inflammatory Disease
    - Endometritis
  - **Inflammatory**
    - Endometriosis
    - Adhesions
    - Chronic PID (Fitz-Hugh-Curtis syndrome)
  - **Trauma**
    - Foreign Body
    - Uterine perforation
  - **Mechanical**
    - Pressure symptoms from ovarian cysts and fibroids
  - **Tumour**
    - Ovarian, endometrial or cervical cancer
    - Degenerating Fibroid
  - **Ischaemic / Haemorrhagic**
    - Ovarian Torsion
    - Haemorrhagic Corpus Luteum Haematoma
    - Pelvic Congestive Syndrome

53

Tip

The uterus and adnexae have the same autonomic nerve supply as the lower gastrointestinal tract (T10–L1), causing similar distribution of lower abdominal pain.

What are the non-surgical causes of acute abdominal pain?

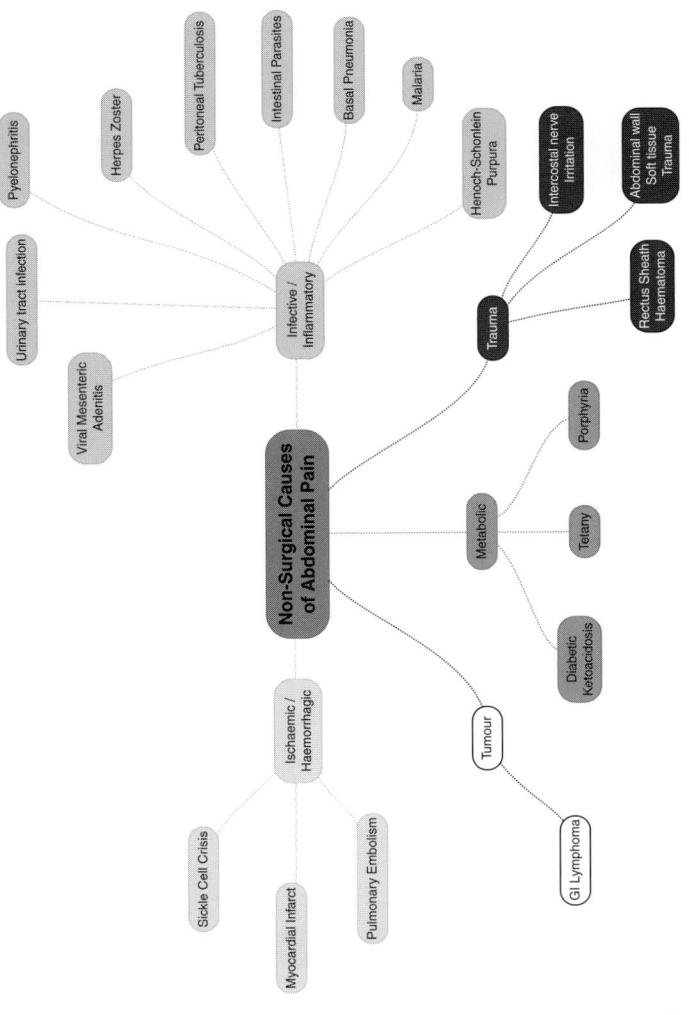

Non-Surgical Causes of Abdominal Pain

Infective / Inflammatory
- Viral Mesenteric Adenitis
- Urinary tract Infection
- Pyelonephritis
- Herpes Zoster
- Peritoneal Tuberculosis
- Intestinal Parasites
- Basal Pneumonia
- Malaria
- Henoch-Schonlein Purpura

Trauma
- Intercostal nerve Irritation
- Abdominal wall Soft tissue Trauma
- Rectus Sheath Haematoma

Metabolic
- Diabetic Ketoacidosis
- Tetany
- Porphyria

Tumour
- GI Lymphoma

Ischaemic / Haemorrhagic
- Sickle Cell Crisis
- Myocardial Infarct
- Pulmonary Embolism

55

What are the causes of bowel obstruction?

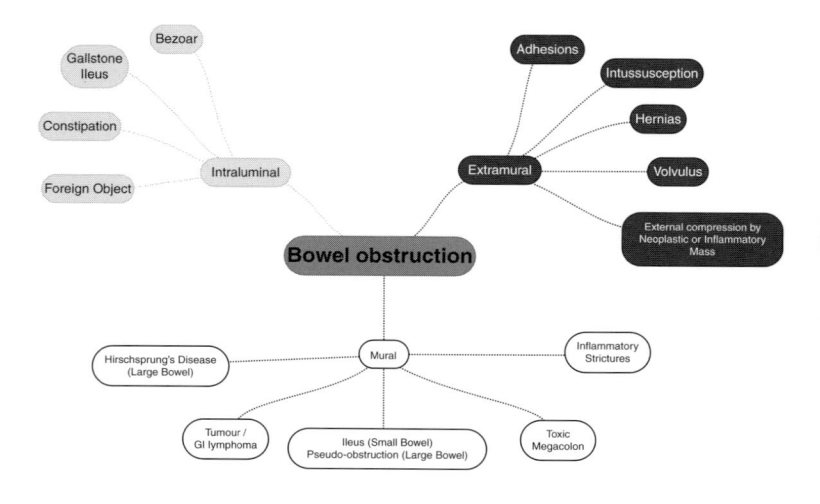

- **Bowel obstruction**
  - **Intraluminal**
    - Bezoar
    - Gallstone Ileus
    - Constipation
    - Foreign Object
  - **Extramural**
    - Adhesions
    - Intussusception
    - Hernias
    - Volvulus
    - External compression by Neoplastic or Inflammatory Mass
  - **Mural**
    - Hirschsprung's Disease (Large Bowel)
    - Inflammatory Strictures
    - Tumour / GI lymphoma
    - Ileus (Small Bowel) Pseudo-obstruction (Large Bowel)
    - Toxic Megacolon

What are the causes of hepatomegaly?

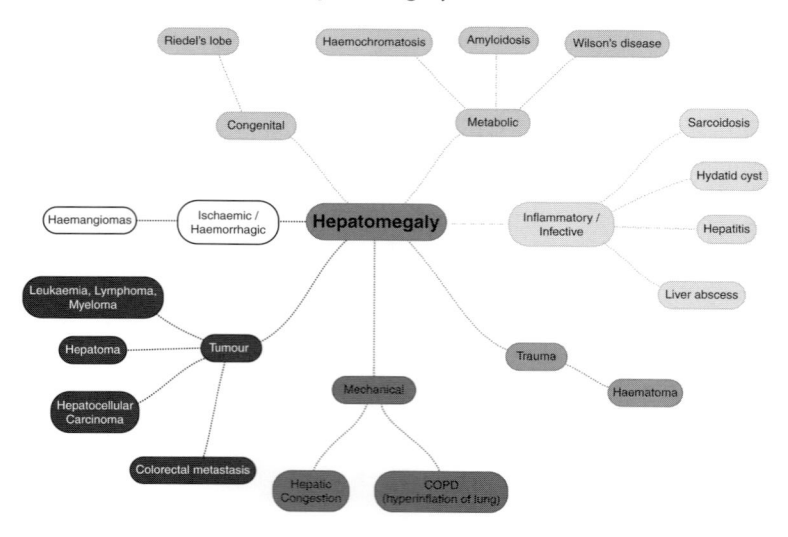

- **Hepatomegaly**
  - **Congenital**
    - Riedel's lobe
  - **Metabolic**
    - Haemochromatosis
    - Amyloidosis
    - Wilson's disease
  - **Inflammatory / Infective**
    - Sarcoidosis
    - Hydatid cyst
    - Hepatitis
    - Liver abscess
  - **Ischaemic / Haemorrhagic**
    - Haemangiomas
  - **Tumour**
    - Leukaemia, Lymphoma, Myeloma
    - Hepatoma
    - Hepatocellular Carcinoma
    - Colorectal metastasis
  - **Mechanical**
    - Hepatic Congestion
    - COPD (hyperinflation of lung)
  - **Trauma**
    - Haematoma

What are the causes of splenomegaly?

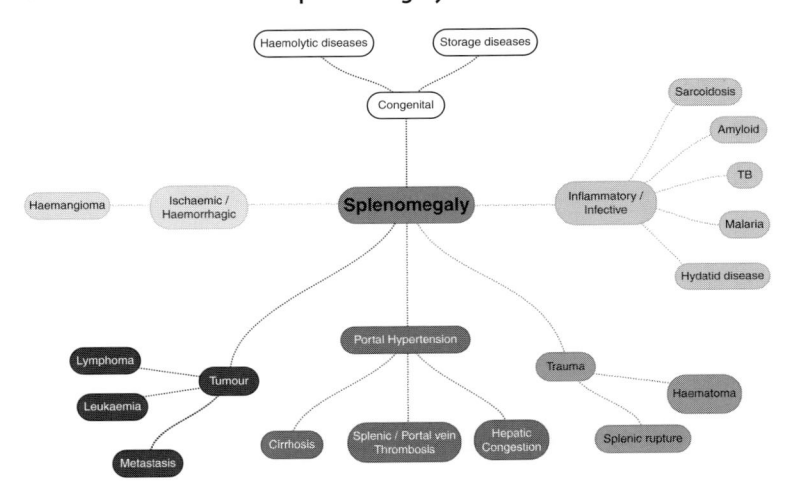

Splenomegaly

- Congenital
  - Haemolytic diseases
  - Storage diseases
- Ischaemic / Haemorrhagic
  - Haemangioma
- Inflammatory / Infective
  - Sarcoidosis
  - Amyloid
  - TB
  - Malaria
  - Hydatid disease
- Portal Hypertension
  - Cirrhosis
  - Splenic / Portal vein Thrombosis
  - Hepatic Congestion
- Tumour
  - Lymphoma
  - Leukaemia
  - Metastasis
- Trauma
  - Haematoma
  - Splenic rupture

What causes ascites?
- Ascites is an abnormal collection of fluid in the peritoneal cavity.
- Ascitic fluid is sampled by paracentesis (percutaneous needle aspiration of the peritoneal cavity).
- Traditionally ascites was classified as an exudate (high protein > 2.5–3 g/dl) or transudate (low protein < 2.5–3 g/dl).
- More recently serum–ascitic albumin gradient (SAAG) has superseded this classification.
- SAAG = serum albumin concentration − ascites albumin concentration.
- A high SAAG (> 1.1 g/dl) suggests ascites secondary to portal hypertension.
- A low SAAG (< 1.1 g/dl) suggests non-portal aetiology.

Ascites classification (diagram)

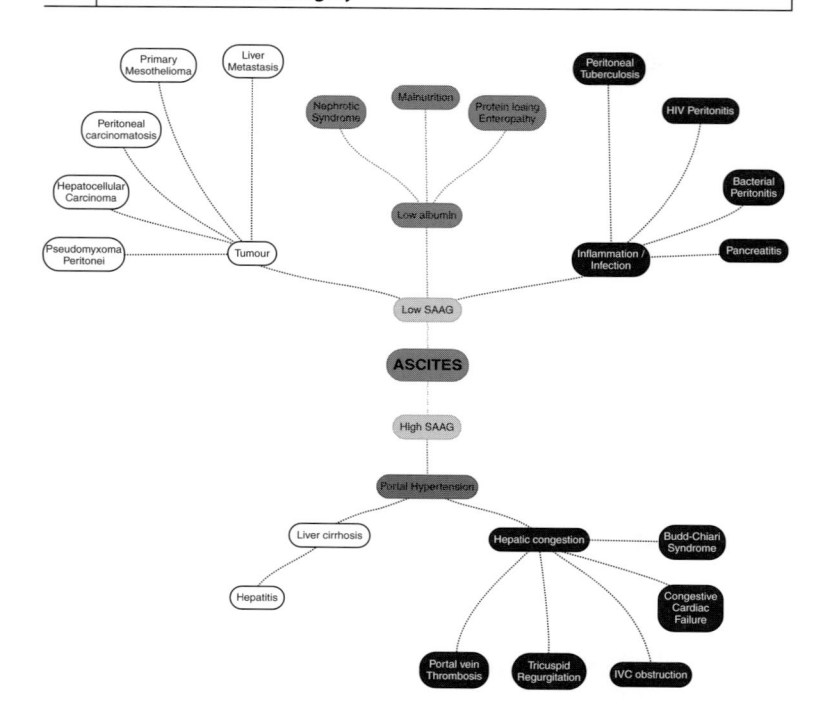

Low SAAG
- Tumour
  - Primary Mesothelioma
  - Liver Metastasis
  - Peritoneal carcinomatosis
  - Hepatocellular Carcinoma
  - Pseudomyxoma Peritonei
- Low albumin
  - Nephrotic Syndrome
  - Malnutrition
  - Protein losing Enteropathy
- Inflammation / Infection
  - Peritoneal Tuberculosis
  - HIV Peritonitis
  - Bacterial Peritonitis
  - Pancreatitis

High SAAG → Portal Hypertension
- Liver cirrhosis
- Hepatitis
- Hepatic congestion
  - Budd-Chiari Syndrome
  - Congestive Cardiac Failure
  - Portal vein Thrombosis
  - Tricuspid Regurgitation
  - IVC obstruction

When can shifting dullness be detected in a patient with ascites?

Ascites > 500 ml

How can low-volume ascites be identified?

Puddle sign: patient is placed on hands and knees and the abdomen is percussed for dullness. This is potentially unreliable and awkward for the patient. An ultrasound scan of the abdomen should rather be performed to identify low-volume ascites.

Chapter 4: Examination of the abdomen

What are the causes of an epigastric mass?

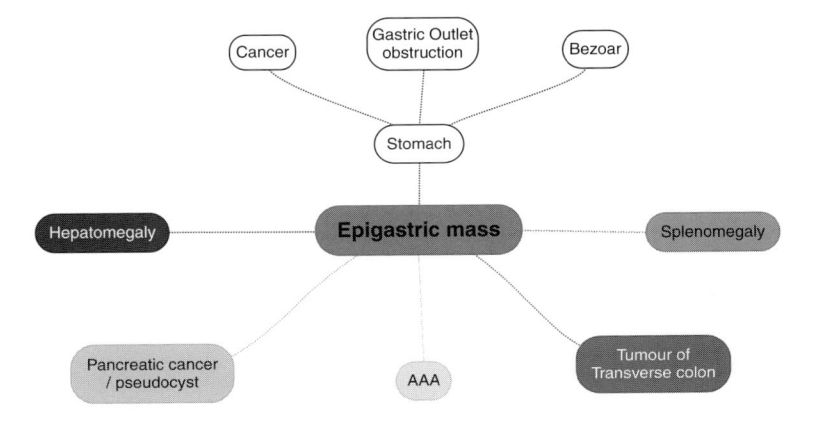

- Epigastric mass
  - Stomach
    - Cancer
    - Gastric Outlet obstruction
    - Bezoar
  - Hepatomegaly
  - Splenomegaly
  - Pancreatic cancer / pseudocyst
  - AAA
  - Tumour of Transverse colon

What are the causes of an iliac fossa mass?

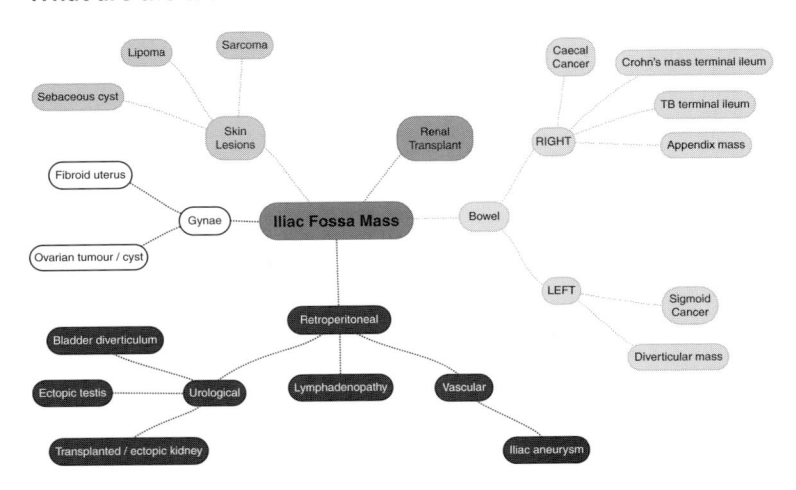

- Iliac Fossa Mass
  - Skin Lesions
    - Lipoma
    - Sarcoma
    - Sebaceous cyst
  - Renal Transplant
  - Bowel
    - RIGHT
      - Caecal Cancer
      - Crohn's mass terminal ileum
      - TB terminal ileum
      - Appendix mass
    - LEFT
      - Sigmoid Cancer
      - Diverticular mass
  - Gynae
    - Fibroid uterus
    - Ovarian tumour / cyst
  - Retroperitoneal
    - Lymphadenopathy
  - Urological
    - Bladder diverticulum
    - Ectopic testis
    - Transplanted / ectopic kidney
  - Vascular
    - Iliac aneurysm

What are the causes of a renal mass?

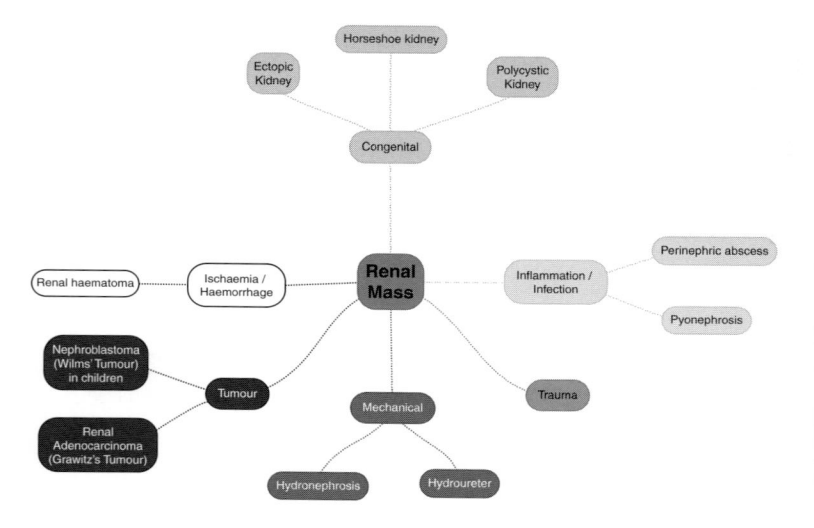

- **Renal Mass**
  - **Congenital**
    - Horseshoe kidney
    - Ectopic Kidney
    - Polycystic Kidney
  - **Ischaemia / Haemorrhage**
    - Renal haematoma
  - **Inflammation / Infection**
    - Perinephric abscess
    - Pyonephrosis
  - **Tumour**
    - Nephroblastoma (Wilms' Tumour) in children
    - Renal Adenocarcinoma (Grawitz's Tumour)
  - **Mechanical**
    - Hydronephrosis
    - Hydroureter
  - **Trauma**

Section 2: General surgery

Chapter 5: Examination of abdominal scars

Petrut Gogalniceanu, Parveen Jayia and Andrew T. Raftery

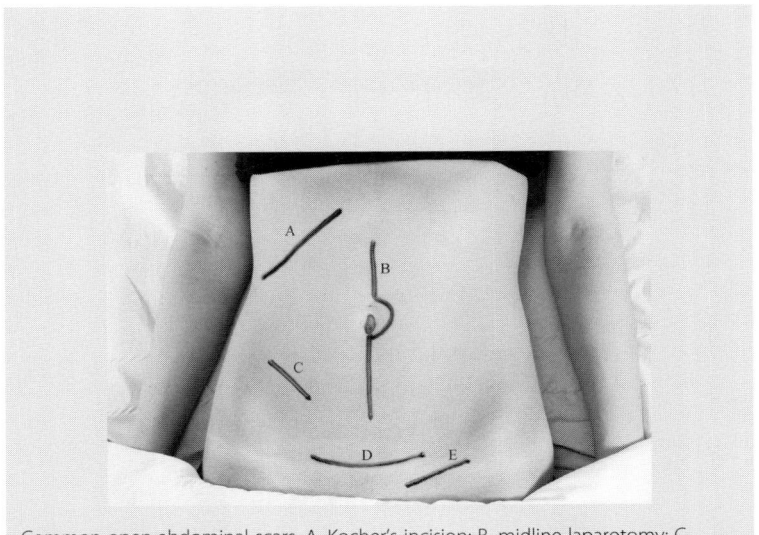

Common open abdominal scars. A, Kocher's incision; B, midline laparotomy; C, McBurney's incision; D, Pfannenstiel incision; E, inguinal hernia repair (the same incision may be used in a high approach for a femoral hernia repair).

Physical Examination for Surgeons, ed. Petrut Gogalniceanu, James Pegrum and William Lynn. Published by Cambridge University Press. © Cambridge University Press 2015.

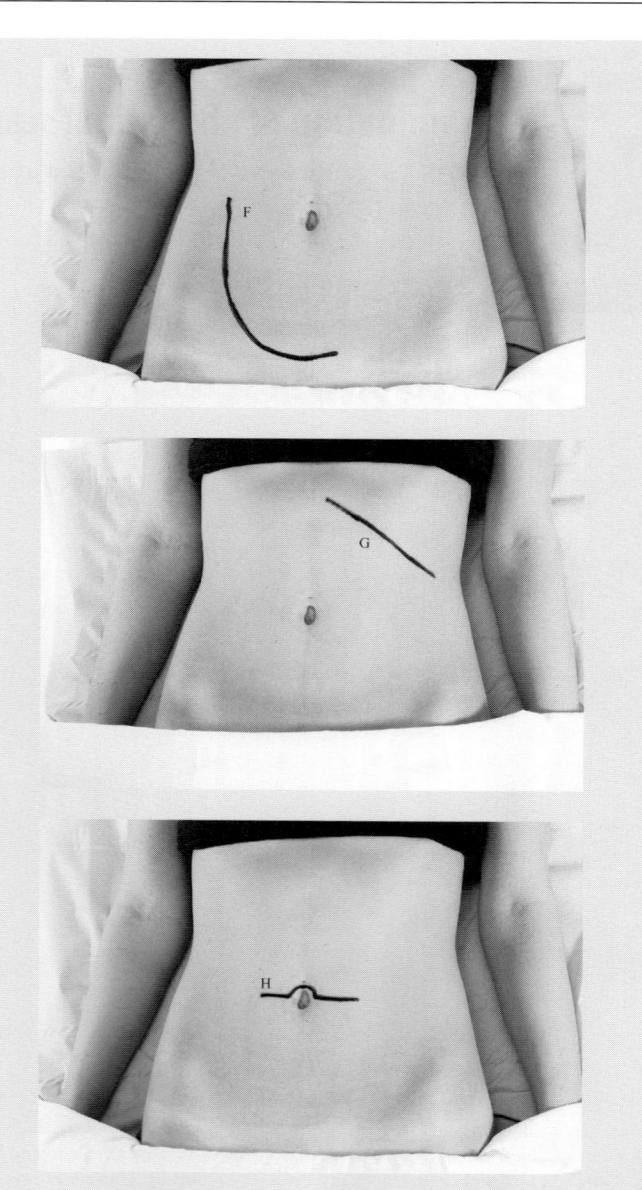

Common open abdominal scars. F, Rutherford Morison incision. G, Left subcostal incision for access to the spleen, left adrenal gland or kidney. H, umbilical or paraumbilical hernia repair.

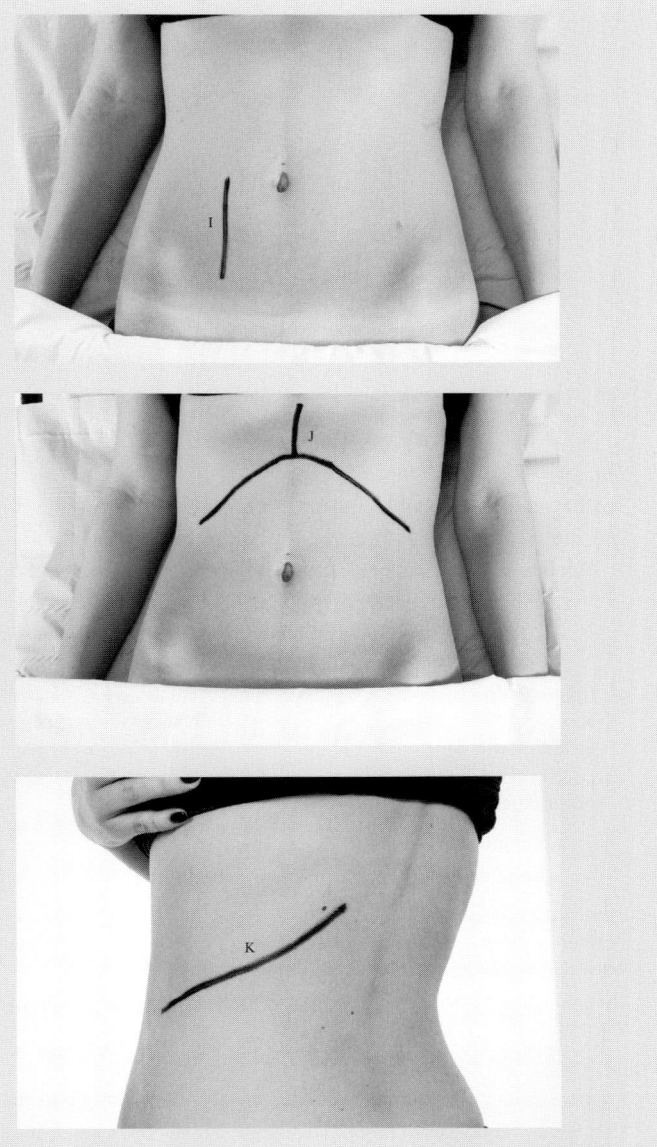

Common open abdominal scars. I, right paramedian incision; J, Mercedes Benz incision. K, left nephrectomy incision.

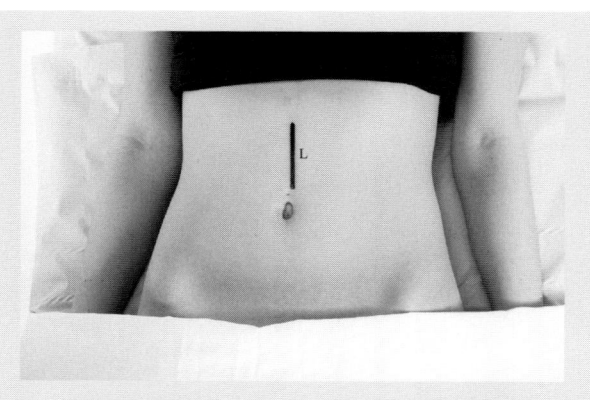

Common open abdominal scars. L, upper midline laparotomy (access to the upper abdomen or epigastric ventral hernias).

Midline laparotomy

Position: vertical incision through the linea alba.

Use: most widely used incision for exploring the abdominal cavity.

- Xiphisternum to pubis incisions are used for major operations, giving access to all peritoneal, retroperitoneal and pelvic organs.
    - e.g. trauma laparotomies, open abdominal aortic aneurysm repairs and total colectomies.
- Upper midline laparotomies (xiphisternum to umbilicus) are used for accessing the upper digestive tract, spleen and gallbladder e.g. perforated gastric ulcer.
- Lower midline laparotomies (umbilicus to pubis) are used for accessing the lower digestive tract.
    - e.g. sigmoid colectomy.

Paramedian incision

Position: vertical incision through the anterior rectus sheath with lateral retraction or splitting of the rectus abdominis muscle.

Use: rarely used nowadays; for access to the duodenum, stomach, spleen or kidneys.

Battle's incision

Position: lower pararectus incision with medial retraction of the rectus muscle.

Use: less commonly used for open appendicectomy; open insertion of CAPD (continuous ambulatory peritoneal dialysis) catheter.

Kocher's incision

Position: oblique subcostal incision in right or left upper quadrant. Transects the rectus abdominis and transversus abdominis muscles.

Use: access to the gallbladder (right side, e.g. open cholecystectomy) or spleen (left side).

Rooftop/chevron incision

Position: bilateral oblique subcostal incisions that are joined subxiphisternally (bilateral Kocher's incisions).

Use: total gastrectomy, oesophagectomy, hepatic resections, liver transplant, bilateral nephrectomy for large polycystic kidneys.

Mercedes Benz incision

Position: a vertical superior component added to the midpoint of the rooftop incision. It may be added for access to the thorax and lower oesophagus.

Use: liver transplant.

Transverse abdominal incision

Position: horizontal incision in the epigastrium. Transects rectus abdominis muscles.

Use: used in adults with short xiphisternum to pubis length for access to stomach and duodenum. Preferentially used in children for access to liver, duodenum, ascending and descending colon.

McBurney's (gridiron) incision

Position: oblique incision at McBurney's point, one-third along a line from ASIS to umbilicus. Muscle-splitting incision, splitting external and internal oblique, as well as transversus abdominis muscle along the line of their fibres. It can be extended laterally if needed.

Use: open appendicectomy, limited right hemicolectomy if extended.

Lanz incision

Position: horizontal incision at or below McBurney's point (bikini line).

Use: open appendicectomy.

Rutherford Morison incision

Position: an oblique incision extending from 2 cm above the ASIS towards the pubic symphysis, dividing external oblique along the line of its fibres and cutting through internal oblique and transversus. A gridiron incision can be extended to make a Rutherford Morison incision.

Use: renal transplant (extraperitoneal), limited right hemicolectomy, complicated appendicectomy.

'Hockey stick' incision (J-shaped Alexandre incision)

Position: a pararectal incision prolonged medially to the midline above the pubic symphysis.

Use: renal transplant, extraperitoneal approach to the iliac vessels.

Lateral thoracolumbar incision

Position: lateral subcostal approach.

Use: nephrectomy.

Pfannenstiel incision

Position: transverse, suprapubic incision at skin. Vertical midline incision of linea alba. Lateral retraction of rectus muscles.

Use: caesarean section, bladder and gynaecological surgery.

Chapter 5: Examination of abdominal scars | 67

Laparoscopic port scars

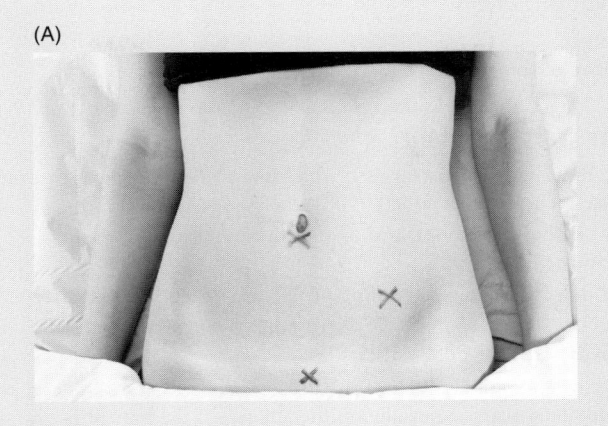

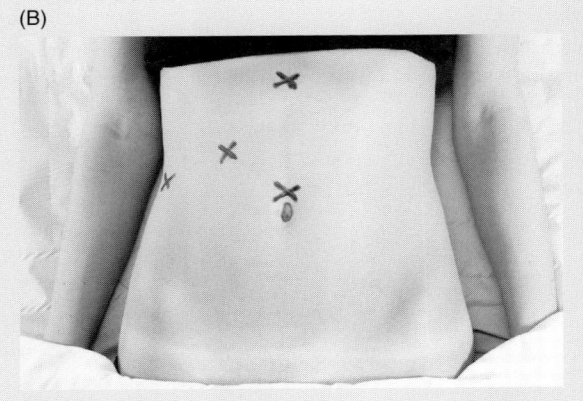

(A)

(B)

Common laparoscopic scars. The underlying operation can never be fully deduced from the position of the laparoscopic ports. 'Typical' port positions for (A) appendicectomy and (B) cholecystectomy are shown.

Position: most procedures involve the insertion of an umbilical port. Other 10 mm or 5 mm ports may be inserted at various sites.

Use: the procedure performed cannot be inferred from the port position. Triangulation of ports may indicate which part of the abdomen has been previously operated on.

Examination notes

How are abdominal incisions classified?
- Vertical/longitudinal
- Oblique
- Horizontal/transverse

Why are scars important?
- They indicate previous surgery, which may guide diagnosis or predict disease recurrence.
- They can have complications (e.g. keloids, incisional hernias, adhesions).
- They may cause pain or healing problems (infection on dehiscence).

What scars can be easily missed?
- Posterior abdominal wall and chest scars: nephrectomy scars and posterior thoracotomy scars, especially on the left side if the patient is examined from the right.
- Groin scars that have healed well in patients with a pendulous abdominal wall: ensure that the groin tissues are exposed and stretched.

Section 2 General surgery

Chapter 6 Examination of the groin

Petrut Gogalniceanu, William Lynn and Andrew T. Raftery

Checklist

WIPER
- Patient standing, trousers removed, groin and genitals exposed. Chaperone as required.

Physiological parameters

Inspection
- Evidence of raised intra-abdominal pressure: nicotine stains, barrel chest in COPD, abdominal distension
- Masses: groin lumps
- Scars: laparoscopic port access, groin scars
- Scrotal asymmetry: absent testicle, inguinoscrotal hernias
  Ask: 'Have you noticed a lump in your groin? Please show me where it is.'
  Ask: 'Can you cough please?'

Palpation
Patient standing:
  Ask: 'Do you have pain in the groin?'
  - Define anatomy: ASIS, pubic tubercle, inguinal ligament.
  - Feel the mass: Tender? Cough reflex? Borborygmi?[6] Pulsatile?
  - Locate mass: Finger on pubic tubercle and *ask patient to cough*.
  - Is it superior/medial or inferior/lateral?

---

[6] Rumbling or gurgling suggestive of a bowel-containing hernia.

Physical Examination for Surgeons, ed. Petrut Gogalniceanu, James Pegrum and William Lynn. Published by Cambridge University Press. © Cambridge University Press 2015.

- Palpate scrotum: Both testes present? Scrotal masses? Cough impulse?
- Palpate contralateral groin: Bilateral hernias?

Patient supine:
Ask patient to reduce hernia.
- Reduce hernia: reducible or irreducible?
- Control hernia: pressure at midpoint of inguinal ligament.

Ask patient to cough.
- Controlled (indirect hernia) or uncontrolled (direct hernia) by pressure?

Percussion
- Bowel gas present?

Auscultation
- Bowel sounds present in mass?
- Transillumination is optional.

To complete the examination...
- Examine the scrotum, contralateral groin and abdomen (if not done).
- Perform a digital rectal examination.

Examination notes

What are the risk factors for hernia formation that may be elicited in the examination?

Any factor that increases intra-abdominal pressure: smoking, chronic cough, constipation or change in bowel habit, chronic urinary retention, pelvic masses, pregnancy or ascites.

How do you prepare for the examination of the groin?

If examining a patient of the opposite sex ask for a chaperone. The patient needs to be standing so as to allow any hernias to become evident under the effect of gravity. Expose the patient's abdomen, groins and upper thighs. Examine from the front. You may kneel to bring the patient's groin to eye level.

What do you look for in inspecting the groin?

- Inspect the abdomen and both groins for scars and masses.
- Inspection of the abdomen is essential in hernia examination, as many hernias are now repaired laparoscopically. The only evidence of previous

hernia surgery and recurrence may be inferred from previous laparoscopic port-site scars. It is important to remember that oblique incisions above the inguinal ligament may represent previous open hernia repairs. Oblique incisions below the inguinal ligament or in the groin crease may represent a previous femoral hernia repair or femoral artery cut-down.
- Look for abdominal distension. Any cause of raised intra-abdominal pressure, such as ascites or pelvic tumours, may lead to herniation through the inguinal or femoral canals. Similarly, symptoms and signs of chest pathology, such as a chronic cough in a COPD sufferer, will lead to increased intra-abdominal pressure and increased risk of herniation. Nicotine staining on the fingers may therefore be a relevant sign.
- If an obvious groin lump is present ask the patient to cough to determine whether there is a cough impulse.
- Look at the scrotum to determine whether the mass extends inferiorly, suggesting the presence of an inguinoscrotal hernia.
- If no mass is evident, ask the patient to point out the perceived mass or painful area.

What do you palpate in the examination of the groin?
1. Define the anatomy of the inguinal canal

Define the anatomy of the inguinal canal to demonstrate understanding of the clinical signs about to be demonstrated. For a right groin examination, palpate the ASIS with the left hand. Palpate the pubic tubercle with the right hand. Outline the path of the inguinal ligament running between the two.

If needed, explain that the middle of a line running between the ASIS and the **pubic tubercle** (inguinal ligament) is the **midpoint of the inguinal ligament**. This corresponds to the deep inguinal ring of the inguinal canal. Indirect hernias emerge through this deep inguinal ring.

Also explain that the **midinguinal point** is a completely different landmark, which corresponds to the middle of a line running from the ASIS to the **pubic symphysis**. It corresponds to the inferior epigastric artery intraoperatively or as a superior marker of the femoral pulse (found lower in the groin in the same vertical plane). Intraoperatively, direct hernias occur medial to the inferior epigastric artery (and the midinguinal point).

The midinguinal point is therefore more medial than the midpoint of the inguinal ligament.

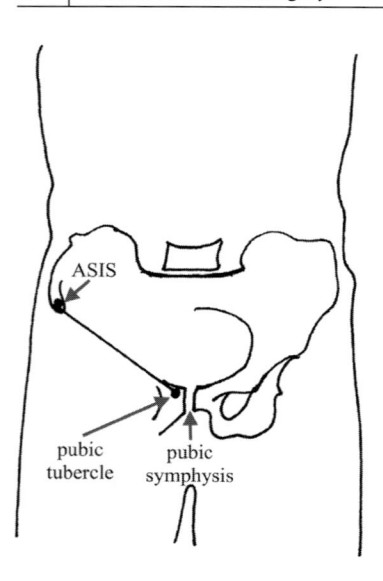

The **inguinal ligament** runs between the ASIS and the pubic tubercle.

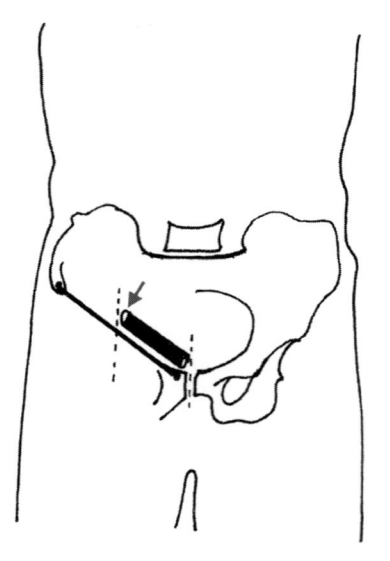

The **midpoint of the inguinal ligament** is the middle of a line running between the ASIS and the pubic tubercle. This coincides with the deep inguinal ring, which is the origin of indirect inguinal hernias (arrow).

Chapter 6: Examination of the groin

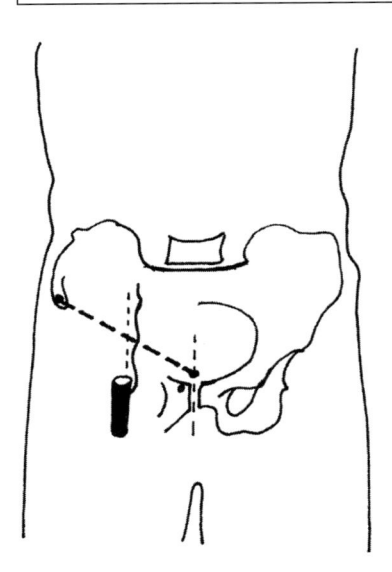

The **midinguinal point** is the middle of a line running between the ASIS and the pubic symphisis. This corresponds to the femoral pulse / common femoral artery, and more proximally to the inferior epigastric artery. The inferior epigastric artery arises from the external iliac artery and ascends medial to the deep inguinal ring.

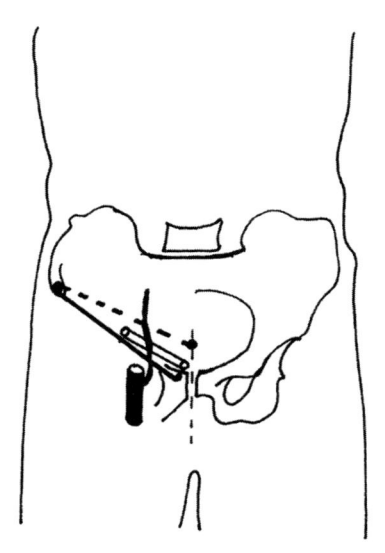

The midpoint of the inguinal ligament is lateral to the midinguinal point. This means that the deep ring of the inguinal canal lies lateral to the inferior epigastric artery. As a result, indirect inguinal hernias are lateral to the inferior epigastric artery and direct ones are found medial to it.

2. Is it a hernia?

First determine if the mass is a hernia. Check if the mass if painful before touching it. Ask the patient to cough to identify a cough impulse, suggestive of a hernia. A pulsatile mass may suggest the presence of a femoral artery aneurysm. A long saphenous vein varix at the saphenofemoral junction may also have a cough impulse, but its location is different from that of a hernia (see later).

3. Is it an inguinal or femoral hernia?

Place two fingers of the right hand on the pubic tubercle and ask the patient to cough.

Inguinal hernias travel through the inguinal canal and may emerge through the superficial inguinal ring. An inguinal hernia will thus manifest as a mass above the inguinal ligament and medial to the pubic tubercle (where the inguinal canal terminates as the superficial ring). Inguinal hernias will therefore be superior and medial to the pubic tubercle.

Femoral hernias travel through the femoral canal. This is inferior to the inguinal ligament. Femoral hernias will therefore emerge as a lump inferior and lateral to the pubic tubercle.

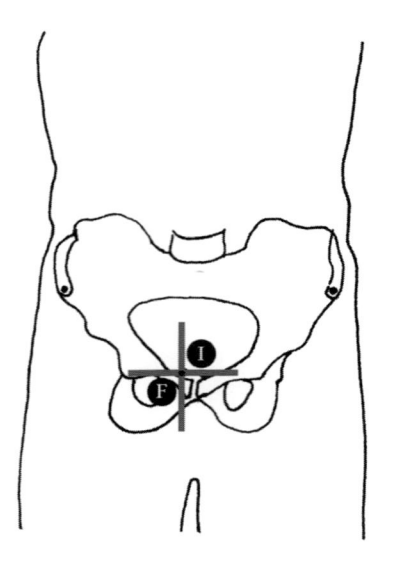

Differentiating between an inguinal and a femoral hernia. Draw an imaginary cross through the ipsilateral pubic tubercle and ascertain the position of the lump in relation to this. I, inguinal hernia; F, femoral hernia.

4. Is it an inguinal or inguinoscrotal hernia?

Palpate the scrotum to determine if the hernia extends inferiorly into the scrotum. Inguinoscrotal hernias may be more difficult to repair, especially if a laparoscopic approach is used. At this stage also determine if both testes are present, clearly defined and normal. An undescended testis in the inguinal canal may mimic an inguinal hernia. Its absence from the scrotum must therefore be identified. A hydrocoele of the cord may also be confused with an inguinoscrotal hernia. Proceed to a formal scrotal examination if any abnormalities are detected.

5. Is it a reducible hernia?

Place the patient in the supine position.

Observe if the hernia reduces spontaneously. Never force a hernia back into the abdominal cavity. Ask the patient to reduce the hernia. If unable to do so, attempt to gently massage the hernia back into the abdominal cavity. If unable to do so, the hernia is irreducible or incarcerated.

6. Is it a direct or indirect inguinal hernia?

There is a lack of consensus whether direct or indirect inguinal hernias can be differentiated on physical examination. This must be stated when attempting to differentiate them on clinical examination.

The hernia must be reduced while the patient is lying flat. The deep inguinal ring is occluded by applying pressure superior to the midpoint of the inguinal ligament. The patient is asked to cough.

If the pressure controls/prevents the hernia from recurring it suggests that this is an indirect hernia (it emerges through the deep ring). If the hernia recurs it suggests that its origin is not the deep ring, and therefore it is assumed to be a direct hernia emerging through a weakness in the posterior wall of the inguinal canal/Hesselbach's triangle. Hesselbach's triangle is an area of weakness in the posterior wall of the inguinal canal. A defect in this area leads to a direct inguinal hernia. The borders of Hesselbach's triangle are the inferior epigastric artery (laterally), the lateral edge of the rectus abdominis muscle (medially) and the inguinal ligament (inferiorly).

7. Is it strangulated?

An incarcerated/irreducible hernia that is tender or is associated with symptoms or signs of bowel obstruction must be treated as a strangulated hernia. Changes to the overlying skin, such as erythema, may suggest compromise of the underlying tissues.

Do you percuss and auscultate when examining the groin?

The presence of a resonant percussion tone or bowel sounds may suggest that the hernia contains bowel.

What else needs to be done before completing your examination?

A digital rectal examination may be needed to rule out anal cancer in patients with suspected inguinal lymphadenopathy, or to assess the size of the prostate in those with chronic bladder obstruction.

Risk factors leading to hernia formation affect both groins, and examination of the contralateral groin is mandatory to rule out a second hernia.

It is also advisable to offer to examine the abdomen for any masses or causes of increased intra-abdominal pressure. If a laparoscopic hernia repair is considered, always examine the umbilical area for potential umbilical or paraumbilical hernias which would have to be negotiated when inserting the laparoscopic umbilical port.

Why are femoral artery cut-downs performed?

These are used in a peripheral arterial bypass operation or endovascular aneurysm repair (EVAR). A vertical scar in the groin is highly suggestive of previous exposure of the femoral artery for a vascular procedure.

How do you differentiate between different groin scars?

- Inguinal hernia repair scars are above the inguinal ligament and medial to the pubic tubercle.
- Femoral hernia repair scars can be above or below the ligament depending on whether a high (McEvedy) or low (Lockwood) approach is used. Alternatively, these can be repaired through an incision through the inguinal canal as for an open inguinal hernia repair (Lotheissen approach).
- SFJ incisions may be through the groin crease: the groin skin must be stretched to visualise this.
- Femoral cut-down incisions can be (a) vertical (above and below inguinal ligament), (b) oblique (may cross groin crease, unlike incisions for inguinal hernias) or (c) hockey-stick-shaped (vertical with a curved component at one end).
- For femoropopliteal or femorodistal bypasses, look for scars in the groin associated with ipsilateral scars above or below the knee, respectively.
- For EVAR and crossover bypass grafts look for similar scars in the contralateral groin.

> **Tips**
>
> An incarcerated hernia is one that cannot be reduced. An incarcerated hernia may also be described as an irreducible hernia.
> A strangulated hernia is an incarcerated hernia with a compromised blood supply. This leads to infarction and necrosis of the herniated tissue.

Chapter 6: Examination of the groin | 77

> **Tips**
>
> The midpoint of the inguinal ligament corresponds to the deep inguinal ring (halfway between ASIS and pubic tubercle).
>
> The midinguinal point corresponds to the femoral artery (halfway between ASIS and pubic symphysis).
>
> The midinguinal point is more medial, whilst the midpoint of the inguinal ligament is more lateral.

Differential diagnoses

What are the causes of a groin lump?

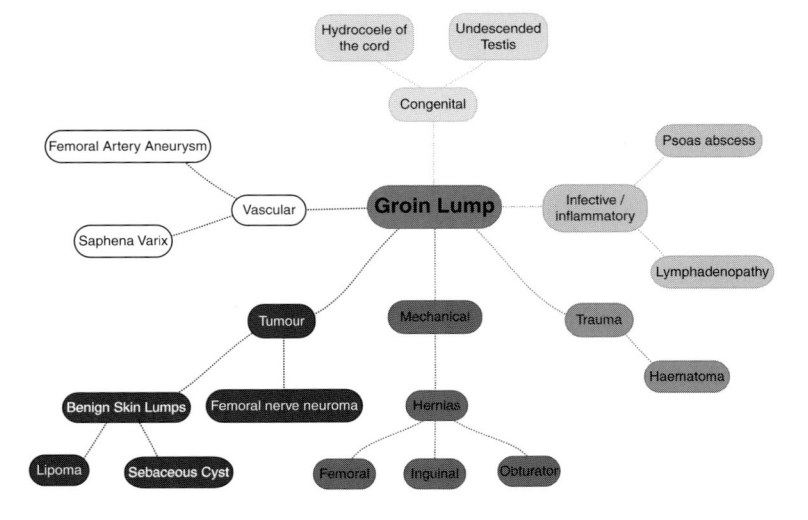

Groin Lump

- Congenital
  - Hydrocoele of the cord
  - Undescended Testis
- Vascular
  - Femoral Artery Aneurysm
  - Saphena Varix
- Infective / inflammatory
  - Psoas abscess
  - Lymphadenopathy
- Trauma
  - Haematoma
- Mechanical
  - Hernias
    - Femoral
    - Inguinal
    - Obturator
- Tumour
  - Benign Skin Lumps
    - Lipoma
    - Sebaceous Cyst
  - Femoral nerve neuroma

What are the causes of groin scars?

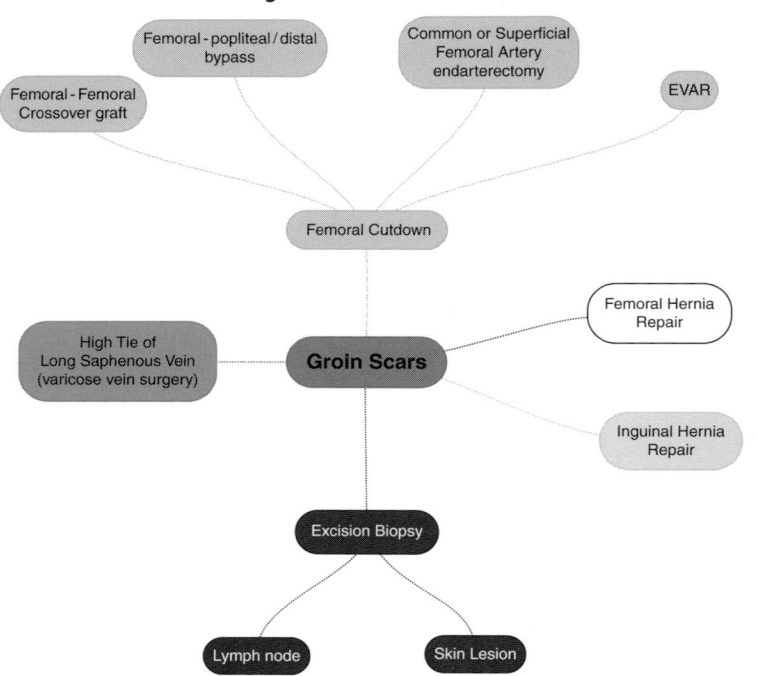

- **Groin Scars**
  - Femoral Cutdown
    - Femoral - Femoral Crossover graft
    - Femoral - popliteal / distal bypass
    - Common or Superficial Femoral Artery endarterectomy
    - EVAR
  - High Tie of Long Saphenous Vein (varicose vein surgery)
  - Femoral Hernia Repair
  - Inguinal Hernia Repair
  - Excision Biopsy
    - Lymph node
    - Skin Lesion

How can hernias be classified?

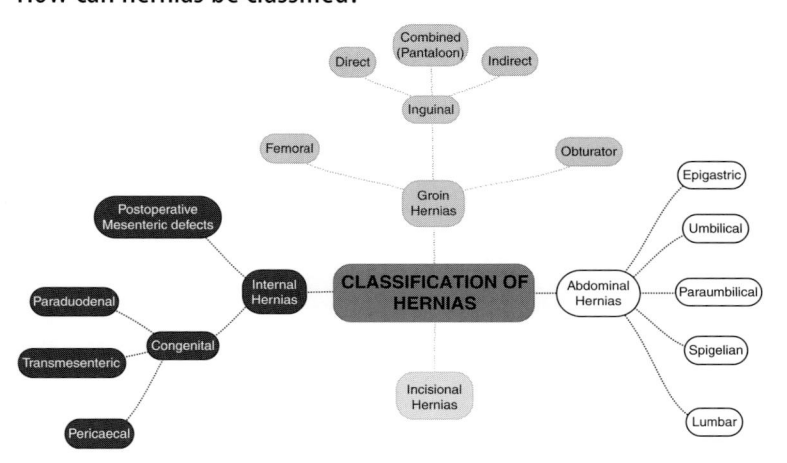

CLASSIFICATION OF HERNIAS

- Groin Hernias
  - Inguinal
    - Direct
    - Combined (Pantaloon)
    - Indirect
  - Femoral
  - Obturator
- Abdominal Hernias
  - Epigastric
  - Umbilical
  - Paraumbilical
  - Spigelian
  - Lumbar
- Internal Hernias
  - Postoperative Mesenteric defects
  - Congenital
    - Paraduodenal
    - Transmesenteric
    - Pericaecal
- Incisional Hernias

Section 2 General surgery

Chapter 7

Examination of a stoma
William Lynn, Petrut Gogalniceanu and Andrew T. Raftery

Checklist

WIPER

Physiological parameters

Inspection

Scars:
- Midline laparotomy
- Laparoscopic scars
- No scars and stoma: trephine colostomy
- Linear or purse-string scar in RIF or LIF: reversed stoma

Stoma character:
- Site: RIF vs. LIF
- Spouted vs. flush
- Size of lumen
- Number of lumens
- Stoma bridge
- Bag contents:
  - urine (urostomy)
  - small bowel contents: liquid (ileostomy)
  - formed faeces (colostomy)

Stoma complications:
- Parastomal mass (hernia)
- Dusky or ischaemic mucosa
- Surrounding skin excoriated

Physical Examination for Surgeons, ed. Petrut Gogalniceanu, James Pegrum and William Lynn. Published by Cambridge University Press. © Cambridge University Press 2015.

- Stoma edge dehiscence
- Stoma retraction

Palpation
- Palpate around stoma and ask patient to cough to exclude parastomal hernia.
- Digitate stoma with a well-lubricated finger (only if required).

Percussion
- Hyper-resonance: bowel obstruction

Auscultation
- Hyperactive bowel sounds in bowel obstruction
- Quiet bowel sounds in ileus

To complete the examination...
- Ask to examine the perineum to determine if the anal orifice is present.
- Perform a full examination of the abdomen.

Examination notes

What is the definition of a stoma?
A stoma is a surgically created communication between a hollow viscus and the skin.

What are the different types of stomas?
- Ileostomy – ileum
- Colostomy – colon
- Urostomy – ileum anastomosed to ureters

How are stomas constructed?
- End-stoma: single lumen. Suggests that the distal end of the viscus has either been resected or closed and left in the abdomen; e.g. Hartmann's procedure.
- Loop-ileostomy: two lumens may be seen. The distal end of the viscus is present but defunctioned, e.g. to allow an anastomosis to heal.
- A urostomy is formed when the urinary bladder has been excised. A loop of ileum (ileal conduit) is separated proximally and distally. The ureters are anastomosed to one end, and the other end is used to form the stoma (urostomy).

How can the three different stomas be differentiated?

	Urostomy	Ileostomy	Colostomy
Consistency	Clear liquid	Liquid	Solid
Content	Urine	Small bowel content	Faeces
Site	RIF or LIF	Usually RIF	Usually LIF
Spout	Spouted	Spouted	Flush

Why are some stomas spouted?
- An ileostomy has alkaline fluid effluent rich in proteolytic enzymes which can excoriate the skin. Similarly urine can be an irritant. The spout is used to direct the liquid content straight into a bag without contacting skin.

What feature of a stoma might suggest it is a urostomy (not always)?
- The stoma bag might have a tap on it.

What are the complications of a stoma?
Complications may be divided into general and specific. The specific complications may then be further divided into immediate, early and late complications.
- Immediate complications: haemorrhage, retraction, dehiscence, ischaemic necrosis.
- Early complications: electrolyte disturbance secondary to high output, prolapsed, leakage, IBD involvement of stoma, psychological.
- Late complications: parastomal hernia, fistula formation, stenosis, leakage, psychological.

What factors should be considered when planning to give a patient a stoma?
- Patients should be seen preoperatively by a stoma specialist nurse, both for marking and for counseling regarding the stoma.
- The site must be assessed with the patient standing, sitting and lying supine. The patient's resting posture must also be considered (wheelchair).
- Site the stoma away from the midline: lateral border of the rectus muscle.
- Patient preferences regarding clothing positioning: e.g. trousers/belts.
- Care arrangements for the patient: a previously independent person may not be able to cope with the stoma alone (mobility, memory, eyesight).

Differential diagnoses

What are the causes of a discharging defect/stoma/fistula/sinus on the anterior abdominal wall?

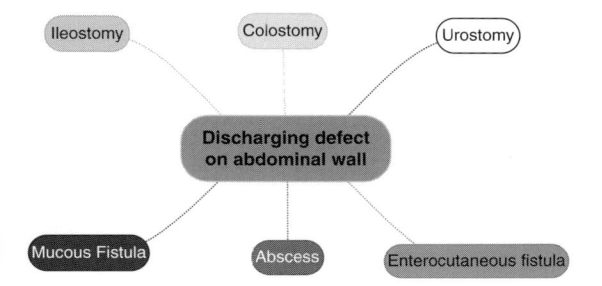

- Ileostomy
- Colostomy
- Urostomy
- Mucous Fistula
- Abscess
- Enterocutaneous fistula

(Discharging defect on abdominal wall)

Section 2: General surgery

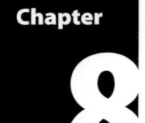

Chapter 8: Renal access and transplant examination

Petrut Gogalniceanu and Andrew T. Raftery

Checklist

WIPER
- Patient supine. Expose both arms completely, as well as chest and abdomen.

Physiological parameters

General
- Fluid status: shortness of breath, audible crackles, dry mucous membranes, facial oedema, peripheral oedema, cyanosis
- Clinical features of immunosuppression or chronic steroid use

Inspection
Arm fistulas:
- Radiocephalic fistula[7] (wrist)
- Brachiocephalic or brachiobasilic fistulas (antecubital fossa)
- Prosthetic straight or loop grafts (PTFE)

Fistula complications:
- Non-functioning/thrombosed fistulas
- Haematomas or ecchymosis from needling
- Aneurysmal changes: tight or shiny skin
- Hand ischaemia from fistula: steal syndrome or embolization

---

[7] Also known as a Cimino–Brescia fistula.

Physical Examination for Surgeons, ed. Petrut Gogalniceanu, James Pegrum and William Lynn. Published by Cambridge University Press. © Cambridge University Press 2015.

Neck and chest (subclavian and internal jugular veins):
- Raised JVP (fluid overload)
- Dilated neck veins: central vein stenosis from long-term central dialysis lines
- Temporary non-tunnelled haemodialysis intravenous catheters (VasCath)
- Long-term tunnelled haemodialysis intravenous catheters (PermCath)

Abdomen:
- Peritoneal dialysis (PD) catheter[8]
- Scars: nephrectomy scars in flanks, midline scars for PD catheters, suprapubic catheter scars, iliac fossae scars for renal transplant (Rutherford Morison incision, 'hockey-stick' incision), laparoscopic scars for nephrectomy (donor)

Leg:
- Prosthetic PTFE loop graft.

Palpation
- Skin turgor: fluid status
- Fistula (if present): thrill or pulse, palpable stenosis
- Pulses (if fistula present): radial, ulnar, brachial, axillary, subclavian
- Abdomen:
    - ascites
    - peritonitis (if PD catheter present)
    - ballotable masses (polycystic kidneys)
    - iliac fossa masses (transplanted kidney)

Percussion
- Percuss any iliac fossa mass to confirm it is dull (kidney) rather than cystic.

Auscultate
- Fistula: bruit (continuous 'machinery' bruit)
- Chest: crackles, effusions (fluid overload)

To complete the examination...
- Examine groins (femoral lines) and lower limbs (fistulas and grafts).

Examination notes
What are the three most likely clinical scenarios?
1. End-stage renal failure patient on dialysis:
   a. peritoneal dialysis
   b. dialysis via fistula

---

[8] Also known as a Tenckhoff catheter.

c. dialysis via intravenous line
  d. haemofiltration via intravenous line
2. Low-clearance patient approaching need for renal replacement with a fistula created in advance; still passes urine
3. Renal transplant patient:
   a. transplant working: not on dialysis but on immunosuppressive therapy
   b. transplant failed: recommenced dialysis; transplanted kidney may be in situ or removed

What are the basic history points that need to be established in assessing for fistula formation?

- Is the patient left- or right-handed?
- Is the patient already on dialysis or has the fistula been created in advance?
- Any pain, cyanosis or loss of function of the hand (steal syndrome) in those with fistulas?
- Is the patient still producing urine?
- Has there been a change in the bruit or shape of the fistula recently (thrombosis or aneurysmal change)?

How do you differentiate between different fistulas?

- Radiocephalic AVF: at the wrist; longitudinal incision.
- Brachiocephalic AVF: transverse incision at the antecubital fossa; thrill palpable on **lateral** aspect of arm; superficial.
- Brachiobasilic AVF (first-stage): transverse incision at the antecubital fossa; thrill palpable on **medial** aspect of arm; deep.
- Brachiobasilic AVF (second-stage; superficialised): transverse incision at the antecubital fossa extending longitudinally up on the medial side of the arm; thrill palpable superficially on the anterior/central aspect of the arm.

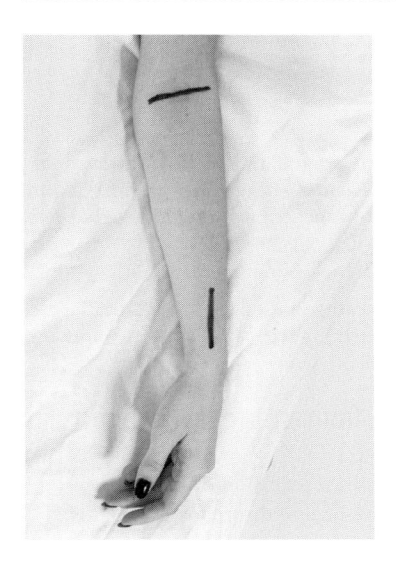

Radiocephalic (Cimino–Brescia) arteriovenous fistula at the wrist; brachiocephalic or first-stage brachiobasilic fistula in the antecubital fossa.

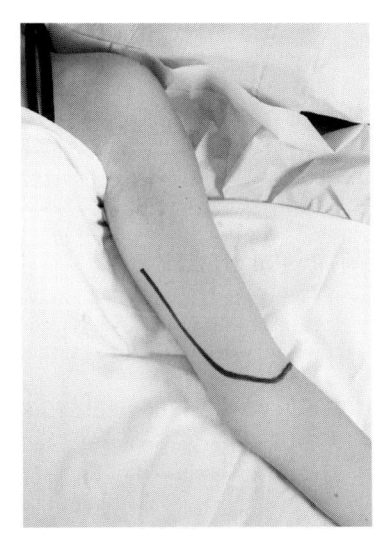

Second-stage brachiobasilic arteriovenous fistula, also known as a basilic vein transposition and superficialisation; palpate for a possible prosthetic graft (PTFE or Dacron) in case the fistula has been revised.

What are the features of a transplanted kidney?
- Renal transplants are most commonly placed in the right or left iliac fossa.
- Non-functioning native kidneys are usually left in situ. Consequently, nephrectomy scars will not always be present in patients with end-stage renal failure. Indications for nephrectomy in patients with renal failure include infected polycystic kidneys or renal carcinoma.
- Beware of small incisions used in laparoscopic nephrectomy.
- A smooth, non-tender, kidney-shaped, dull mass may be palpable in the iliac fossa.

What investigation may be necessary in patients planning to have a fistula formed?
- A bedside/outpatient ultrasound scan may be performed to assess the position and calibre of the peripheral arteries and veins.

- A venogram may be performed to assess the calibre and patency of peripheral and central limb veins.

What is a VasCath?
- VasCaths are large-bore, double-lumen (arterial and venous) intravenous catheters used for haemodialysis in the acute setting. They are inserted in the internal jugular veins. They are not tunnelled but secured with sutures.

What is a PermCath?
- A PermCath is a tunnelled intravenous catheter used for long-term dialysis. It is inserted in the subclavian or internal jugular vein. It has two lumens travelling through one intravenous line.

How can you test for steal syndrome from an arteriovenous fistula?
- Arm elevation causes blanching of digits.
- Temporary occlusion of the fistula causes reperfusion of fingers.
- NB: care must be taken not to damage or cause thrombosis of the fistula.

What are the features of an arteriovenous fistula?
- It is a firm and palpable subcutaneous vascular structure.
- It has a palpable thrill.
- It has a bruit on auscultation.

> **Tips**
>
> A pulsatile fistula signifies low-volume flow.
> A thrill in a fistula signifies adequate flow volume.

What are the common arteriovenous fistula complications that can be encountered in an exam?
- Anastomotic stenosis (low flow)
- Thrombosis (no/low flow)
- Aneurysmal change (high flow/steal syndrome/bleeding)
- Steal syndrome

Section editor: Petrut Gogalniceanu
Senior author: Michael Douek

Section 3 — Breast surgery

Chapter 9 — Examination of the breast

Petrut Gogalniceanu, Yezen Sheena and Michael Douek

Checklist

WIPER

- A chaperone will help the patient get changed into an examination gown in a private area.
- The patient is positioned sitting on the edge of the bed with hands resting on hips.
- The breasts are exposed only when the examination begins.

Physiological parameters

General

- Weight loss
- Radiotherapy tattoos or Hickman line scar (for chemotherapy)
- Donor site scars: TRAM or DIEP flap (lower abdomen), LD flap (back) or other scars (e.g. gluteal or transverse myocutaneous gracilis)[9]
- Bra: prosthetic or cosmetic inserts suggestive of breast asymmetry, bra cup size

---

[9] TRAM, transverse rectus abdominis myocutaneous; DIEP, deep inferior epigastric perforator; LD, latissimus dorsi.

Physical Examination for Surgeons, ed. Petrut Gogalniceanu, James Pegrum and William Lynn. Published by Cambridge University Press. © Cambridge University Press 2015.

Inspection
- Chest wall/spine/shoulder: symmetry/deformities (crucial to apparent breast appearance)
- Breast: volume, symmetry, shape, projection, chest wall position
- Nipples: deviation, retraction, inversion, discharge, Paget's disease, eczema
- Skin: scars, mammary fistulas, erythema
- Soft tissues: lumps, skin dimpling, peau d'orange, cancer en cuirasse, ulceration
- Haagensen manoeuvre: press arms on hips, lift hands behind head, slowly lower arms
- Axillae: masses, SLNB or ANC scars[10]
- Supraclavicular fossae: swelling/masses
- Arms: lymphoedema (comment on any compression garment), muscle wasting

Palpation
- Breast: masses, tenderness:
  - four breast quadrants (upper/lower, outer/inner)
  - nipple and retroareolar tissues
  - axillary tail of Spence
- Nipple: discharge
- Axilla: lymphadenopathy (five sites per side), accessory breasts
- Lateral chest wall: port sites for breast expander implants

To complete the examination...
- Neck/supraclavicular fossae: lymphadenopathy
- Spine: tenderness
- Abdomen: hepatomegaly
- Chest: pleural effusions

Examination notes
How are breast lumps assessed?
Any new breast lump requires triple assessment. Symptomatic patients should be assessed in a one-stop breast clinic.

What does the triple assessment involve?
1. Clinical: examination by a surgeon

---

[10] SLNB, sentinel lymph-node biopsy; ANC, axillary node clearance.

2. Imaging: breast ultrasound (women under 40 years) or mammography (women 40 years or older)
3. Histology: fine-needle aspiration (FNA) or core biopsy

Each is scored 1–5 (1 = low, 5 = very high risk). Younger women with suspicious lumps should be offered an additional mammogram. Older women with suspicious lumps should be offered an additional ultrasound of the breast and axilla.

How is the axilla examined?

To palpate the left axilla, the surgeon's left arm supports the patient's flexed left forearm. The left axilla is palpated with the surgeon's right hand. Likewise, when examining the right axilla, the surgeon uses his/her right forearm to support the patient's right forearm, and the left hand is used for palpation.

Palpate the apex, lateral (humerus), medial (thoracic), posterior (latissimus dorsi) and anterior (pectoralis muscles) walls of the axilla.

What is the rationale behind the focused systemic examination at the end of the breast exam?

The focused systemic examination aims to identify potential sites of metastases from breast cancer in the regional lymph nodes (axillae), neck, spine, liver and chest.

What are the different breast scars?

Patients with breast cancer will have undergone a wide local excision or mastectomy, with their respective scars. They might have undergone immediate or indeed delayed breast reconstruction, commonly by means of implant only, LD +/− implant, or DIEP flap.

Breast scars and incisions.

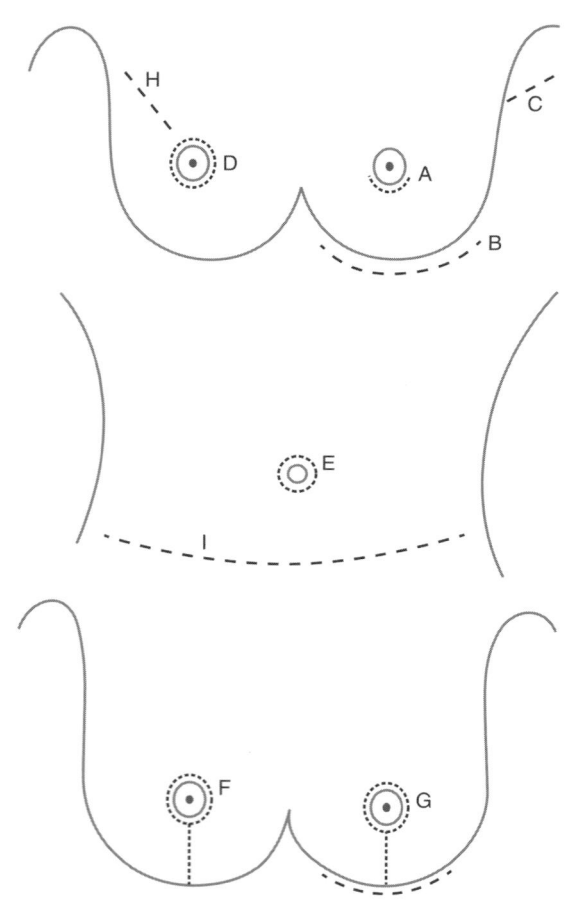

Key Incisions of the breast

A   Periareolar incision
B   Inframammary incision
C   Trans - Axillary incision
D   Circumareolar incision
E   Periumbilical incision
F   Vertical mammoplasty incision
G   Wise pattern incision
H   Radial scar
I   TRAM/DIEP flap harvest site

The commonest scars for non-cancer procedures are those following lumpectomy of benign lumps or following breast augmentation (cosmetic, or for breast asymmetry).

The common procedures for breast augmentation are IMF[11] scars. Sometimes periareolar, transaxillary or even periumbilical access incisions are used. Mastopexy (breast lift) and reduction surgery may be performed through periareolar, vertical or Wise-pattern 'anchor-shaped' scars.

What are the specific features of certain breast implants?

Some implants, namely expanders, have an internal (integrated) or external (subcutaneous) port to allow transcutaneous inflation with saline in clinic. They are generally replaced with a definitive implant once the desired size is achieved, but some, such as the Becker Adjustable Implant, allow the injection port to be pulled out via a small incision, leaving a self-sealing valve within the main implant that can be left as a definitive device.

> **Tip**
> Capsular contracture is the body's over-scarring around breast implants, and should be documented in patients with breast implants. Baker classified capsular contractures as class I (normal), II (palpable), III (visible), IV (painful).

What is peau d'orange?

The characteristic 'orange-peel' skin appearance overlying a breast is caused by lymphatic obstruction by invasive carcinoma (i.e. it represents malignant lymphoedema). It signifies a T4 tumour.

What is Paget's disease of the breast?

Paget's disease is an eczematous change in the appearance of the nipple thought to be caused by ductal carcinoma in situ cells that migrate into the nipple. It is sometimes associated with an underlying breast cancer.

What is SLNB?

Sentinel lymph-node biopsy (SLNB) is a technique whereby axillary lymph nodes are identified using dyes injected into the breast (radiocolloid and blue dye) and removed for surgical tumour staging. A positive biopsy will usually lead to total axillary lymph-node clearance at the time of surgery or as a

---

[11] Inframammary fold.

separate procedure. A negative biopsy avoids unnecessary axillary node clearance, reducing the risk of procedural morbidity, such as arm lymphoedema.

What is the commonest type of post-mastectomy breast reconstruction?

The commonest type of reconstruction used is implant reconstruction. In some countries in Southeast Asia, without access to breast implants, TRAM flaps are the most common type of breast reconstruction.

What is an implant reconstruction?

Implant reconstruction is the commonest form of breast reconstruction. An implant is inserted into a submuscular (subpectoral) pocket. The inferior pole is usually covered with muscle (in small-breasted women), with the patient's own skin (dermal flap – in large-breasted women) or increasingly with acellular dermal matrix (ADM).

What is an ADM?

An ADM (acellular dermal matrix) is an implant derived from human, bovine or porcine tissue. The tissue is processed to remove cells and leave a collagen-rich matrix. ADMs are used to create an internal bra, providing lower pole implant cover between the raised pectoralis major muscle (superomedially) and the chest wall (inferolaterally). This avoids a partly subcutaneous portion of the implant (thought to increase complications) and improves ptosis at the inframammary fold.

What is a TRAM flap?

The transverse rectus abdominis myocutaneous (TRAM) flap can be used for autologous breast reconstruction as a pedicled (based on the superior epigastric vessels) or free flap (based on the larger inferior epigastric vessels). The rectus muscle has two main pedicles – superior epigastric from the internal mammary, and inferior epigastric from the external iliac – and the flap will survive off either. The donor site is generally closed as a Pfannenstiel abdominoplasty, leaving a cosmetically acceptable result. Complications include abdominal weakness, bulges and hernias (5%), umbilical or abdominal flap necrosis, seromas, wound infection and breakdown. Long-term numbness and pain is sometimes seen. Pedicled TRAM flaps are often used for breast reconstruction in Southeast Asia. In the West, DIEPs are now used. The most serious complication of a free TRAM or DIEP is failure of the flap, which occurs in 1–2% of cases.

What is a DIEP flap?
This autologous breast reconstruction method is a muscle-preserving variation on the free TRAM flap. The deep inferior epigastric perforator (DIEP) flap has reduced donor site morbidity such as abdominal bulges or hernias (incidence 1%). The pedicle is the same as in free TRAM, but perforator(s) are dissected individually, leaving rectus muscle intact, and fascia is also repaired in layers. Although potentially less bulky than a TRAM, the DIEP provides sufficient tissue to reconstruct the breast without requiring a prosthesis.

What is an LD flap?
The latissimus dorsi (LD) flap is based on the thoracodorsal pedicle, a continuation of the subscapular artery, which in turn arises from the third part of the axillary artery. The flap may be taken as muscle only, with skin paddle (of varying shape, size and orientation) or as a muscle-sparing thoracodorsal artery perforator (TAP) flap. It is commonly used as a pedicled flap in breast reconstruction with or without (extended LD) an implant to augment volume. It can be used as a free flap to reconstruct any defect on trunk, extremities or head and neck. It generates a cosmetically pleasing breast reconstruction leaving a transverse (bra line) or oblique (RSTL) scar on the ipsilateral back. Depending on the indication, like TRAM/DIEPs, it can be used bilaterally for example to reconstruct the breast after skin-sparing mastectomy for risk reduction in BRCA carriers.

Why are these flaps easily missed?
- TRAM and DIEP flaps are harvested from a lower abdomen/bikini-line access incision. The resulting suprapubic scar can be missed if it is not actively sought by exposing the suprapubic area in patients with a breast skin paddle and no evidence of an ipsilateral back scar (LD flap).
- Flap skin paddles post skin-sparing mastectomy may be rather small and restricted to a normal sized/positioned areola region (that you may well not easily notice if nipple reconstruction/tattooing has been completed).
- The LD flap can be placed in the bra line posteriorly and can be misinterpreted as a bra skin impression.

> **Tip**
> Multiple small stab incision scars around the breast, abdomen/flanks or thighs may indicate previous fat transfer with liposuction and filling to remodel the breast. This is performed to refine the result or deal with tethered scars, contour defects (e.g. after fat necrosis in a flap) or post-radiotherapy changes.

Differential diagnoses

What are the causes of a breast lump?

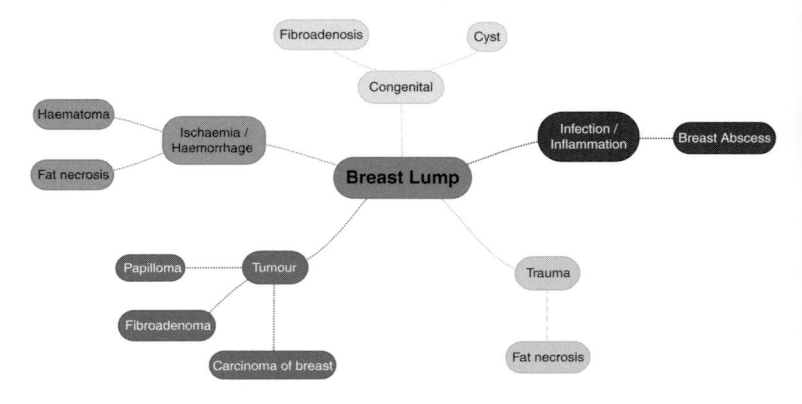

- **Breast Lump**
  - Congenital
    - Fibroadenosis
    - Cyst
  - Ischaemia / Haemorrhage
    - Haematoma
    - Fat necrosis
  - Infection / Inflammation
    - Breast Abscess
  - Tumour
    - Papilloma
    - Fibroadenoma
    - Carcinoma of breast
  - Trauma
    - Fat necrosis

What are the causes of gynaecomastia?

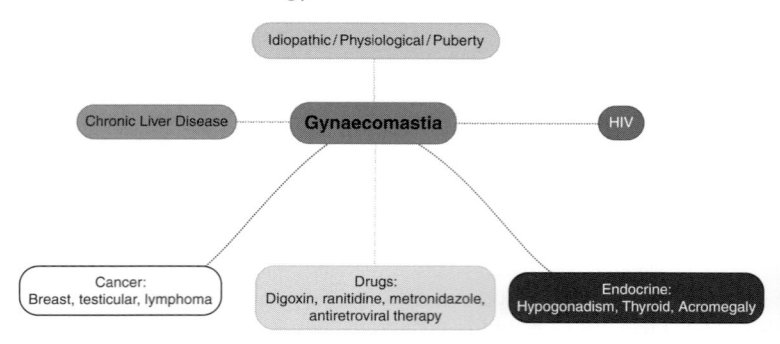

- **Gynaecomastia**
  - Idiopathic / Physiological / Puberty
  - Chronic Liver Disease
  - HIV
  - Cancer: Breast, testicular, lymphoma
  - Drugs: Digoxin, ranitidine, metronidazole, antiretroviral therapy
  - Endocrine: Hypogonadism, Thyroid, Acromegaly

What are the causes of nipple discharge?

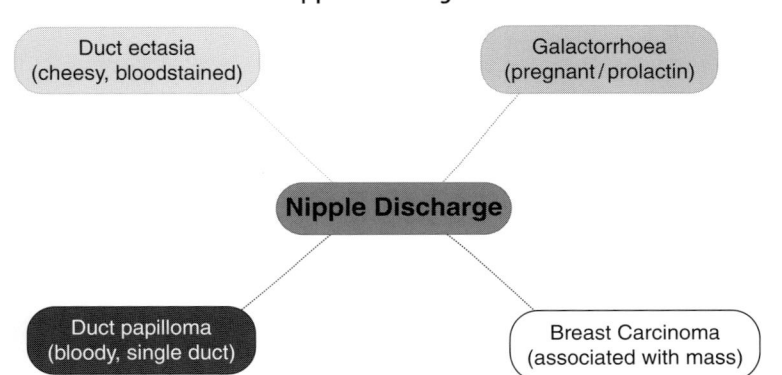

- Duct ectasia (cheesy, bloodstained)
- Galactorrhoea (pregnant / prolactin)
- Duct papilloma (bloody, single duct)
- Breast Carcinoma (associated with mass)

→ **Nipple Discharge**

Section editor: Petrut Gogalniceanu
Senior authors: Andrew T. Raftery, Wai Yoong, Justin Vale

Section 4: Pelvis and perineum

Chapter 10: Examination of the anus

Petrut Gogalniceanu, William Lynn and Andrew T. Raftery

Checklist

WIPER
- Chaperone and good light source
- Gloves and lubricating gel
- Patient on couch, left lateral position, knees up towards the chest

Physiological parameters

General
- Perineal excoriation or dermatitis
- Abnormal discharge at the anal verge: pus, blood, faeces

External
- Inspection of gluteal cleft: pilonidal disease (sinus or abscess)
- Inspection of perineum:
  - erythema, abnormal moisture or purulent discharge
  - haemorrhoids, abscesses, fissures, fistulas, skin tags
  - scars or wounds from previous abscess drainage
  - setons
  - anorectal prolapse (ask patient to cough)
- Palpation:
  - anal sphincter contour

Physical Examination for Surgeons, ed. Petrut Gogalniceanu, James Pegrum and William Lynn. Published by Cambridge University Press. © Cambridge University Press 2015.

- perianal sensation
- perianal fluctuance

Internal (digital rectal examination)
- Pain
- Anal sphincter tone
- Pelvic peritoneal irritation
- Pelvic abscess
- Masses in anus
- Prostate/uterine cervix (anteriorly)
- Areas of induration or fluctuance: fissures, haemorrhoids, fistulas
- Blood on examining finger

Special tests
- Faecal occult blood testing
- Proctoscopy
- Rigid sigmoidoscopy (10–20 cm)

To complete the examination...
- Examine groins for inguinal lymphadenopathy

Examination notes

Tips

Always have a chaperone in the room, irrespective of patient's or examiner's gender.

Have adequate lighting.

Stretch the anal skin with the fingers of the non-examining hand to reveal subtle lesions, such as anal fissures or sentinel tags.

Absence of blood on the examining finger does not exclude lower gastrointestinal bleeding. Microscopic bleeding can be identified with bedside occult bleeding testing kits.

What are the basic history points that need to be established?
- Pain
- Prolapse
- Pruritus
- Incontinence
- Abnormal discharge: pus, mucus, blood
- Anal trauma or intercourse
- Past medical history of Crohn's disease

> Mnemonic for findings on external inspection of the anus: **HAFFSSS**
> **H**aemorrhoids, **A**bscesses, **F**issures, **F**istulas, **S**kin tags, **S**cars, **S**etons

What is Goodsall's rule?
- With the patient in the lithotomy position, an imaginary transverse line is drawn horizontally (from 9 to 3 o'clock) to bisect the anus – the transverse anal line.
- A fistula that opens at the skin anterior to this line is likely to communicate with the anal canal via a straight tract.
- A fistula that opens at the skin posterior to this line is likely to communicate with the anal canal via a curved tract. The internal opening of the fistula is in the posterior midline of the anal canal.

What is a seton?
- A seton is a thick ligature or plastic sling inserted through a fistula and tied in a loop.
- A loose seton aims to keep the fistula tract open and allow drainage of pus.
- A tight or cutting seton aims to provide drainage of pus, as well as superficial migration of a deep fistula. Once the fistula is superficial to the sphincter muscles it can be incised open to allow healing.

What prostatic signs should be noted?
- Size: enlarged
- Position: 'high riding' in membranous urethral trauma
- Tenderness: prostatitis
- Contour: presence or loss of midline raphe; irregular or craggy contour

Section 4 Pelvis and perineum

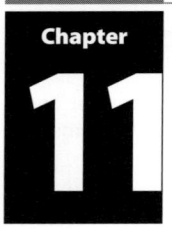

Chapter 11

Examination of the pudendum and vagina

Maria Memtsa and Wai Yoong

Checklist

WIPER
- Patient lying down, undressed from the waist down. Chaperone as required.

Physiological parameters

Inspection
- Hair distribution: measure of sexual development
- Rash/coloured areas: infection, atrophy
- Ulcers: *see notes below for differential diagnosis*
- Lumps: painful or painless
- Sinus openings: fistula
- Scars/asymmetry: previous surgery

  Gently separate the labia.

- Inspect for all the above: do not forget to look at the medial aspect of the labia
- Size and shape of clitoris
- Urethra: urethral caruncle/prolapse
- Presence of discharge from urethral orifice and/or vaginal outlet

  Ask the patient to bear down.

- Presence of lump/bulge: cystocoele/rectocoele/uterine prolapse

  Ask the patient to cough.

- Leakage of urine: stress incontinence

Physical Examination for Surgeons, ed. Petrut Gogalniceanu, James Pegrum and William Lynn. Published by Cambridge University Press. © Cambridge University Press 2015.

Cusco's and Sims' speculum examination
- To visualise the vaginal walls and cervix
- To obtain specific samples (for cytology, microbiology)

Palpation/digital bimanual examination
- Lumps: Bartholin's cyst or abscess
- Vaginal walls
- Cervix: shape, consistency, regularity, mobility, tenderness
- Uterus: size, shape, consistency, position, mobility
- Adnexae: presence of any masses; if any determine characteristics
- Uterosacral ligaments in the pouch of Douglas: regularity, tenderness

To complete the examination...
- Examine the abdomen: remember, if an enlarged pelvic organ is palpable abdominally, you cannot get below it.
- Examine the groins: lymphadenopathy (if vulval pathology is present).
- Perform a rectal examination: identify pelvic masses/tenderness and distinguish between enterocoele and rectocoele.

Examination notes
Essential history points
A focused gynaecological history should be obtained prior to examination. As an absolute minimum, the examining clinician ought to determine:
- LMP (first day of last menstrual period)
- Parity
- Pregnancy status in women of childbearing age
- Vaginal discharge or bleeding
- Abdominal pain
- Methods of contraception

How do you prepare for the gynaecological examination?
Any internal examination is potentially frightening for the patient, so it is imperative to ensure privacy, explain in simple language what you are going to do and ask for the patient's permission. Always ask for a chaperone to be present throughout the examination, and document her presence. The patient should have an empty bladder. The patient lies supine on the examination couch with hips and knees flexed, heels close together and legs apart (lithotomy position). The left lateral position is reserved for patients who are unable to lie flat, or when a clear view of the anterior vaginal wall is required (in case

of cystocoele or vesicovaginal fistula). Cover the abdomen and mons pubis with a sheet. Ensure adequate lighting with a direct light source and wear disposable gloves on both hands.

Does it matter if I do the speculum examination after the digital bimanual examination?

Yes, it does. By doing the speculum examination first, you have the opportunity to obtain microbiology swabs from the fornices (i.e. high vaginal swabs) that are not contaminated by lower vaginal flora. Accurate sampling maximises the potential to culture possible organisms that cause pelvic inflammatory disease (PID).

How do you perform a speculum examination?

- A bivalve (Cusco's) speculum is the instrument most commonly used to visualise the vaginal walls and the cervix, as well as to obtain microbiology and cytology samples.
- The speculum should be warmed and lubricated (if intending to obtain samples, use water as a lubricant as gels may interfere with the analysis of the samples).
- Part the labia with one hand and expose the introitus.
- Make sure the blades are closed and parallel to the labia, gently insert the speculum and rotate it 90°, so that the opening mechanism is positioned anteriorly.
- Slowly open the blades and advance the speculum as far as it goes without causing any pain. The cervix should be visible, but it may need to be readjusted depending on the position of the uterus.
- Once completed, withdraw the speculum under direct vision, ensuring the cervix is completely clear of the blades before closing them.
- The Sims' speculum is used to visualise vaginal wall prolapse by pressing on the opposite vaginal wall, with the patient in the left lateral position and bearing down.

How do you perform a digital bimanual examination?

- Ensuring that both hands are gloved and lubricated, part the labia with the thumb and forefinger of one hand and gently insert the index and middle finger of the other hand in the vagina. The thumb is abducted and the ring and little fingers are flexed to maximise the length of the index and middle finger.
- Gently feel for the cervix. Assess its mobility by placing the fingers in the posterior fornix (i.e. below the cervix) and gently move it.

- To assess the uterus, place the palmar aspect of your free hand on the abdomen in the suprapubic area, pressing it downwards, and with the other hand elevate the cervix (as before). Move your fingers to the right and the left of the cervix to assess the right and left adnexae in turn. Continue to apply gentle pressure with your other hand.
- Assess the uterosacral ligaments by feeling posteriorly to the cervix.
- Look at the glove at the end of the examination for the presence of blood or discharge.

What do you look for on inspection of the external female genitalia?

Define the anatomy and proceed systematically. Examine the labia majora, labia minora, introitus, urethra and clitoris. Part the labia and inspect again.

- **Hair distribution** and the size and shape of the clitoris provide important information about sexual development.
- **Rashes and skin discolourations**. The mucosa in post-pubertal pre-menopausal women is light pink and moist. After the menopause, the labial adipose tissue reduces in size, and the skin loses its turgor and moisture, causing it to have a darker pink appearance. These atrophic changes are normal and due to the lack of hormones, mainly oestrogen. Itchy red rash in the inner aspects of the thighs accompanied by thick white discharge is a sign of candidiasis. Sclerotic white areas in the labia, clitoris and perineum suggest leukoplakia, which is a potentially pre-malignant condition.
- **Scars or asymmetry**. The perineum of multiparous women may reveal an episiotomy scar, especially mediolaterally on the right. Rarely the scarring is more extensive, in cases of necrotising fasciitis post-delivery. In older women, scarring may be due to vulval surgery in case of previous carcinoma. In such cases, do not forget to look at the groin for scars following lymph-node clearance.
- **Swellings** (see differential diagnosis below). Due to the presence of hair the vulva is a common site for furuncles (boils), which present as red painful lumps. In contrast, sebaceous cysts are non-tender, yellowish in colour, firm and well-defined.
- **Ulcers** are very common in the genital area and are most frequently infective in origin. A chronic ulcer with an everted edge is suggestive of vulval carcinoma. These tend to metastasise early to the inguinal lymph nodes, and the primary lesion may be hidden in the labia folds.
- **Fistulas** are infrequent in the Western world but still very common in the developing world as a result of traumatic childbirth. The patient usually complains of a continuous discharge, which betrays the underlying pathology, although it can be tricky to identify the lesion.

- **Urethra**. A urethral caruncle is common in post-menopausal women and is a bright red tender granulomatous area arising from the mucosa of the urethral orifice. It should be differentiated from a urethral prolapse, which appears purple in colour, and carcinoma.
- **Uterine and vaginal prolpase** can be determined by increasing the intra-abdominal pressure. These can range from minimal descent to complete procidentia.
- Inspection of the vaginal walls and cervix is made possible by using a Cusco's speculum. Again, look for lesions, ulcers and scarring which may be present following obstetric trauma or post-radiotherapy for cervical carcinoma.
- On **cervical inspection**, look for the colour, regularity and smoothness of the cervix. If if in doubt or suspect carcinoma, refer to colposcopy clinic, as in case of ulceration or fungating growths.

What do you palpate in the pelvic examination?

- Feel the **labia majora** between your thumb and index finger. The tissue should be soft.
- Next examine **Bartholin's glands** by gently inserting the index finger in the lower vagina and keeping your thumb on the perineum. Bartholin's gland is located on the posterolateral aspect of the vagina near the fourchette and it should not be palpable, unless enlarged by a collection. Erythema, tenderness and feeling hot are signs of an **abscess**, while a fluctuant, non-tender lump is most probably a **cyst**.
- Continue with the digital bimanual palpation. First feel the **vaginal walls** and assess for any scar tissue, a result of perineal trauma during childbirth. Reach for the cervix. Cervical excitation is tenderness when moving the cervix. It is a sign of infection or inflammation in the pelvic organs (for example, PID) or ruptured ectopic pregnancy in pregnant women.
- Next assess the **uterus**. If enlarged and palpable abdominally, try to determine whether it moves together with the cervix as a unit. Fibroids (leiomyomas) are a common cause of an enlarged uterus.
- Feel for **adnexal fullness**, indicative of pathology in the tubes or ovaries. Ovarian cysts are the commonest cause of enlarged ovaries. Tenderness on palpation of the lateral fornices is a sign of tubal pathology, e.g. acute salpingitis.
- Finally, feel the **uterosacral ligaments**. Do they feel thickened? Is there tenderness? It may be due to the presence of endometriosis.

What else needs to be done to complete the examination?

- A complete gynaecological examination starts at the supraclavicular lymph nodes and ends at the ankles.

- Detailed breast examination is covered in Chapter 9.
- Examine the abdomen if you suspect ovarian, tubal or uterine pathology. In fact, the majority of patients seen in gynaecological clinics present with abdominal symptomatology, so it is imperative to perform a thorough abdominal examination (as described in Chapter 4).
- Due to the proximity of the pelvic organs to the rectum, a lot of information can be obtained by performing a digital rectal examination. A bidigital examination (examining the vagina and the rectum simultaneously) can be invaluable in cases of cervical malignancy, and is preferably performed with the patient under anaesthesia.

Differential diagnoses

What are the causes of masses in the external female genitalia?

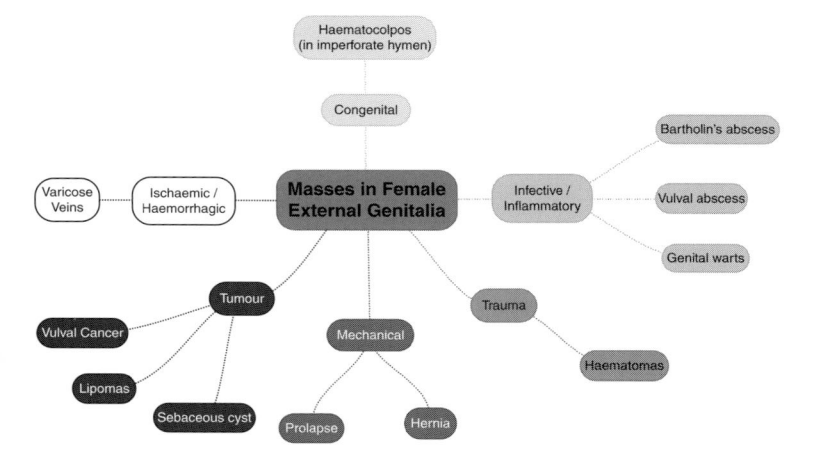

Masses in Female External Genitalia:

- Congenital
  - Haematocolpos (in imperforate hymen)
- Ischaemic / Haemorrhagic
  - Varicose Veins
- Infective / Inflammatory
  - Bartholin's abscess
  - Vulval abscess
  - Genital warts
- Tumour
  - Vulval Cancer
  - Lipomas
  - Sebaceous cyst
- Mechanical
  - Prolapse
  - Hernia
- Trauma
  - Haematomas

What are the causes of vulval ulceration?

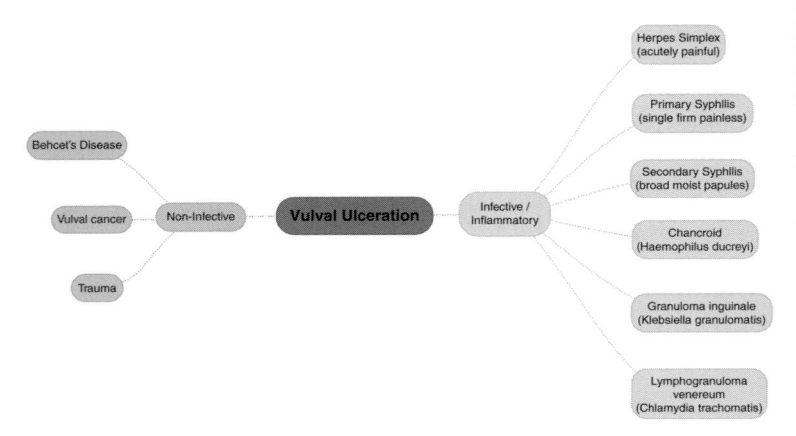

- **Vulval Ulceration**
  - **Non-Infective**
    - Behcet's Disease
    - Vulval cancer
    - Trauma
  - **Infective / Inflammatory**
    - Herpes Simplex (acutely painful)
    - Primary Syphilis (single firm painless)
    - Secondary Syphilis (broad moist papules)
    - Chancroid (Haemophilus ducreyi)
    - Granuloma inguinale (Klebsiella granulomatis)
    - Lymphogranuloma venereum (Chlamydia trachomatis)

| Section 4 | **Pelvis and perineum** |

| Chapter 12 | **Examination of the penis** |

Paul Erotocritou, Vassilios Memtsas, Petrut Gogalniceanu and Justin Vale

Checklist

WIPER
- Patient supine. Trousers removed. Groins and genitals exposed. Chaperone as required.

Physiological parameters

Inspection
- Penile shape: chordae, priapism
- Presence or absence of foreskin (circumcision)
- Retract foreskin (if uncircumcised): phimosis, paraphimosis, tight frenulum
- Position of external meatus: normal, hypospadias, epispadias
- Lesions on glans: carcinoma, papillomata acuminata, balanitis, ulcers (chancre)
- Lesions on inner or outer foreskin: as above

Palpation
- Open external meatus to assess size of urethral opening:
    - discharge (urinary incontinence, pus, blood)
    - erythema/ulceration
    - pinhole meatus

- Palpate glans and shaft of penis: evidence of Peyronie's disease.
- Palpate urethra: urethral stricture, carcinoma, diverticulum or abscess.

To complete the examination...
- Palpate inguinal lymph nodes: particularly in the presence of a penile lesion.

Physical Examination for Surgeons, ed. Petrut Gogalniceanu, James Pegrum and William Lynn. Published by Cambridge University Press. © Cambridge University Press 2015.

- Perform a scrotal, perineal and rectal examination.
- Urine dipstick.

Examination notes

What are the essential history points prior to a penile examination?
- Nature of lesion
- Circumcised or not
- Effect of erection on lesion
- Sexual history including erectile function and risk of sexually transmitted infections

What do you look for on inspection?
Assess whether the patient is circumcised. If the patient is not circumcised it is important to retract the foreskin to expose the glans. This allows inspection of the glans as well as the inner surface of the prepuce for any suspicious lesions. One needs to assess the position of the external urethral meatus.

What do you palpate in a penile examination?
Assess the actual diameter of the urethral opening deep to the external meatus, as a pinhole meatus may be present despite an apparently large external orifice. This is best performed by gently squeezing the tip of the glans in the anteroposterior axis, which encourages the slit-like urethra to open into a circular orifice.

The glans and shaft of the penis need to be palpated. There may be palpable fibrotic plaques on the penile shaft suggestive of Peyronie's disease. Gross urethral lesions in the penile shaft may also be palpable.

What else needs to be done before completing your examination?
To complete the penile examination assess the groins for lymphadenopathy, as penile lymphatics drain to the inguinal nodes. Proceed to examining the scrotum, perineum and prostate as described in Chapters 13, 10 and 6.

Differential diagnoses

What are the causes of haematuria?

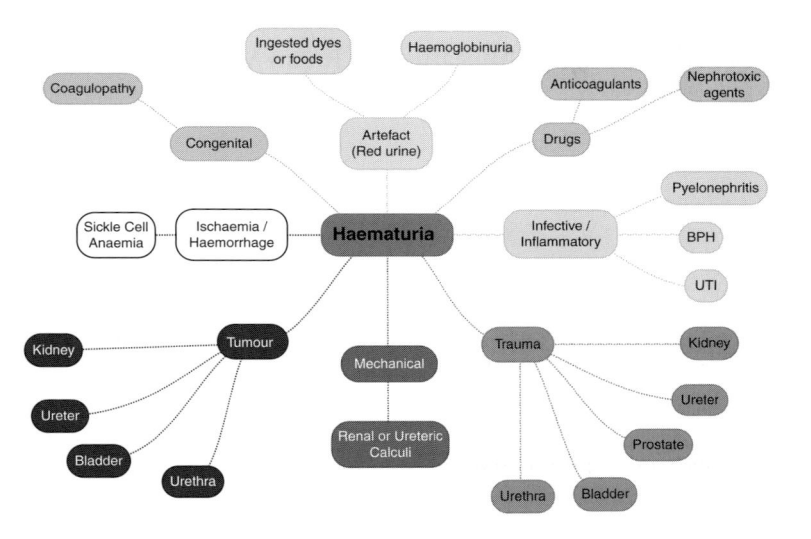

- **Haematuria**
  - Artefact (Red urine)
    - Ingested dyes or foods
    - Haemoglobinuria
  - Congenital
    - Coagulopathy
  - Drugs
    - Anticoagulants
    - Nephrotoxic agents
  - Ischaemia / Haemorrhage
    - Sickle Cell Anaemia
  - Infective / Inflammatory
    - Pyelonephritis
    - BPH
    - UTI
  - Tumour
    - Kidney
    - Ureter
    - Bladder
    - Urethra
  - Mechanical
    - Renal or Ureteric Calculi
  - Trauma
    - Kidney
    - Ureter
    - Prostate
    - Bladder
    - Urethra

What are the causes of penile lesions?

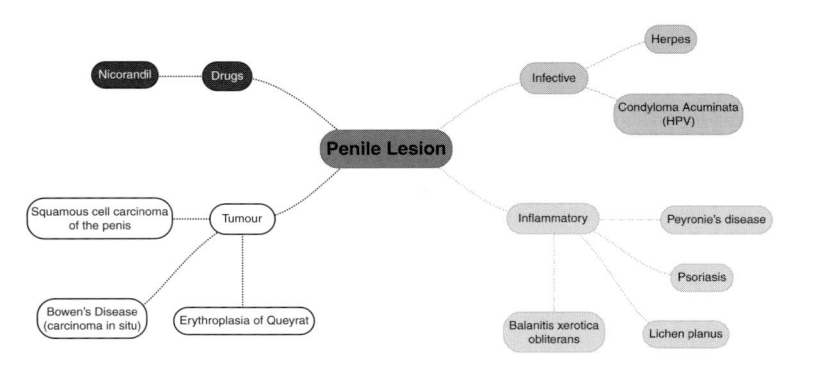

- **Penile Lesion**
  - Drugs
    - Nicorandil
  - Infective
    - Herpes
    - Condyloma Acuminata (HPV)
  - Inflammatory
    - Peyronie's disease
    - Psoriasis
    - Lichen planus
    - Balanitis xerotica obliterans
  - Tumour
    - Squamous cell carcinoma of the penis
    - Bowen's Disease (carcinoma in situ)
    - Erythroplasia of Queyrat

| Section 4 | Pelvis and perineum |

Chapter 13: Examination of the scrotum

Paul Erotocritou, Vassilios Memtsas, Petrut Gogalniceanu and Justin Vale

Checklist

WIPER
- Patient standing. Trousers removed. Exposure from nipple to knee. Chaperone as required.

Physiological parameters

Inspection
- Scrotal asymmetry: pathology within hemiscrotum:
    - absent testicle: failure of scrotal development or testicular descent, or orchidectomy
    - scrotal mass
- Skin:
    - oedema, cellulitis, Fournier's gangrene
    - scars from previous scrotal surgery or orchidopexy
- Groin: scars (hernia repair) and masses (undescended testis)

Palpation
Patient standing:

Ask: 'Do you have any pain?'

- **Anatomy**: define (a) superficial inguinal ring, (b) spermatic cord and vas deferens, (c) testicle, (d) epididymis. Compare left and right sides.
- **Scrotal skin lumps**: sebaceous cysts, abscesses and furuncles.

Physical Examination for Surgeons, ed. Petrut Gogalniceanu, James Pegrum and William Lynn. Published by Cambridge University Press. © Cambridge University Press 2015.

- **Testicle**: presence, contour, masses, size. If absent testicle, palpate groin and see if able to manipulate testicle into scrotum.
- **Epididymis** (posterior aspect of testis): tender or swollen.
- If **scrotal mass** felt:
  - Can you get above it?
  - Can you define testis and epididymis separately?
  - Does the mass transilluminate (hydrocoele)?
  - Is there a cough impulse (hernia/varicocoele)?

Patient supine:

- Re-examine the scrotum. Assess if any palpable abnormality becomes less prominent, as in the case of a varicocoele or hernia. Always ensure the scrotum is lifted up to inspect the posterior aspect of the scrotum and perineum.

To complete the examination...
- Examine the abdomen, especially if the testicle feels abnormal.
- Examine groin, penis and perineum: identify hernias, undescended or ectopic testes.

Examination notes

What are the essential history points for a scrotal mass?

History as for any mass (see Chapter 39, *Examination of skin lesions and lumps*). Specific points to elucidate:

- Previous scrotal operations
- Risk factors for testicular malignancy (undescended testis, family history, infertility, small testis)

What do you look for on inspection of the scrotum?

- Assess scrotal symmetry and development. Scrotal asymmetry together with the history may indicate the underlying pathology: e.g. a patient with a recent history of an inguinal hernia repair who has a smaller testicle on the same side would suggest testicular atrophy following hernia repair (ischaemic orchitis).
- Failure of scrotal development suggests that there has been a failure of testicular descent. It is thus important to assess the perineum and groin in case the patient has an ectopic testis.
- Assess both the scrotum and the groins for scars. A scar in the groin may suggest a previous orchidopexy, while a scar on the scrotum suggests previous scrotal surgery.

What do you palpate in the examination of the scrotum?

Define the anatomy: testicle, epididymis and vas deferens.

- Palpate the testicles to ensure they have a smooth surface.
- The epididymis is palpable posterior to the testis as a distinct ridge of tissue.
- If a firm, irregular testis is palpated and there is suspicion of testicular cancer one should also perform an abdominal examination, as well as an examination of the groins and supraclavicular areas for lymphadenopathy.
- Arising superiorly from the testis is the spermatic cord, which contains the vas deferens. This is palpable as a cord-like structure.
- If the vas is absent bilaterally one should screen the patient for cystic fibrosis.
- If there is unilateral absence of the vas an ultrasound of the kidneys should be performed, as there is an association with unilateral renal agenesis.

Is there a swelling confined to the scrotum?

A scrotal mass can arise from scrotal structures or extend into the scrotum through the inguinal canal. Determining whether or not it is possible to get above the mass can differentiate between the two.

- If one is unable to get above the swelling, the swelling is not confined to the scrotum and is likely to be an inguinoscrotal hernia or hydrocoele of the cord.
- If one is able to get above the swelling, this suggests it has arisen from within the scrotum (testis, vas or epididymis).

Are the testis and epididymis palpable separately?

- If unable to palpate the testis and epididymis separately, in the absence of marked tenderness, the scrotal mass is most likely to be a hydrocoele. This can be confirmed by transilluminating the hydrocoele around the testis.
- If unable to palpate the testis and epididymis separately, and the mass is tender, the patient may be suffering from epididymo-orchitis or a haematocoele (if there is a history of trauma).
- If the testis and epididymis are separately palpable it is important to assess which structure the swelling originates from:
    - A swelling arising from the epididymis with the testis palpable separately is usually an epididymal cyst and should transilluminate. Solid tumours of the epididymis, such as an adenomatoid tumour, are rare.
    - A mass arising distinctly from the testis may represent a testicular tumour.

- If able to palpate the testis and epididymis separately and the mass feels like 'a bag of worms' it is likely that the patient has a varicocoele. This can be confirmed by asking the patient to lie down. Reduction in the size of the scrotal mass may confirm the presence of a varicocoele, but may also be seen in reducible inguinoscrotal hernias. If the patient has a varicocoele it is also necessary to examine the abdomen, as in 1% of cases a renal cell cancer may present with a varicocoele.

Are you able to diagnose testicular torsion from clinical examination alone?

There are a number of findings that would suggest torsion on examination (**3 Hs**):

- **H**igh-riding testicle
- **H**orizontal lie
- Pre**h**n's sign: elevation of the testicle relieves the pain of epididymo-orchitis, but not pain caused by torsion

It is important to realise that the only way to exclude a diagnosis of torsion in a young male with history of sudden-onset testicular pain is through a testicular exploration.

What else needs to be done to complete examination?

- If you suspect testicular cancer, it is important to examine the abdomen, as well as the inguinal and supraclavicular regions, for lymphadenopathy.
- In the presence of a varicocoele you should perform an abdominal examination, to look for palpable renal masses.
- If a patient has only a single palpable testis in the scrotum you should assess the groin and perineum to look for an undescended or ectopic testis respectively.
- One must also remember that the scrotal skin is a hair-bearing area and may commonly be a site for sebaceous cysts. These cysts will be palpable in the scrotal skin separate from the testis.
- In patients with bilateral testicular atrophy or failure of development, inspect for gynaecomastia to rule out an underlying endocrinological cause or oestrogen therapy for prostate cancer.

Differential diagnoses

What are the causes of loin-to-groin pain?

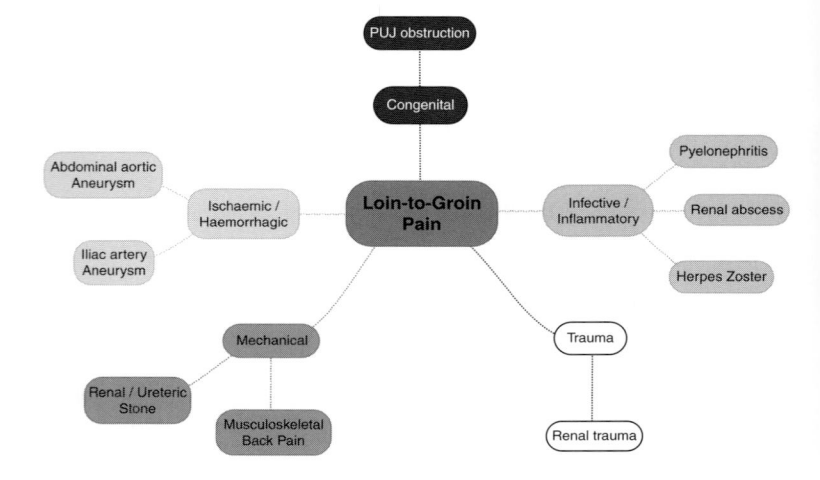

- **Loin-to-Groin Pain**
  - **Congenital**
    - PUJ obstruction
  - **Infective / Inflammatory**
    - Pyelonephritis
    - Renal abscess
    - Herpes Zoster
  - **Trauma**
    - Renal trauma
  - **Mechanical**
    - Renal / Ureteric Stone
    - Musculoskeletal Back Pain
  - **Ischaemic / Haemorrhagic**
    - Abdominal aortic Aneurysm
    - Iliac artery Aneurysm

What are the causes of a scrotal mass?

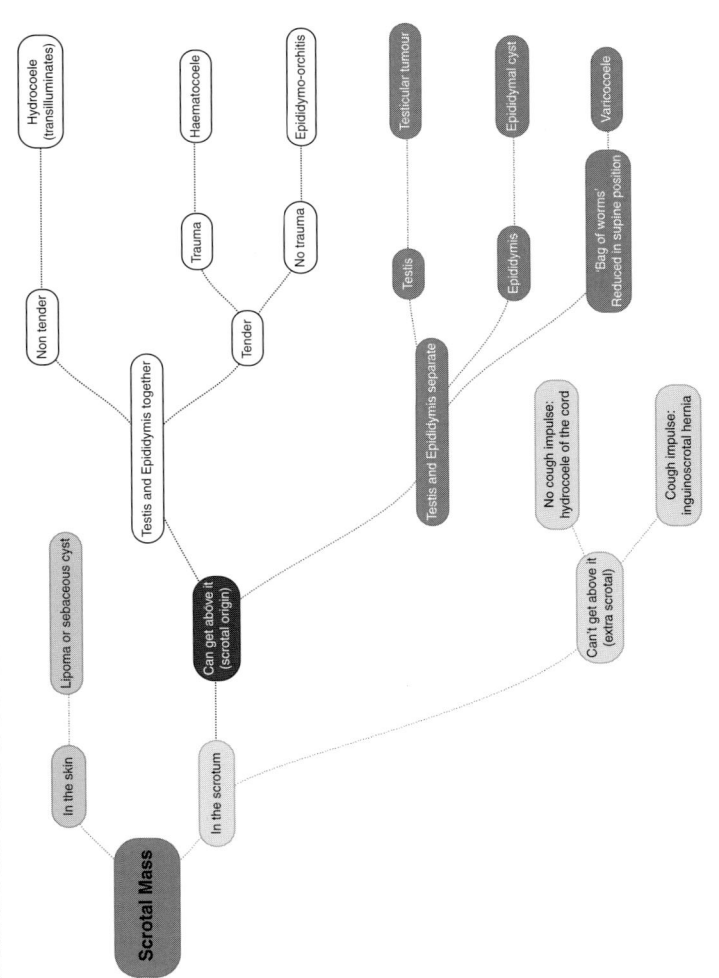

Scrotal Mass

- **In the skin**
  - Lipoma or sebaceous cyst
- **In the scrotum**
  - **Can get above it (scrotal origin)**
    - **Testis and Epididymis together**
      - Non tender → Hydrocoele (transilluminates)
      - Tender
        - Trauma → Haematocoele
        - No trauma → Epididymo-orchitis
    - **Testis and Epididymis separate**
      - Testis → Testicular tumour
      - Epididymis → Epididymal cyst
      - 'Bag of worms' Reduced in supine position → Varicocoele
  - **Can't get above it (extra scrotal)**
    - No cough impulse: hydrocoele of the cord
    - Cough impulse: inguinoscrotal hernia

117

Scrotal mass (by pathology)

- Congenital: hydrocoele, epididymal cyst
- Inflammatory/infective: epidiymo-orchitis, scrotal abscess
- Vascular: varicocoele
- Trauma: haematocoele
- Tumour: testicular cancer, sebaceous cyst
- Mechanical: inguinoscrotal mass, testicular torsion

What are the causes of testicular atrophy?

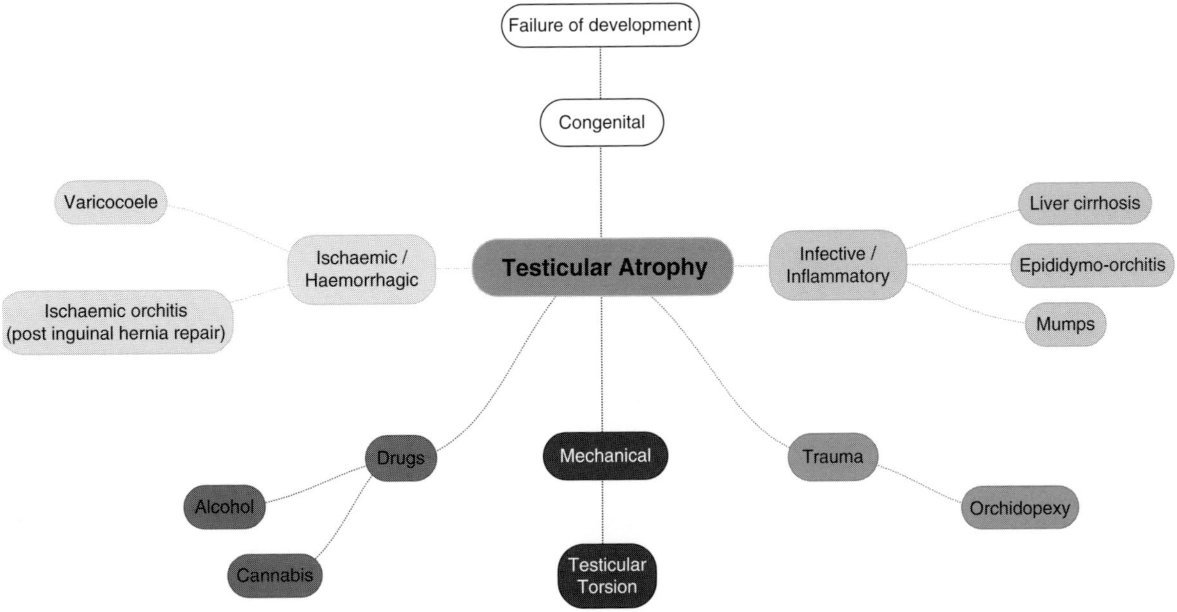

- **Testicular Atrophy**
  - **Congenital**
    - Failure of development
  - **Infective / Inflammatory**
    - Liver cirrhosis
    - Epididymo-orchitis
    - Mumps
  - **Trauma**
    - Orchidopexy
  - **Mechanical**
    - Testicular Torsion
  - **Drugs**
    - Alcohol
    - Cannabis
  - **Ischaemic / Haemorrhagic**
    - Varicocoele
    - Ischaemic orchitis (post inguinal hernia repair)

What are the causes of scrotal pain?

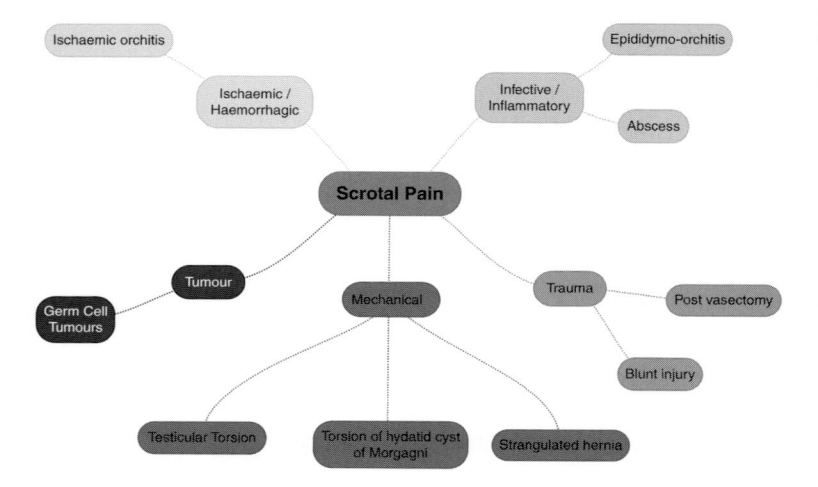

- **Scrotal Pain**
  - Ischaemic / Haemorrhagic
    - Ischaemic orchitis
  - Infective / Inflammatory
    - Epididymo-orchitis
    - Abscess
  - Tumour
    - Germ Cell Tumours
  - Mechanical
    - Testicular Torsion
    - Torsion of hydatid cyst of Morgagni
    - Strangulated hernia
  - Trauma
    - Post vasectomy
    - Blunt injury

Section editors: James Pegrum
Senior author: Chris Lavy

Section 5 — **Orthopaedic surgery**

Chapter 14

Generic joint examination

James Pegrum, Petrut Gogalniceanu and Chris Lavy

Checklist

WIPER
- Bilateral limb exposure
- Exposure of joint above and joint below
- Aids, orthotics and soles of footwear

Physiological parameters

Gait
- Specific gait
- Symmetry and pattern of movement
- Posture

Tape (measure)
- Length or diameter discrepancies between limbs (true or apparent)

Look
- Skin: scars, erythema, ecchymosis, sinuses (SEES)
- Soft tissues: wasting, swelling
- Bone: deformity, asymmetry, amputations

Feel
- Skin: temperature, tenderness

Physical Examination for Surgeons, ed. Petrut Gogalniceanu, James Pegrum and William Lynn. Published by Cambridge University Press. © Cambridge University Press 2015.

- Soft tissues: muscles, tendons, induration, fluctuance, pulses, capillary refill, sensation
- Bone: bone and joint contours

Move
- Active (and range of movement)
- Passive
- Resisted

Test
- Special joint provocation tests

X-ray
- X-rays of joints (2 views, 2 joints, 2 limbs, 2 points in time)

To complete the examination...
- Say you would like to ask the patient questions about impact on lifestyle.
- Examine the joint above and the joint below – with limb pain, consider examining the neck/back for referred pain.

Examination notes

A structured, consistent and universal approach is needed in the orthopaedics examination in order to avoid missing pathology irrespective of the joint examined.

The typical algorithm used in orthopaedics involves seven four-letter words:

GAIT	LOOK	TEST
TAPE	FEEL	X-RAY
	MOVE	

The *look* and *feel* parts of the examination are subdivided into three further categories: SKIN, SOFT (tissues) and BONE. These are easily remembered, as they are also four-letter words.

Intial observation and gait

The initial observation of the patient and any adjuncts such as walking aids, slings, heel or shoe raises, orthotics or prosthetics helps identify potential pathology. At this time ask the patient to walk. If there is lower limb pathology this is an ideal opportunity to assess smoothness and symmetry of gait. It is also important to assess the presence of an antalgic (painful) gait or walking pattern typical of a particular central or peripheral neurological pathology (e.g. foot drop or cerebral palsy). In the examination of the lower limb and spine, examine the soles of the feet for callosities and shoes for the pattern of wear. Gait examination provides the clinician with 'thinking time' to establish and identify gross pathology in order to formulate an answer. Typical gait patterns are shown in the following table.

Typical gait patterns seen in clinical practice

Gait pattern	Clinically	Cause
Spastic gait	Adducted internally rotated arm with flexed hip and plantarflexed foot	Hemiparesis
Antalgic gait	Reduced time spent on weight-bearing side ('dot–dash' gait)	Trauma, infection, arthritis
Ataxic gait	Wide-based unsteady gait	Unsteadiness from cerebellar or Friedreich's ataxia
Trendelenburg gait	Weak hip abductors cause tilting of the pelvis away from the standing leg, i.e. normal side sags	Perthe's disease, slipped capital femoral epiphysis, developmental dysplasia of the hip, hip arthritis, spina bifida, cerebral palsy and spinal cord injury, gluteal nerve injury or poor muscle balancing in hip replacements
Circumducting gait	Exaggerated hip abduction during leg swing	Hemiplegia, leg length discrepancy, unilateral spasticity
High-stepping gait	Exaggerated hip flexion to allow clearance of foot during swing phase of gait	Foot drop, spina bifida, polio, peripheral neuropathies
Tiptoe walking gait	Plantarflexed or equinus foot position	Common in children; differentials include diplegia cerebral palsy or lysosomal storage disorder

Tape

Establish limb length discrepancy or subtle muscle atrophy (limb circumference changes) as a means of diagnosis and operative planning.

- **Apparent leg length** is measured from the xiphisternum to the inferior surface of the medial malleolus. Discrepancy in apparent leg length (not true leg length) is caused by a pelvic tilt, scoliosis or hip fixed flexion deformity.
- **True leg length** is measured from the anterior superior iliac spine (ASIS) to the inferior surface of the medial malleolus on the ipsilateral side. Discrepancy in true leg length is a result of shortening of the tibia or femur. If there is a discrepancy in true leg length, Galleazi's test assesses which bone is involved (see Chapter 21, *Examination of the hip*).

Look

How should the patient be generally observed?

Inspect the patient systematically and thoroughly. Start with a 360° circumferential inspection; this is performed with the clinician standing still and the patient moving around 90° at a time. The lack of movement from the clinician allows time to discover pathology and compose a logical and concise response. Inspect the skin, the soft tissues and then the bony contours. The same systematic approach is easily transferable to the palpation stage.

How should specific points be identified on skin inspection?

- Identify scars from previous surgery. Note small (1 cm) wounds from previous arthroscopy.
- Look for subtle signs of infection or inflammation: erythema, cellulitis, sinuses or fistulas discharging pus. Identify non-surgical pathologies such as gout or rheumatoid arthritis.

How should the soft tissues be inspected?

The inspection of soft tissues can identify two signs of disease:

- Swelling – can be caused by a variety of mechanisms, such as tumours, haematomas, abscesses or effusions.
- Wasting – caused by tissue loss following trauma/surgery, or from muscle wasting secondary to inactivity caused by pain, nerve damage, immobilisation or joint pathology.

How should bones be inspected?

Look for:

- Congenital deformities (absence or duplication).

- Acquired asymmetries caused by a current fracture, malunion of old fractures, varus or valgus deformity, arthritic joint pathologies or amputations.

> **Tip**
>
> **Varus** refers to a medial deviation from the midline of the *distal bone*.
> **Valgus** describes a lateral deviation from midline of the *distal bone*.
> This can be remembered by the fact that **valgus** contains an **L**, as does **Lateral**.

Feel
What should be palpated in the skin?
Assess the temperature using the dorsum of hand and identify any tenderness. Look at the patient's face to identify discomfort.

What should be palpated in the soft tissues?
- Identify effusions or abscesses.
- Tenderness over the origins and insertions of tendons.
- Assess muscle bulk, as well as compartmental tenderness or turgidity indicative of ischaemic pain or compartment syndrome.

What should be palpated in the bones?
- Palpate bony contours for step deformities or fractures.
- Assess superficial joint lines for tenderness or presence of osteophytes.

Move
- Initial assessment of joint movement is best carried out actively by the patient. This quickly establishes the range of movement possible without causing undue distress to the patient. Look for symmetry, smoothness and ease of active movement.
- There are some movements that are not possible to perform actively, and this is when the examiner passively controls the joint to produce the movement: for example, knee hyperextension.
- Finally, resisted movements are important for particular muscle groups, to assess any form of weakness and reproduction of discomfort.
- The absolute values of joint movement are hugely variable in the literature and are rarely useful to remember verbatim. What is more useful is to

compare the contralateral side as the 'normal' value. A useful point in documenting joint range of movement is to use angles that are easy to visualise: i.e. right angle (90°), half a right angle (45°) and a third of a right angle (30°), which can be visually calculated without a goniometer. The documentation of range of movement using values such as 10° or 105° without a goniometer is less credible, but multiples of 30° or 45° will be.

> **Tip**
>
> **Active movement** is the movement carried out by the patient.
> **Passive movement** is carried out by the examiner.
> Remember: A comes before P in the alphabet, and also in the examination of patients.

Special tests

There are numerous special tests for each joint, and these are explained in detail in the relevant chapter. Special tests are performed to assess stability and function of the joint, and are carried out to reproduce the symptoms experienced by the patient in a controlled manner.

Special tests are reported using the '**RTP**' system:

- **Rationale** – what is the test trying to elicit / what is the clinical importance of a positive test?
- **Technique** – how is the test performed?
- **Positive** test – what clinical finding indicates the test to be positive?

To complete the examination...

All joint examinations are completed by examining the joint above and the joint below, which should be actively encouraged in an OSCE situation if there is sufficient time.

A quick neurovascular exam should be performed in all orthopaedic examinations, but at the end of the examination one should mention that a 'full vascular and neurological examination should be performed to complete my examination'.

- Distal upper limb pulses: radial and the ulnar arteries.
- Lower limb pulses: dorsalis pedis and posterior tibial arteries.
- Capillary refill time (usually <3 seconds).
- Palpate muscle compartments to identify compartment syndrome in the context of limb ischaemia or trauma. This is essential in day-to-day clinical

examination, but you will not be faced with this situation in an exam setting.
- Dermatomal sensation to touch (upper limb: C5–8, T1–2; lower limb: L2–5 and S1).

Finally, organise appropriate investigations. In orthopaedics it is easy and cost-effective to say 'I will organise an anterior–posterior and lateral radiograph.' However, when assessing soft tissue injuries radiographs are useless and an ultrasound scan or MRI with or without contrast is diagnostic. For the principles and interpretation of different radiological examinations, see Section 11, *Surgical radiology*.

Section 5 Orthopaedic surgery

Chapter 15

Examination of gait

James Pegrum and Chris Lavy

Overview of the gait cycle

1. **Stance phase** – 60% of cycle
   - Heel strike – flat foot – mid-stance – heel off – toe off
2. **Swing phase** – 40% of cycle
   - Acceleration – mid-swing – deceleration

What is the lower limb biomechanical assessment used for?

A lower limb biomechanical assessment analyses the link between the structure, function, strengths and weaknesses of the lower limb joints and muscles. Lower limb pain can be caused or referred from a number of joints. A comprehensive examination is needed to identify the numerous contributing pathological processes, which may need to be treated concurrently with physiotherapy, orthotics, injections or surgery.

What is the difference between open and closed kinetic chains?

In open kinetic chain assessment the joint is able to move freely, either by active movement or by passive movement by the examiner. Closed kinetic chain is the assessment of gait and lower limb function whilst it is in contact with the ground.

What is the normal gait cycle?

A gait cycle is the sequence that starts with the heel strike of one foot and ends with the subsequent floor contact of the same foot. The gait is defined as a series of rhythmical and alternating movements of the trunk and lower limbs that result in forward progression of the centre of gravity.

Physical Examination for Surgeons, ed. Petrut Gogalniceanu, James Pegrum and William Lynn. Published by Cambridge University Press. © Cambridge University Press 2015.

During increasing walking speeds and running the swing phase increases and the stance phase decreases until the ratio of stance to swing phase reverses.

What are the commonly used terms?

- A **step length** is the distance from one heel strike to the contralateral heel strike.
- A **stride length** is the distance between two heel contacts of the same foot, and in a normal gait it is double the step length.

Section 5

Orthopaedic surgery

Chapter 16

Examination of the cervical and thoracic spine

James Pegrum and Chris Lavy

Checklist

WIPER
- Patient standing in shorts or underwear. Access is required to the neck and thoracic cage.

Physiological parameters

Gait and balance
- Smoothness and symmetry
- Sagittal balance

Look
- **Skin**: erythema, scars (posterior and anterior), alignment of skin creases
- **Soft tissues**: swelling; wasting of paraspinal muscles, intervertebral spaces
- **Bone**: scoliosis, kyphosis, lordosis, rib cage asymmetry, shoulder girdle

Feel
- **Skin**: temperature, tenderness, sensation
- **Soft tissues**: paraspinal muscle bulk and spasm
- **Bone**: spinous processes, facet joints, sacroiliac joints, coccyx

Move
- **Active**:
  - flexion/extension of spine

Physical Examination for Surgeons, ed. Petrut Gogalniceanu, James Pegrum and William Lynn. Published by Cambridge University Press. © Cambridge University Press 2015.

- side flexion of spine
- rotation of spine

Special tests (* = essential tests)
- Spurling's nerve root compression test*
- Axial compression test*
- Disc test: Valsalva manoeuvre*
- Neurological examination*
- Thoracic outlet syndrome (see Chapter 26)
- Waddell's behavioural signs

To complete the examination...
- Examine the shoulder, lumbar spine and sacroiliac joint.
- Check full neurovascular status of the lower limb.
- Order appropriate radiographs and further imaging.

Examination notes

What do you look for during gait and initial observations?

Look at the sagittal and coronal planes of the patient. In the sagittal plane a vertical line should be drawn through the ear, shoulder, hip, knee and ankle. This quick screening test helps identify any spinal deformity, for example found in ankylosing spondylitis.

What signs should be identified in examining the skin?

The skin needs to be assessed for signs of systemic disease:
- Café-au-lait spots found in neurofibromatosis.
- Psoriasis, cutaneous vasculitis or nodules found in rheumatoid arthritis.
- Evidence of steroid use with striae, telangiectasia, skin thinning and bruising.
- Scars: evidence of previous cervical spine surgery via a posterior or an anterior approach (where a scar is found in the skin crease medial to the sternocleidomastoid).

How should the soft tissues be inspected?

The symmetry of the surrounding soft tissues and muscles are assessed:
- Anteriorly: the scalene, sternocleidomastoid and pectoralis muscles.
- Posteriorly: the paraspinal muscles (levator scapulae, trapezius, rhomboid and trapezius muscles) are palpated.

How should the bony contours of the cervical spine be inspected?
- C6 and C7 spinous processes are easily visualised in slim patients.
- Coronal plane: pelvic tilt (indicates either scoliosis or leg length discrepancy).
- Sagittal plane: abnormal kyphosis or lordosis.
- Note symmetry and degree of chest expansion. This can be altered in patients with scoliosis or ankylosing spondylitis.
- Scapulae: position and the shape may be altered in scoliosis.

Observation and inspection of the cervical and thoracic spine

Skin	Manifestations of systemic disease, scars, asymmetrical skin creases, erythema, hairy patch, café-au-lait spots
Soft tissues	Muscle wasting and bulk, abscess
Bone	Scoliosis, lordosis, kyphosis, scapula, pelvic tilt, chest expansion

How is the cervical and thoracic spine palpated?
- The skin surrounding the cervical and thoracic spine is palpated for warmth and altered sensation.
- The muscles are assessed for bulk and spasticity: the sternocleidomastoid, scalene, nuchal cervical extensor muscle group, trapezius, levator scapulae and rhomboids.
- Cervical lymph nodes may also be examined (see Chapter 36, *Examination of the neck and thyroid*).
- Bony prominences of C6/7 spinous processes, as well as the spaces between the spinous process, which correspond to intervertebral ligaments.
- Facet joints can be palpated 2.5 cm lateral to the midline.

How is movement of the cervical and thoracic spine assessed?
- Assess flexion, extension, side flexion and rotation, which occur predominantly at the C1/2 junction.
- Passive movement evaluates muscle lengths:
  - The scalene muscles are assessed on lateral side flexion.
  - The trapezius is stretched by placing the patient's hands behind his or her head and flexing the chin towards the chest.
  - The levator scapulae is assessed by a combination of side and forward cervical flexion, by asking the patient to place his or her nose towards the axilla.

- Chest expansion can be assessed by measuring the chest wall during full expiration and inspiration at the 4th intercostal space. The typical chest expansion is 4–7 cm and varies between males and females. This decreases with age.

What is Spurling's test?*

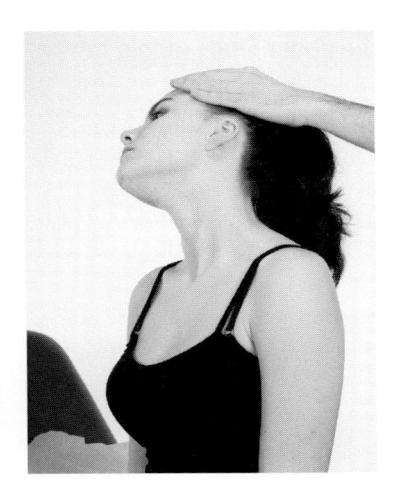

Rationale: This test helps to reproduce the neuropathic pain felt in nerve root compression.
Technique: The head is extended and side flexed.
Positive test: A positive test causes radicular pain down the arm. Dizziness, blurring of vision or slurring of speech may indicate vertebrobasilar insufficiency.

How do you perform an axial compression test?*

Rationale: To rule out the pathological significance of cervical neck pain in the malingering patient.
Technique: Axial compression of the cervical spine by placing axial pressure through the top of the head whilst the patient is sitting or standing.
Positive test: Reproduction of pain in this instance is rarely pathological.

How is disc prolapse pain diagnosed?*

Rationale: Disc prolapse pain is exacerbated by a Valsalva manoeuvre.

Technique: This is carried out by exhalation against a closed airway. Alternative methods include blowing into a test tube, blowing up a balloon, sneezing or coughing.

Positive test: Reproduction of the patients' symptoms or discomfort.

What neurological examination of the upper limbs should be performed?*

Rationale: Cervical myelopathy can cause upper motor neuron signs.

Technique: Assess the dermatomes, myotomes and reflexes described in the tables below.

- Hoffmann's sign involves flicking the patient's middle-finger nail plate. In patients with myelopathy there is a reflex flexion at the distal interphalangeal joint of the index finger.

Positive test: e.g. a C6 nerve root compression secondary to a disc causes diminished sensation in the lateral forearm, index finger and thumb, with weakness to elbow flexion and absent brachioradialis reflex.

What are Waddell's signs?

Rationale: A set of tests and clinical findings that *may* indicate a non-organic cause of back pain.

Technique: the following features have been reported by Waddell *et al.*:[12]

- Superficial or diffuse non-anatomical spinal tenderness.
- Axial loading.
- Repeating straight leg raise during the hip examination or with the patient sitting not reproducing the initial clinical signs.
- Non-anatomical weakness or sensory disturbance.
- Over-reaction in the patient's demeanour.

---

[12] Waddell G, McCulloch JA, Kummel E, Venner RM. Nonorganic physical signs in low-back pain. Spine (Phila Pa 1976) 1980; **5**: 117–25.

Positive test: Multiple inconsistent clinical findings should raise suspicion, but need to be interpreted carefully.

Upper limb neurology

Disc	Root	Myotomes	Dermatomes	Reflex
C4–5	C5	Shoulder abduction/deltoid	Lateral arm	Biceps
C5–6	C6	Elbow flexion/biceps	Lateral forearm, thumb and index finger	Brachioradialis
C6–7	C7	Elbow extension/triceps	Middle finger	Triceps
C7–T1	C8	Wrist flexion/long finger flexors	Medial forearm	—
T1–2	T1	Finger abduction/finger intrinsics	Medial arm	—

Lower limb neurology

Disc	Root	Myotomes	Dermatomes	Reflex
L1–2	L2	Hip flexion/iliopsoas (femoral nerve)	Medial thigh	—
L2–3	L3	Knee extension/quadriceps (femoral nerve)	Medial knee	—
L3–4	L4	Ankle dorsiflexion/tibialis anterior (deep peroneal nerve)	Medial ankle	Patella
L4–5	L5	Great toe extension/extensor hallucis longus (deep peroneal nerve)	Dorsum of foot	—
L5–S1	S1	Foot plantarflexion/Achilles tendon (tibial nerve)	Lateral ankle	Achilles tendon
Cauda equina	S2–4	—	Perianal sensation (saddle anaesthesia)	Anal wink, bulbocavernosus

Tips

Pain in the cervical spine can be referred from the shoulder in up to one-third of cases.

Assessment for red flags is essential to avoid missing infection, cancer or acute cord compression.

What are the causes of cervical pain?

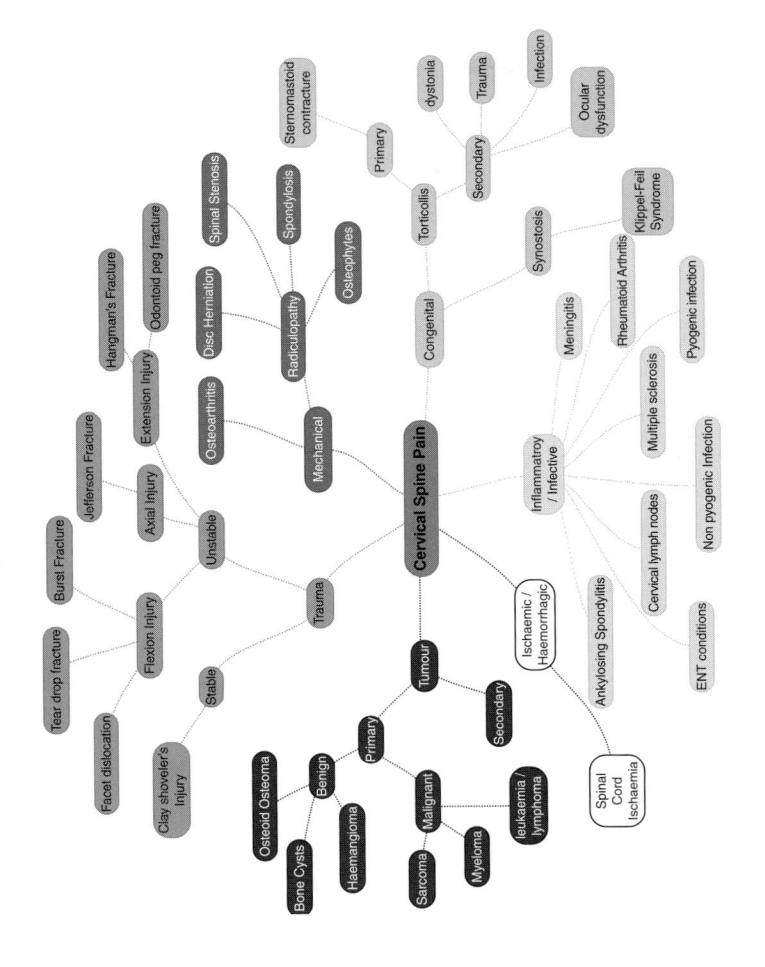

- **Cervical Spine Pain**
  - **Trauma**
    - Unstable
      - Burst Fracture
      - Jefferson Fracture
      - Extension Injury
        - Hangman's Fracture
        - Odontoid peg fracture
      - Axial Injury
      - Flexion Injury
        - Tear drop fracture
        - Facet dislocation
    - Stable
      - Clay shoveler's Injury
  - **Mechanical**
    - Osteoarthritis
    - Radiculopathy
      - Disc Herniation
      - Spinal Stenosis
      - Spondylosis
      - Osteophytes
  - **Congenital**
    - Torticollis
      - Primary
        - Sternomastoid contracture
      - Secondary
        - dystonia
        - Trauma
        - Infection
        - Ocular dysfunction
    - Synostosis
      - Klippel-Feil Syndrome
  - **Inflammatroy / Infective**
    - Rheumatoid Arthritis
    - Meningitis
    - Pyogenic infection
    - Multiple sclerosis
    - Non pyogenic Infection
    - Cervical lymph nodes
    - ENT conditions
    - Ankylosing Spondylitis
  - **Ischaemic / Haemorrhagic**
    - Spinal Cord Ischaemia
  - **Tumour**
    - Primary
      - Benign
        - Osteoid Osteoma
        - Bone Cysts
        - Haemangioma
      - Malignant
        - Sarcoma
        - Myeloma
        - Leukaemia / lymphoma
    - Secondary

Section 5

Orthopaedic surgery

Chapter 17

Cervical spine injury: assessment in trauma

James Pegrum and Chris Lavy

Rules
- All trauma patients have a C-spine injury until proven otherwise.
- Patient's neck can be cleared by radiographic or clinical means.

Clinical clearance requires:

1. No high-risk factors regarding the injury, such as:[13]
   a. diving or axial injury
   b. fall from height >3 feet (90 cm)/five steps
   c. high-speed car collision >60 mph (97 km/h)
   d. bike or recreational vehicle collision

2. No high-risk factors regarding the patient:
   a. age >65 or <16
   b. intoxicated or altered mental status
   c. GCS <15
   d. abnormal neurology
   e. no distracting injuries
   f. midline cervical tenderness

---

[13] Canadian C-Spine Rules: Stiell IG, Clement CM, Grimshaw J, *et al.* Implementation of the Canadian C-Spine Rule: prospective 12 centre cluster randomised trial. *BMJ* 2009; **339**: b4146.

Physical Examination for Surgeons, ed. Petrut Gogalniceanu, James Pegrum and William Lynn. Published by Cambridge University Press. © Cambridge University Press 2015.

Clinical clearance system

1. Completion of ATLS primary survey.
2. History regarding the event and evaluation of the patient for risk factors.
3. Assessment for the presence of distracting injuries (presence of distracting injuries requires cervical imaging).
4. Full neurological examination.
5. In-line immobilisation of C-spine and removal of collar.
6. Second assessor palpates cervical spine. If there is no pain the patient is then asked to actively rotate the head left and right.
7. If there is still no neck pain or numbness/tingling in the limbs the cervical spine can be cleared without radiographic evaluation.

Radiographic clearance system

- Cervical spine radiographs (See Chapter 49, *Cervical spine x-ray*):
    - AP and lateral views.
    - All C1–7 and superior aspect of T1 vertebrae must be visualised.
    - Swimmer's view or traction on arms (if traumatic injury permits) are needed if standard views are inadequate.
- Current recommendations are for computed tomography (CT) imaging.[14]

---

[14] British Orthopaedic Association Standards for Trauma (BOAST). BOAST 2: Spinal clearance in the trauma patient, November 2008. http://www.boa.ac.uk/publications/boast-2.

Section 5 Orthopaedic surgery

Chapter 18
Examination of the shoulder
James Pegrum, Petrut Gogalniceanu and Chris Lavy

Checklist

WIPER
- Patient standing in shorts or underwear with shoulder girdle exposed (bra to remain on in women).
- Expose upper limb and cervical spine.

Physiological parameters
- Observe for spinal lordosis, kyphosis or scoliosis.

Look
- **Skin**: erythema, scars, sinuses, symmetry of skin creases or skin elevation from underlying fracture
- **Soft tissues**:
  - joint and soft tissue swelling
  - wasting of deltoid, biceps, supraspinatus and infraspinatus muscles
- **Bone**: prominence of acromion, clavicular asymmetry or deformity

Feel
- **Skin**: temperature, tenderness, sensation
- **Soft tissues**:
  - muscle mass: trapezius, deltoid, triceps, biceps and biceps tendon
  - ligaments: coracoclavicular ligaments
  - radial and ulnar pulses, capillary refill time
  - sensation in 'regimental badge' area (axillary nerve) and in hand

---

Physical Examination for Surgeons, ed. Petrut Gogalniceanu, James Pegrum and William Lynn. Published by Cambridge University Press. © Cambridge University Press 2015.

- **Bone**:
  - sternoclavicular joint
  - clavicle: deformity or malunion
  - acromioclavicular joint
  - coracoid process
  - spine and borders of the scapula
  - greater tuberosity of humerus
  - margins of glenoid cavity
  - cervical spine

Move

- **Active and passive**:
  - flexion/extension
  - internal/external rotation
  - abduction/adduction

- **Resisted**:
  - deltoid
  - serratus anterior (winging of the scapula)
  - pectoralis major
  - trapezius

Special tests (= essential tests)*

- Acromioclavicular test*
- Impingement test*
- Instability and apprehension test*
- Rotator cuff test*
- Biceps tendon test
- SLAP test
- Thoracic outlet syndrome tests

To complete the examination...

- Examine the joint above (cervical spine: up to 30% of shoulder pain is referred from the cervical region) and the joint below (elbow).
- Check full neurovascular status of the upper limb.
- Order appropriate radiographs and further imaging.

Examination notes

What do you look for during initial observations?

- Assess the skin quality and contours of the shoulder girdle, clavicle and scapula.
- The soft tissues mass and muscle bulk are evaluated for evidence of muscle loss from disuse atrophy, found around the scapular from rotator cuff atrophy or pectoral muscles anteriorly. Deltoid muscle atrophy can also be found in axillary nerve injury.
- The bony contours:
  - Rule out shoulder dislocation, suggested by squaring of the lateral aspect of the shoulder.
  - Scapular winging is caused by serratus anterior weakness due to long thoracic nerve damage.
  - Assess the clavicle and acromioclavicular joint for steps suggestive of previous injury or malunion.
  - Assess the curvature of the spine for scoliosis or spinal deformity, as these will impact on shoulder symmetry and movement.

What structures form the shoulder joint?

The shoulder joint is a complex interaction between four joints: the sternoclavicular, acromioclavicular, scapulothoracic and glenohumeral joints. All four need to be assessed.

How should anterior structures of the shoulder be palpated?

- Anteromedially, the sternum and sternoclavicular joint are assessed for scars, steps or tenderness.
- The clavicle is assessed for evidence of previous surgery, resection, malunion with asymmetrical deformities or acute injuries signified by swelling bruising and pain.
- The lateral aspect of the clavicle articulates with the acromion in the acromioclavicular joint (ACJ). This joint would typically be injured from falling onto the point of the shoulder, as commonly occurs after being tackled in rugby. Bruising, swelling, clinical deformity and pain signify an ACJ disruption.
- The coracoid is immediately distal and medial to the ACJ and has important ligamentous attachments stabilising the lateral aspect of the clavicle.
- The muscle bulk of pectoralis major and deltoid is assessed.

How should lateral structures of the shoulder be palpated?

- The proximal aspect of the humerus is assessed for bruising or swelling.
- The greater tuberosity of the humerus and bicipital groove are assessed for tenderness from long head of biceps tendinopathy or acute injury.
- Palpate the margins of the glenoid cavity.

- The lateral bony edge to the shoulder is rounded by the presence of the acromion and deltoid muscle.
  - Squaring to the lateral aspect of the shoulder signifies an anterior shoulder dislocation until proven otherwise.
  - Altered sensation over the regimental badge area from axillary nerve injury is noted.

> **Tip**
>
> The bicipital groove is found by holding the proximal aspect of the humerus between thumb and index finger, whilst gently internally and externally rotating the proximal humerus to find the trough between the greater and lesser tuberosities.

How should posterior structures of the shoulder be palpated?

- Stand at the side of the patient to maintain eye contact and avoid causing undue discomfort.
- Assess the muscle bulk of the supraspinatus and infraspinatus, which are found above and below the spine of the scapula, respectively.
- Palpate the spine of the scapula.
- Palpate superior, inferior and lateral borders of the scapula.
- The cervical spine and associated paraspinal muscles should also be palpated to avoid missing a cause of referred pain.

How is movement of the shoulder joint assessed?

Actively assess forward flexion, extension, abduction, adduction and external rotation by keeping the elbow adducted into the side of the body. These movements are repeated with the patient facing away from the examiner to assess scapula movement. Internal rotation is best assessed by seeing how far the patient can reach up his or her back and comparing against the contralateral side; the dominant side is often stiffer in internal rotation when compared to the contralateral side. The table below shows an anticipated range of movement; comparison with the contralateral side is more clinically relevant.

Range of movement of the shoulder joint

Shoulder movement	Typical range of movement
Flexion	180°
Extension	60°
Internal rotation	90°
External rotation	60–90°
Adduction	0°
Abduction	180°

How are individual shoulder muscles tested?

Resisted movement to test muscle power is important to establish subtle weaknesses.

- The deltoid is assessed with the arm in 90° abduction, thumbs pointing towards the ceiling, and asking the patient to resist abduction against the examiner.
- Serratus anterior is tested by asking the patient to perform a press-up with arms on the wall. Winging of the scapula is seen in long thoracic nerve injury.
- Pectoralis contraction and muscle bulk can be assessed by asking the patient to place hands on hips and squeeze.
- Trapezius muscle is tested by asking the patient to shrug the shoulders, checking power against resistance.

What muscles form the rotator cuff?

The rotator cuff is a group of four muscles surrounding the glenohumeral joint (**SITS** mnemonic):

- **S**upraspinatus – initiates and assists abduction of the humerus (first 30° of abduction)
- **I**nfraspinatus – external rotator of the shoulder
- **T**eres minor – external rotator of the shoulder
- **S**ubscapularis – internal rotator of the shoulder

What are the causes of failure of shoulder abduction?

The range of the movement of the shoulder is variable, and comparison is best made with the contralateral side (see table, above).

- Supraspinatus tear or tendinopathy causes:
  - failure to initiate shoulder abduction
  - pelvic swing to initiate shoulder abduction
  - sudden drop in the arm during the last 30° of adduction
- Subacromial impingement causes painful abduction between 60 and 120°.

How are the rotator cuff muscles tested?*

Testing the rotator cuff involves testing four muscles, using three manoeuvres.

Chapter 18: Examination of the shoulder | 145

How is the supraspinatus muscle tested?

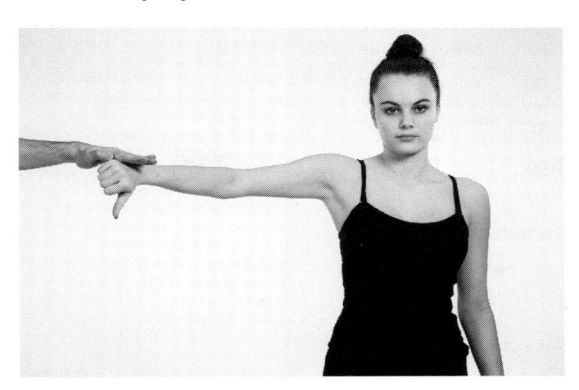

Rationale: Assesses the patient for acute tears or tendinopathy and aids shoulder stability.

Technique: This rotator cuff muscle is assessed with the 'empty can test'. This involves abducting the shoulder to 90°, forward flexion of 30° and the thumbs pointing towards the floor as if pouring out a drink can. Downward pressure is applied by the examiner.

Positive test: Reproduction of the patient's discomfort or weakness indicates pathology.

How are the infraspinatus and teres minor muscles tested?

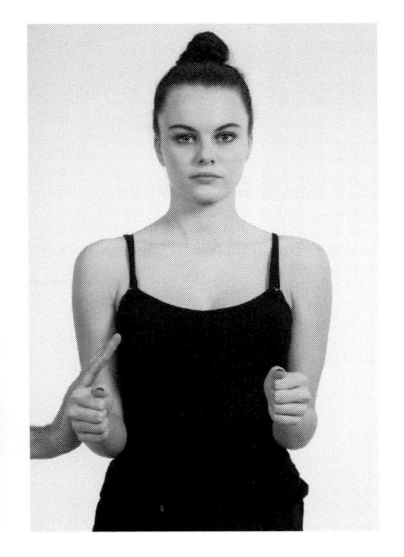

Rationale: Assesses the patient for acute tears or tendinopathy and aids shoulder stability.

Technique: The patient is asked to stand in a 'ski pole' position with the elbows tucked in and flexed to 90°, and the forearms in neutral rotation. Resisted external rotation tests both infraspinatus and teres minor.

Positive test: Reproduction of the patient's discomfort or weakness indicates pathology.

How is the subscapularis muscle tested?

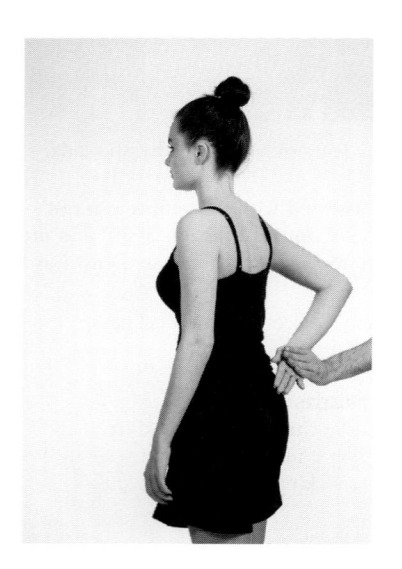

Rationale: Assesses the patient for acute tears or tendinopathy and aids shoulder stability.

Technique: Gerber's lift-off test also tests subscapularis. The patient places the dorsum of the hand on the gluteal region and lifts the hand off the back against resistance.

Positive test: Reproduction of the patient's discomfort or weakness indicates pathology.

How is the acromioclavicular joint tested?*

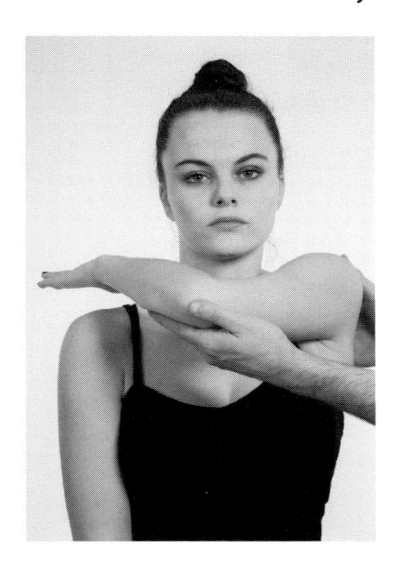

Rationale: Identifies a patient with acute ACJ injury or arthritis.

Technique: The 'scarf test', as its name suggests, involves flexing the shoulder and adducting the arm across the contralateral shoulder, as if wrapping a scarf around the neck. A further test involves interlocking the fingers of both hands at chest height and asking the patient to pull them apart.

Positive test: Reproduction of the patient's discomfort.

How are the shoulder impingement tests performed?*

Rationale: Perform this test with any patient presenting with a painful arc. It assesses abutment of the greater tuberosity of the humerus against the under surface of the acromion.

Technique: Numerous tests are available in the literature. It is important to perform one test well.

- Hawkins–Kennedy test: 90° forward flexion of the shoulder with 90° elbow flexion. The shoulder is then internally rotated.

- Neer's test involves forward flexion of a straight arm in internal rotation (with the thumb pointing towards the ground). Pain is reproduced when the greater tuberosity abuts against the underside of the acromion.

Positive test: Reproduction of the patient's discomfort.

How is shoulder instability assessed?*

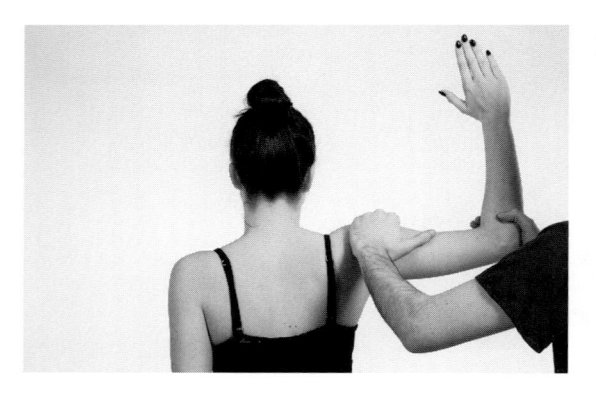

Apprehension testing of the shoulder

Rationale: The shoulder can become unstable in different planes, and the patient becomes apprehensive when the head of the humens subluxes anteriorly.

Technique: For the anterior apprehension test the patient is supine with the arm in 90° abduction, approaching a 'stop sign' position, and apprehension is noted.

Positive test: Asymmetrical apprehension compared to the contralateral side.

How is the biceps tested?

Rationale: Assesses the integrity of the long head of biceps muscle.

Technique: In Speed's test, the shoulder is flexed at 60° with the arm fully supinated and the elbow extended, and resisted forward flexion is carried out against the examiner.

Positive test: A positive test is confirmed by pain exacerbated by resistance.

> **Tip**
>
> A positive biceps test can also occur from a SLAP tear.

How are superior labrum anterior to posterior (SLAP) tears tested?

Rationale: The long head of biceps attaches onto the glenoid labrum. Labral or biceps injuries cause shoulder weakness, mechanical symptoms or joint instability.

Technique: The most diagnostic test, from recent evidence, is the biceps load 2 test.[15] This involves shoulder abduction to 120°, maximum shoulder external rotation, elbow flexion to 90°, and forearm supination.

Positive test: Active elbow flexion against resistance reproducing the pain is a positive test.

Thoracic outlet syndrome tests

Rationale: These tests assess for neurovascular compromise caused by compression of the cervical nerves and subclavian artery as they travel between the scalene muscles of the neck.

Technique: Examination for thoracic outlet syndrome is described in Chapter 26, *Arterial examination of the upper limbs*.

Positive test: Reproduction of neuropathic pain or absence of the radial artery pulse during the examination.

> **Tip**
>
> Up to 30% of shoulder pain is referred from the neck. A thorough assessment of neck movement and upper limb neurology is required to avoid missing referred pathology.
>
> Non-musculoskeletal causes of shoulder pain include lower respiratory tract infections, myocardial infarction and diaphragmatic irritation.

---

[15] Cook C, Beaty S, Kissenberth MJ, et al. Diagnostic accuracy of five orthopedic clinical tests for diagnosis of superior labrum anterior posterior (SLAP) lesions. *J Shoulder Elbow Surg* 2012; **21**: 13–22.

Differential diagnoses

What causes a reduced range of movement of the shoulder?

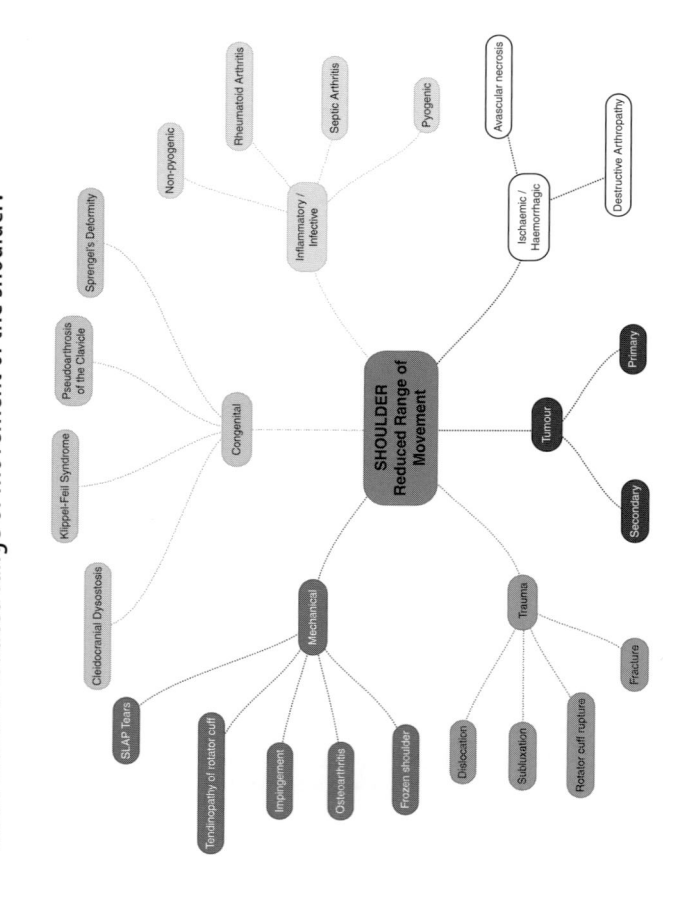

SHOULDER – Reduced Range of Movement

- Inflammatory / Infective
  - Non-pyogenic
    - Rheumatoid Arthritis
  - Septic Arthritis
  - Pyogenic
- Ischaemic / Haemorrhagic
  - Avascular necrosis
  - Destructive Arthropathy
- Tumour
  - Primary
  - Secondary
- Trauma
  - Fracture
  - Dislocation
  - Subluxation
  - Rotator cuff rupture
- Mechanical
  - SLAP Tears
  - Tendinopathy of rotator cuff
  - Impingement
  - Osteoarthritis
  - Frozen shoulder
- Congenital
  - Sprengel's Deformity
  - Pseudoarthrosis of the Clavicle
  - Klippel-Feil Syndrome
  - Cleidocranial Dysostosis

150

Chapter 18: Examination of the shoulder | 151

What are the causes of shoulder pain?

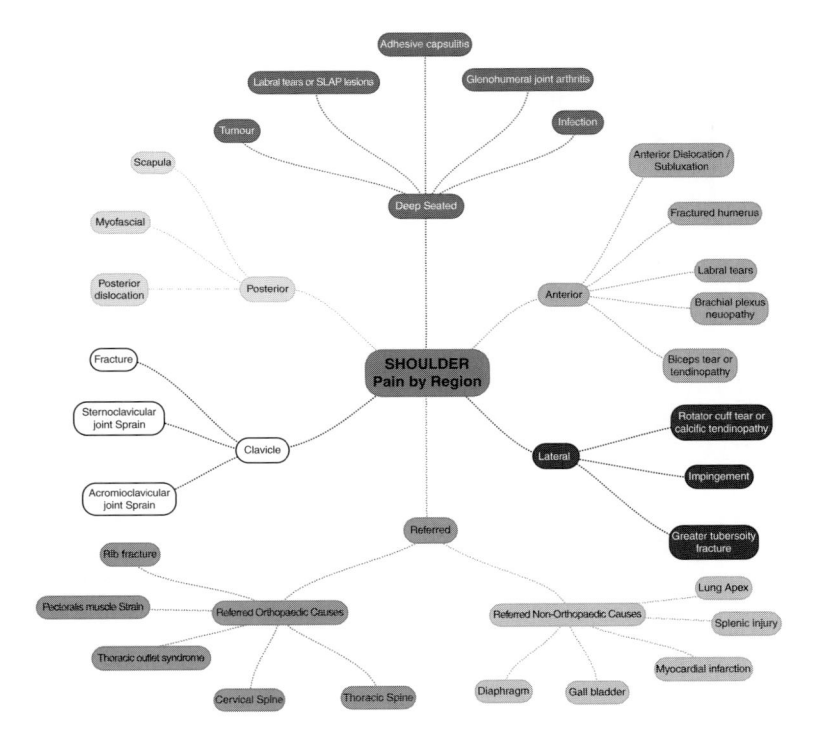

SHOULDER Pain by Region

- **Deep Seated**
  - Adhesive capsulitis
  - Labral tears or SLAP lesions
  - Glenohumeral joint arthritis
  - Tumour
  - Infection

- **Anterior**
  - Anterior Dislocation / Subluxation
  - Fractured humerus
  - Labral tears
  - Brachial plexus neuopathy
  - Biceps tear or tendinopathy

- **Lateral**
  - Rotator cuff tear or calcific tendinopathy
  - Impingement
  - Greater tuberosity fracture

- **Posterior**
  - Scapula
  - Myofascial
  - Posterior dislocation

- **Clavicle**
  - Fracture
  - Sternoclavicular joint Sprain
  - Acromioclavicular joint Sprain

- **Referred**
  - **Referred Orthopaedic Causes**
    - Rib fracture
    - Pectoralis muscle Strain
    - Thoracic outlet syndrome
    - Cervical Spine
    - Thoracic Spine
  - **Referred Non-Orthopaedic Causes**
    - Lung Apex
    - Splenic Injury
    - Myocardial infarction
    - Diaphragm
    - Gall bladder

Section 5: Orthopaedic surgery

Chapter 19: Examination of the elbow

James Pegrum and Chris Lavy

Checklist

WIPER
- Patient standing in shorts or underwear with thorax exposed.

Physiological parameters

Look
- **Skin**: erythema, scars, carrying angle
- **Soft tissues**: biceps and triceps brachii mass, swelling or wasting; common flexor and extensor origins
- **Bone**: asymmetry, epicondyles, valgus/varus deformity

Feel
- **Skin**: temperature, capillary refill time, tenderness, sensation
- **Soft tissues**: pulses, tendons, common flexor and extensor origins, biceps brachii, triceps tendon
- **Bone**: bone and joint contours, epicondyles, radial head, olecranon

Move
- **Active**
    - flexion/extension
    - supination/pronation

Physical Examination for Surgeons, ed. Petrut Gogalniceanu, James Pegrum and William Lynn. Published by Cambridge University Press. © Cambridge University Press 2015.

- **Passive**
  - flexion/extension
  - supination/pronation
- **Resisted**
  - flexion tests biceps brachii muscle and C5/C6 myotome
  - extension tests triceps brachii muscle and C7 myotome
  - supination tests biceps and supinator muscles
  - pronation tests pronator teres and pronator quadratus muscles

Special tests
- Common flexor origin tendinopathy (medial epicondyle – golfer's elbow):
  - resisted wrist flexion with the elbow extended and hand in a supinated position
- Common extensor origin (lateral epicondyle – tennis elbow):
  - resisted middle finger extension with elbow pronated and flexed at 90° tests extensor carpi radialis brevis
  - resisted index finger extension with elbow pronated and flexed at 90° tests extensor carpi radialis longus
- Valgus and varus testing to stress collateral ligaments

To complete the examination...
- Examine the joint above (shoulder) and the joint below (wrist).
- Check full neurovascular status of the upper limb.
- Order appropriate radiographs and further imaging.

Section 5 Orthopaedic surgery

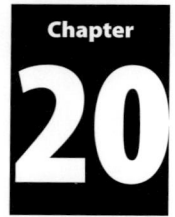

Chapter 20

Examination of the lumbar spine and sacroiliac joint

James Pegrum and Chris Lavy

Checklist

WIPER
- Patient standing in shorts or underwear; access is required to the gluteal region and lumbar spine.

Physiological parameters

Gait and observation
- Gait and posture:
  - half-shut knife position in sciatic irritation
  - flexed hips in ankylosing spondylitis
- Asymmetry of spine
- Neurological screen

Tape
- Leg length
- Spine flexion

Look
- **Skin**:
  - scars, erythema, sinuses and alignment of skin creases
  - dimples, hairy patch, café-au-lait lesions
- **Soft tissues**:
  - swelling, muscle wasting
  - psoas abscess draining in subgluteal fold

Physical Examination for Surgeons, ed. Petrut Gogalniceanu, James Pegrum and William Lynn. Published by Cambridge University Press. © Cambridge University Press 2015.

- **Bone**: scoliosis, kyphosis, lordosis, pelvic tilt

Feel
- **Skin**: temperature, tenderness, sensation
- **Soft tissues**: paraspinal muscles
- **Bone**: midline bony tenderness, bony steps, sacroiliac joint tenderness, and coccyx for coccydynia

Move
- **Active**:
  - flexion and extension
  - side flexion
  - rotation when sitting
- **Passive**:
  - Stork extension test

Special tests (* = essential tests)
- Straight leg raise*
- Hip screen (FABER)*
- Neurology examination*
- Nerve tension tests
- Sacroiliac joint
- Muscle length tests

To complete the examination...
- Examine the joint above (thoracic and cervical spine) and the joint below (hip joint).
- Check full neurovascular status of the lower limb.
- Order appropriate radiographs and further imaging.

Examination notes
What do you look for during gait and initial observations?
Look for an antalgic gait and for high stepping associated with a foot drop. At the same time observe for muscle wasting or scars.

Disc disease typically affects the lower lumbar spine and lumbosacral junction, and this is a good opportunity to carry out a neurological screen of the L4–S1 myotomes and dermatomes.

Quick neurological screen

	Dermatome	Myotome
L4	Medial ankle joint	Foot dorsiflexion
L5	Dorsum of foot	Extensor hallucis longus
S1	Little toe, lateral side of foot and plantar surface	Foot plantarflexion

How is spinal flexion assessed?

Spinal flexion is assessed using Schober's test.

Rationale: To determine the patient's ability to flex the lumbar spine.

Technique: An imaginary horizontal line is drawn between the posterior superior iliac spines with the patient standing upright. Two points are identified, one 10 cm above and one 5 cm below the midpoint of this line (15 cm apart). On flexion of the spine the distance between the two points should increase by a further 5 cm to measure at least 20 cm.

Positive test: Failure of the spine to flex adequately suggests ankylosis of the lumbar spine.

What is the relevance of a lumbar hairy patch?

This may suggest underlying spina bifida.

What is the relevance of café-au-lait patches?

This may suggest a diagnosis of neurofibromatosis.

How do you palpate the lumbar spine?

In the midline, feel the lumbar spinous processes and interspinous ligaments, as well as the paraspinal soft tissues and muscles for spasm and localising pain. The paraspinal bony structures include the facet joints and sacroiliac joints.

How are the sacroiliac joints palpated?

The anatomical landmark for palpation of the sacroiliac joint are the dimples of Venus. These are the paramidline indentations created by short ligament stretching between the posterior superior iliac spines and the skin.

How is movement of the lumbar spine assessed?

- **Flexion**: The patient is asked to touch his or her toes, to assess smoothness and identify hesitancy of spinal flexion. The knees must be

kept straight and locked. The distance between the tips of the fingers and the floor can be measured.
- **Extension**: The patient stands up against a wall. This will identify subtle kyphotic deformity, as the heels, gluteal muscles and occiput should all be able to touch the wall simultaneously. Failure to do so suggests ankylosing spondylitis or spinal kyphosis in the elderly.
- Passive extension of the spine can be assessed with the stork test. The stork test involves the patient standing on one leg with the examiner supporting and pulling the patient into extension. Pain in the lumbar spine exacerbated by this movement can come from a pars defect, facet inflammation or spinal stenosis. Side flexion is assessed by the patient moving the hand down the lateral aspect of the leg, and is assessed in comparison with the contralateral side. Rotation of the spine is rarely clinically useful.

How is the straight leg test performed?*

- **Rationale**: May allow differentiation between neuropathic pain and pain from tight hamstrings.

    See Chapter 21, *Examination of the hip*.

How is the FABER test performed?*

Rationale: Back pain can radiate from the hip or the sacroiliac joint. The test differentiates between the two.

Technique: The hip is placed in Flexion, ABduction and External Rotation (FABER), with the leg in a 'figure of four' cross-legged position.

Positive test:
- Discomfort felt in the groin indicates hip pathology.
- Buttock pain is suggestive of sacroiliac joint dysfunction or gluteal tendon pain.

What neurological assessments need to be made when examining the lumbar spine?*

Rationale: A full neurological examination is required to establish if there is a myotomic and dermatomal pattern of weakness from proximal nerve root impingement.

Technique: Typically a disc prolapse is posterolateral. The nerve root above the disc would have already left the spinal canal, whilst the nerve root distal to this level is adjacent to the posterolateral disc and is vulnerable to compression from a disc herniation.

Positive test: A posterolateral disc herniation at L4/5 would cause L5 nerve root signs such as dorsal foot numbness, weak extensor hallucis longus and absent ankle reflex.

How should muscle tightness be assessed?

Rationale: Leg pain can be misinterpreted as radiculopathy during the examination if muscle tension is not assessed.

Technique: The patient is supine and the hip is flexed to 90°. The knee is then straightened and the angle formed by the popliteal fossa, known as the popliteal angle, is noted. The tightness of the quadriceps muscle is best assessed prone. The knee is flexed until muscle tension is felt, and the angle is noted.

Positive test: Angles and flexibility of the muscles are documented and compared to the contralateral leg.

How should nerve tension tests be performed?

Rationale: This aims to stretch a specific nerve to reproduce neuropathic type pain.

Technique: With the patient sitting, the arms are placed behind the back. The chin is touching the chest.

- The deep peroneal nerve can be stretched with foot dorsiflexion.
- The superficial peroneal nerve is tensioned with foot inversion.
- The obturator nerve is isolated with hip abduction and foot dorsiflexion.
- The sciatic nerve (lumbosacral tension) is assessed with the patient supine, chin touching the chest, then performing a straight leg raise with foot dorsiflexion. The symptoms of the patient should be assessed, and relief on neck extension and foot plantarflexion can indicate a positive test (see Chapter 21, *Examination of the hip*).
- The femoral nerve tension test is carried out with the patient prone. Lifting the hip into extension and then the knee into flexion causes neuropathic pain down the front of the thigh.

Positive test: Reproduction of the patient's neuropathic pain.

How should the sacroiliac joint be examined?

Rationale: Pain in the buttock may indicate referred pain from the sacroiliac joint or lumbar spine. Examination of the sacroiliac joint and lumbar spine is essential to avoid missing referred pain.

Technique: There are four tests, carried out in the following order:

- The thigh thrust test involves flexing the hip and knee to 90° and pushing the hip joint posteriorly.
- The pelvic distraction test involves crossing over the examiner's hands and placing pressure on the ASIS and then pushing away from the midline.
- The pelvic compression test involves pushing on the ASIS, squeezing both hemipelves towards the midline.
- The sacral thrust test involves vertical pressure with the palm of the examiner's hand over the sacroiliac joint, whilst the patient is in a prone position.

Positive test: Sacroiliac joint pain is considered positive when two out of the four tests reproduce the patient's discomfort.

Tips

Groin pain is suggestive of hip pathology, whereas buttock and midline pain typically originates in the sacroiliac joint or lumbar spine.

Red flags or new neurological findings are an indication for further imaging.

Differential diagnoses

What are the causes of reduced ROM of the lumbar spine?

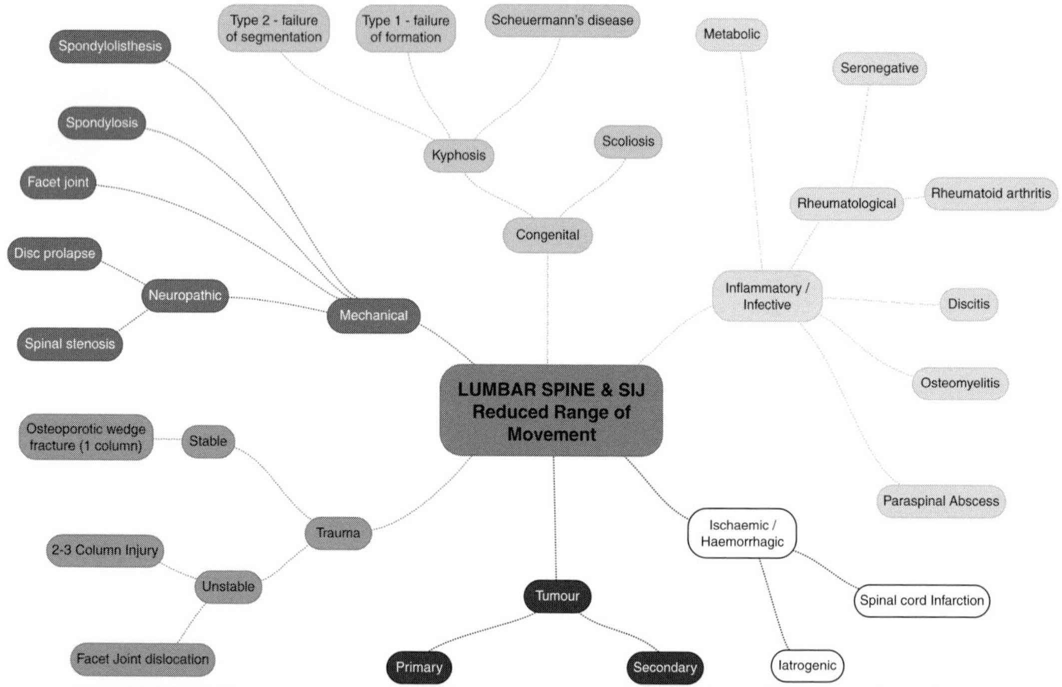

LUMBAR SPINE & SIJ Reduced Range of Movement

- Inflammatory / Infective
  - Metabolic
  - Rheumatological
    - Seronegative
    - Rheumatoid arthritis
  - Discitis
  - Osteomyelitis
  - Paraspinal Abscess
- Ischaemic / Haemorrhagic
  - Spinal cord Infarction
  - Iatrogenic
- Tumour
  - Primary
  - Secondary
- Trauma
  - Stable
    - Osteoporotic wedge fracture (1 column)
  - Unstable
    - 2-3 Column Injury
    - Facet Joint dislocation
- Mechanical
  - Spondylolisthesis
  - Spondylosis
  - Facet Joint
  - Neuropathic
    - Disc prolapse
    - Spinal stenosis
  - Congenital
    - Scoliosis
    - Kyphosis
      - Scheuermann's disease
      - Type 1 - failure of formation
      - Type 2 - failure of segmentation

160

Chapter 20: Examination of lumbar spine and sacroiliac joint

What are the causes of lumbar spine pain?

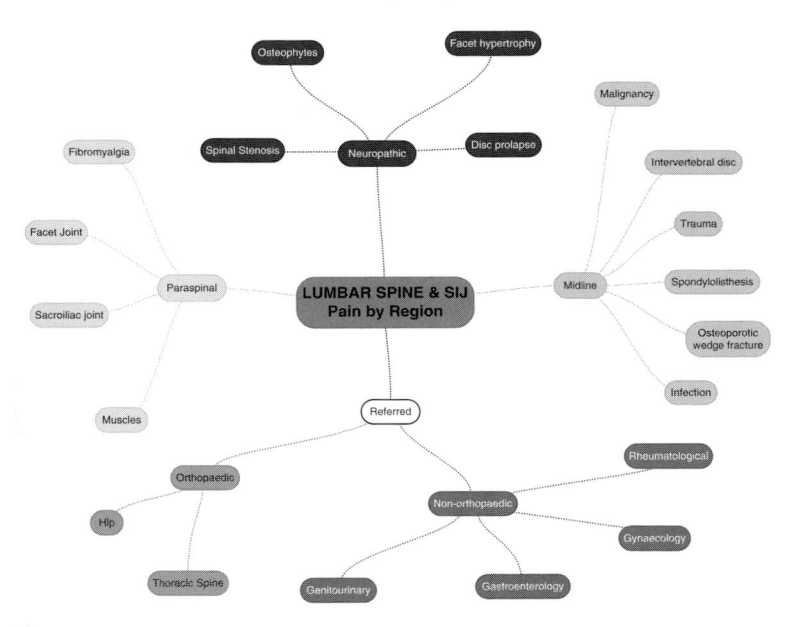

LUMBAR SPINE & SIJ Pain by Region

- **Neuropathic**
  - Osteophytes
  - Facet hypertrophy
  - Spinal Stenosis
  - Disc prolapse

- **Midline**
  - Malignancy
  - Intervertebral disc
  - Trauma
  - Spondylolisthesis
  - Osteoporotic wedge fracture
  - Infection

- **Paraspinal**
  - Fibromyalgia
  - Facet Joint
  - Sacroiliac joint
  - Muscles

- **Referred**
  - Orthopaedic
    - Hip
    - Thoracic Spine
  - Non-orthopaedic
    - Rheumatological
    - Gynaecology
    - Gastroenterology
    - Genitourinary

Section 5 Orthopaedic surgery

Chapter 21

Examination of the hip

James Pegrum, Petrut Gogalniceanu and Chris Lavy

Checklist

WIPER
- Patient standing in shorts or underwear, back and knees exposed.
- Access is required to the groin, thighs and gluteal region.

Physiological parameters

Gait
- Asymmetry of spine
- Gait: antalgic, short leg, Trendelenburg gait
- Walking aids

Test
- Trendelenburg's test

Tape: leg length
- Apparent leg length (xiphisternum to medial malleolus)
- True leg length (ASIS to medial malleolus)

Look
- **Skin**:
  - scars, erythema, ecchymosis
  - sinuses and alignment of skin creases
  - psoas abscess draining in subgluteal fold

Physical Examination for Surgeons, ed. Petrut Gogalniceanu, James Pegrum and William Lynn. Published by Cambridge University Press. © Cambridge University Press 2015.

- **Soft tissues**: swelling or wasting of glutei and quadriceps.
- **Bone**:
    - deformity or asymmetry: shortening of leg; external or internal rotation of hip
    - pelvic tilt
    - valgus or varus knee, lordosis, kyphosis, scoliosis

Feel
- **Skin**: temperature, tenderness, sensation.
- **Soft tissues**:
    - adductor tenderness, bursitis
    - pulses, capillary refill time
    - sensation and movement
- **Bone**:
    - greater trochanter
    - midpoint of inguinal ligament (hip joint)
    - pubic bone and symphysis
    - femoral shaft: tenderness or mobility

Move
- **Active and passive**:
    - flexion/fixed flexion
    - internal rotation (foot moves outwards)
    - external rotation (foot moves inwards)
    - extension (press thigh onto bed)
    - abduction/adduction whilst stabilising pelvis (palpating contralateral ASIS)
- **Resisted**:
    - flexion
    - adduction

Special tests (* = essential tests)
- Thomas's test*
- Impingement sign*
- Straight leg raise*
- FABER test
- Sciatic nerve stretch test
- Ober's test

Section 5: Orthopaedic surgery

> *To complete the examination...*
> - Examine the joint above (back and sacroiliac joint) and the joint below (knee).
> - Check full neurovascular status of the lower limb.
> - Order appropriate radiographs and further imaging.

Examination notes

What do you look for during gait and initial observations?
- Look for an antalgic gait or the use of any walking aids.
- Inspect the soles of the shoes for the pattern of wear.
- In the setting of possible neck of femur fracture, gait and weight-bearing activities should not be examined.

How is a Trendelenburg's test performed and why?

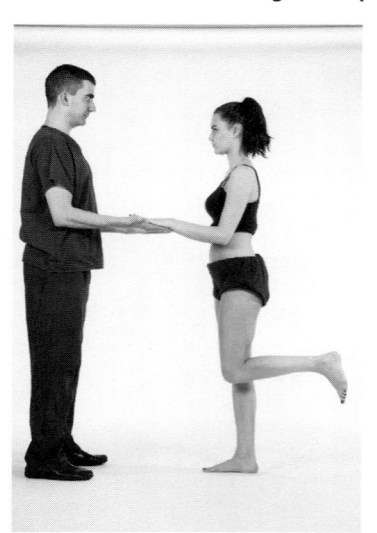

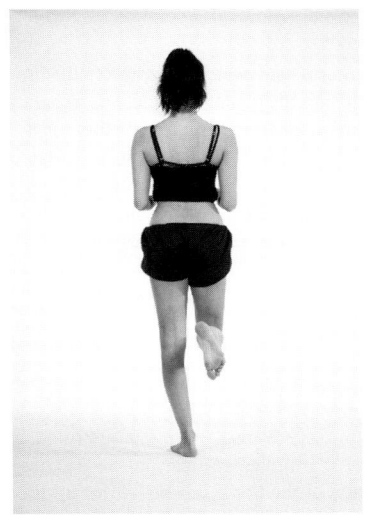

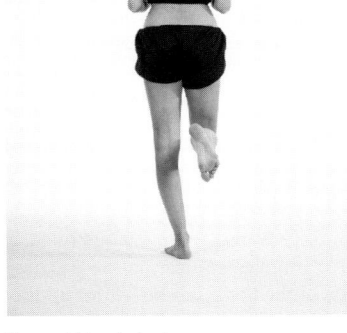

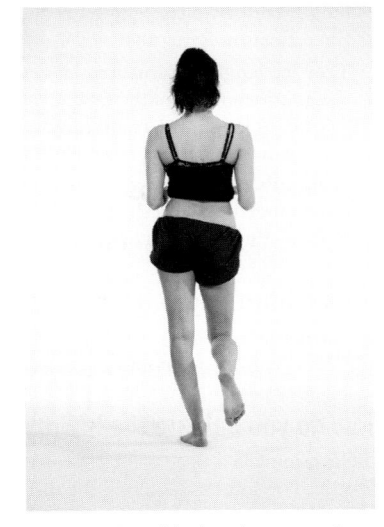

Normal hip abductors.

Positive Trendelenburg's test: weakness of hip abductors on the left side.

Rationale: A Trendelenburg's test (orthopaedic) identifies weakness of the abductors of the hip.

Technique: The patient is standing facing the examiner. The patient places his or her hands (palms down) on the examiner's hands (palms up). The patient is asked to 'stand on one leg'.

Positive test: A contralateral dip of the pelvis or increasing weight placed through the contralateral hand are indicators of weak hip abductors on the standing (ipsilateral) leg. Tilting of the pelvis during walking is known as a Trendelenburg gait.

Example

Trendelenburg's test:

- Patient stands on left leg; right leg is flexed at knee and hip.
- If the pelvis tilts to the right or the patient presses down with right hand, i.e. **'the sound side sags'**, the abductors on the left side (the standing leg) are weak.

How do you assess for leg length discrepancy?

- **Apparent leg length** is measured from the xiphisternum to the inferior surface of the medial malleolus. Discrepancy in apparent leg

length (not true leg length) is caused by a pelvic tilt, scoliosis or hip fixed flexion deformity.
- **True leg length** is measured from the anterior superior iliac spine (ASIS) to the inferior surface of the medial malleolus on the ipsilateral side. Discrepancy in true leg length is a result of shortening of the tibia or femur. If there is a discrepancy in true leg length, Galleazi's test assesses which bone is involved.
- **Galleazi's test** is carried out with the patient supine. The heels and knees are placed together, with the knees flexed to 90°. A mismatch in symmetry between thigh and calf length identifies whether the femur or the tibia is short.

What features do you look for during the hip examination?

A systematic approach assessing skin, soft tissues and then bone alignment will help avoid missing pathology.

How do you palpate the hip joint?

The hip joint is a deep joint covered by large muscles and cannot be palpated directly. The soft tissues along the medial side of the thigh can be felt for adductor tenderness. Tenderness over the greater trochanter would suggest bursitis or gluteal tendinopathy, whilst tenderness over the pubic symphysis may indicate osteitis pubis. Pain in the groin (during movement) may indicate pain arising from the femoral head or acetabulum; direct palpation of these structures is usually not possible. Keep in mind other causes of pain in the groin, such as inguinal or femoral hernias, femoral artery aneurysms or femoral vein thrombosis.

How is movement of the hip joint assessed?

The range of movement of the hip joint is described in the table below. The absolute range of movement of the hip is variable. The most important assessment is comparison with the contralateral side.

Range of movement of the hip joint

Hip movement	Typical range of movement
Flexion	120–140°
Extension	30°
Internal rotation	30–60°
External rotation	30–60°
Adduction	30°
Abduction	45°

How is hip flexion tested?

Asking the patient to 'hold onto your knee and pull it into your chest' actively assesses range of flexion. It is important to note any discomfort experienced by the patient from changes in facial expressions.

How is hip rotation tested?

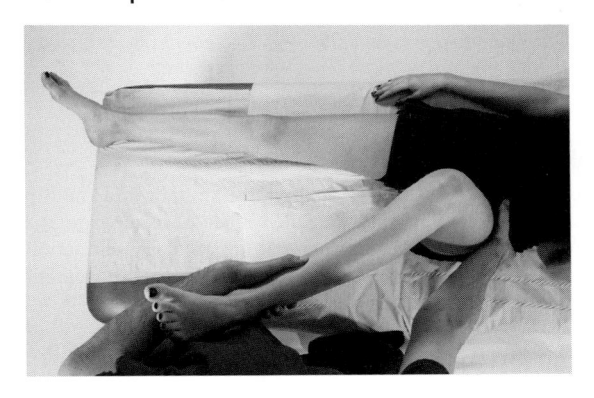

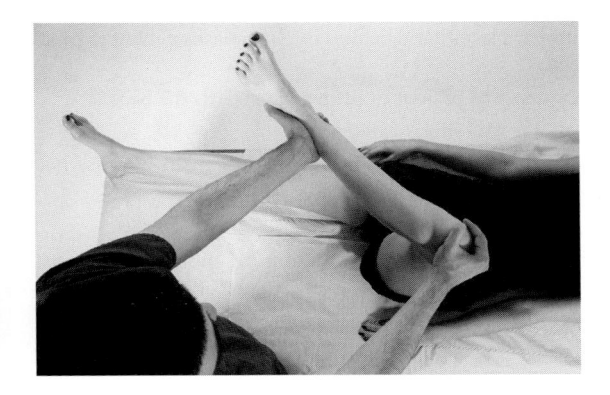

Passive movement is carried out whilst looking for early signs of discomfort in the patient's face. Internal and external rotation of the hip is assessed with the hip flexed to 90°, using the tibia as a protractor. Turning the ankle away from the body (upper image) assesses internal rotation of the hip, and turning the ankle across the body (lower image) assesses external hip rotation.

> **Tip**
>
> Turning the ankle away from the body assesses internal rotation of the hip, whilst turning the ankle across the body assesses external hip rotation.

> **Tip**
>
> Asymmetrical loss of internal rotation is an early sign of osteoarthritis, but can occur in femoral acetabular impingement, or femoral retroversion.

How are hip abduction and adduction tested?

Abduction and adduction are performed with the knee straight and the hip flexed at 20–30°. The spare hand of the examiner must be placed on the contralateral ASIS to stabilise the pelvis and prevent apparent leg abduction from pelvic movement. Hip abduction and adduction is the movement obtained before the movement of the pelvis is felt.

How is hip extension tested?

Hip extension is not routinely useful in clinical examination. Three methods can be used:

1. Patient supine: examiner places hand behind thigh and asks patient to press thigh down onto bed.
2. Patient prone: examiner asks patient to lift leg backwards off bed.
3. Patient is on his/her side and hip is extended.

How are resisted movements of the hip examined?

Useful resisted movements are those of flexion and adduction. The short adductors are tested by asking the patient to 'squeeze the examiner's fist between your knees' with the knees flexed to 90°. The long adductors are examined by squeezing the examiner's fist between the knees with the legs straight on the couch.

> **Tips**
>
> Weakness or pain in resisted hip flexion may indicate weakness in the L2 myotome, iliopsoas tendinopathy, femoral nerve pathology or the presence of iliopsoas abscess.
>
> Adductor pain is commonest amongst athletes and suggests tendinopathy.

What is Thomas's test?*

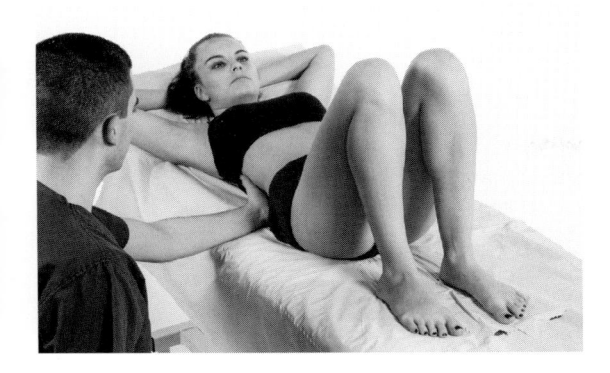

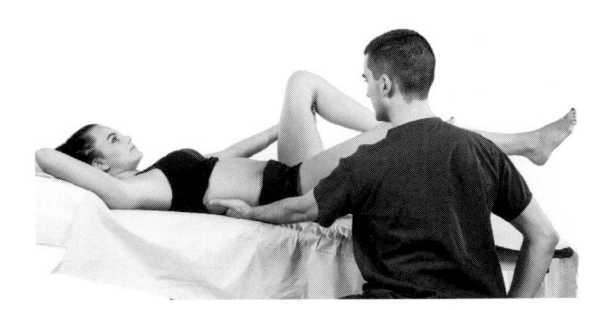

Rationale: Indicates a fixed flexion deformity in a patient with either arthritis or tight iliopsoas tendon.

Technique: A fixed hip flexion can be masked by an over-lordotic lumbar spine. The examiner's hand is placed between the lumbar spine and the examination couch with the patient in the supine position. To flatten the lumbar spine the patient is asked to 'bend both knees to 90° and place your feet flat on the couch.' This is confirmed by the examiner's hand being squeezed between the patient and the couch. The patient is asked to straighten the legs one at a time onto the couch.

Positive test: Inability to place the leg completely flat on the couch confirms a fixed flexion deformity of the hip.

What is the impingement sign?*

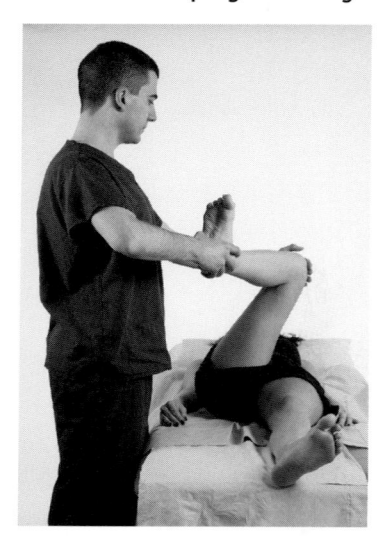

Rationale: Pain indicates acetabular impingement or a labral tear.
Technique: The hip is flexed, adducted and internally rotated.
Positive test: Reproduction of the patient's discomfort.

What is the straight leg raise test?*

Rationale: May allow differentiation between neuropathic and pain from tight hamstrings.

Technique: With the patient supine, ask the patient to 'lift your leg straight up off the bed as high as it can go'. The angle of elevation and description of pain is noted.

Positive test:

- Pain in the groin is indicative of hip or muscle pathology.
- Burning or shooting pain is neuropathic in nature.
- Posterior pulling or tightness suggests hamstring pathology.

What is the FABER test?

Rationale: Discomfort may indicate sacroiliac joint, femoral acetabular impingement or psoas muscle pathology.

Technique: The leg being examined is crossed over the contralateral side to form a 'figure of four'. The hip is now Flexed, ABducted and Externally Rotated (FABER).

Positive test: Discomfort.

For sacroiliac joint assessment see Chapter 20, *Examination of the lumbar spine and sacroiliac joint*.

What is the sciatic nerve stretch test?

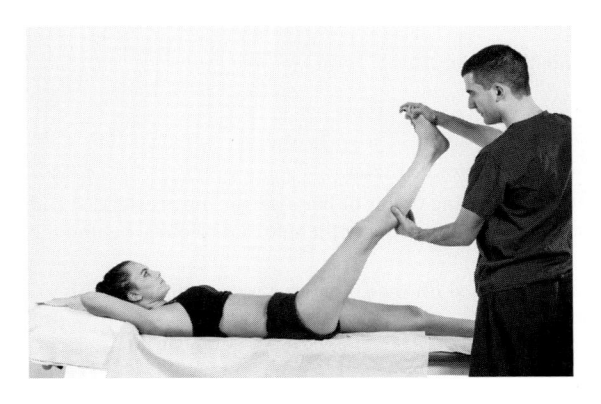

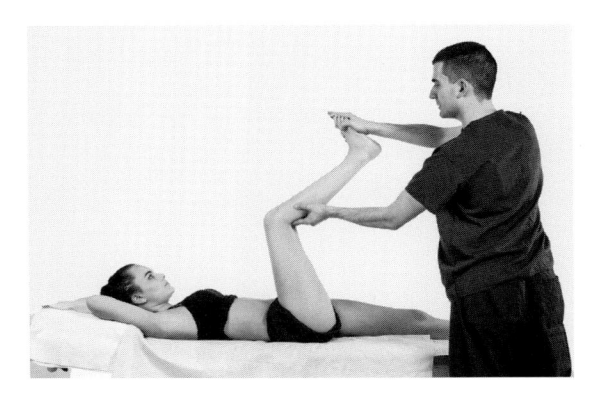

Rationale: This test helps to differentiate between the pulling pain of hamstring tightness and the burning (neuropathic) pain caused by nerve irritation.

Technique: The neuropathic pain is only sciatic in nature when it is reproduced by a straight leg raise and worsened by foot dorsiflexion. The sensitivity of the test can be further improved by reproduction of the pain by compression of the popliteal fossa with the hip flexed to 90° and then extending the knee until the patient feels some discomfort. A negative discriminator consists of pain on compressing the hamstring tendons with the knee flexed, which does not reproduce sciatic symptoms. Worsening pain on foot dorsiflexion and popliteal compression, with no pain exacerbated by hamstring tendon compression, is referred to as 3/3 nerve tension signs positive. This has improved diagnostic accuracy for radiculopathy.

Positive test: Neuropathic pain.

What is Ober's test?

Rationale: A test for a tight iliotibial tract.

Technique: With the patient lying on his or her side, the hip is extended and the knee flexed to allow the leg to overhang the side of the couch, behind the patient.

Positive test: If the leg is raised off the couch in a resting position, this suggests a tight iliotibial band.

Differential diagnoses
What causes hip pain?

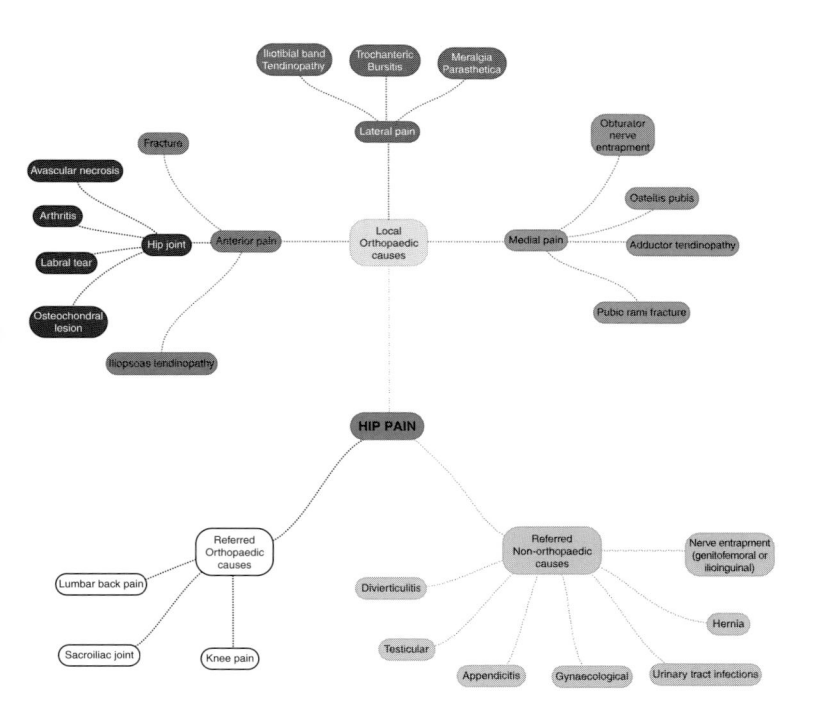

HIP PAIN

- **Local Orthopaedic causes**
  - **Anterior pain**
    - Hip joint
      - Avascular necrosis
      - Arthritis
      - Labral tear
      - Osteochondral lesion
    - Fracture
    - Iliopsoas tendinopathy
  - **Lateral pain**
    - Iliotibial band Tendinopathy
    - Trochanteric Bursitis
    - Meralgia Parasthetica
  - **Medial pain**
    - Obturator nerve entrapment
    - Osteitis pubis
    - Adductor tendinopathy
    - Pubic rami fracture

- **Referred Orthopaedic causes**
  - Lumbar back pain
  - Sacroiliac joint
  - Knee pain

- **Referred Non-orthopaedic causes**
  - Diverticulitis
  - Testicular
  - Appendicitis
  - Gynaecological
  - Urinary tract infections
  - Hernia
  - Nerve entrapment (genitofemoral or ilioinguinal)

What causes reduced ROM of the hip?

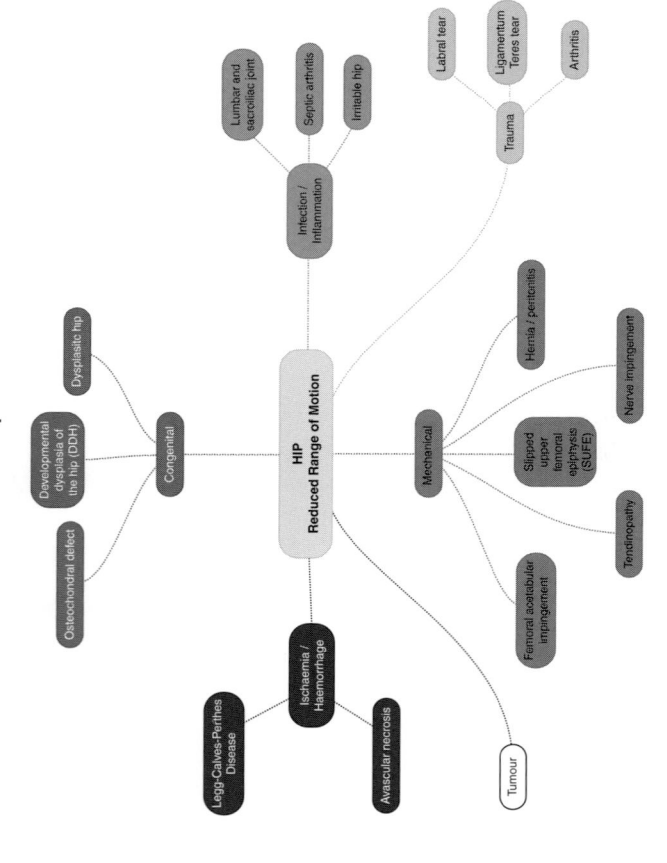

HIP — Reduced Range of Motion

- **Congenital**
  - Osteochondral defect
  - Developmental dysplasia of the hip (DDH)
  - Dysplastic hip
- **Infection / Inflammation**
  - Lumbar and sacroiliac joint
  - Septic arthritis
  - Irritable hip
- **Trauma**
  - Labral tear
  - Ligamentum Teres tear
  - Arthritis
- **Mechanical**
  - Hernia / peritonitis
  - Nerve impingement
  - Slipped upper femoral epiphysis (SUFE)
  - Tendinopathy
  - Femoral acetabular impingement
- **Ischaemia / Haemorrhage**
  - Legg-Calves-Perthes Disease
  - Avascular necrosis
- Tumour

174

Section 5

Orthopaedic surgery

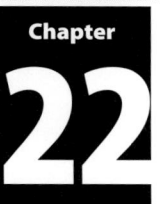

Chapter 22

Examination of the knee

James Pegrum, Petrut Gogalniceanu and Chris Lavy

Checklist

WIPER
- Patient standing in shorts or underwear; hip and ankle joints exposed.

Physiological parameters

Gait
- Asymmetry of spine and pelvis
- Antalgic gait and walking aids
- Soles of footwear

Tape
- Quadriceps diameter: muscle bulk

Look
- **Skin**: scars, erythema, ecchymoses, sinuses, skin creases
- **Soft tissues**: wasting of quadriceps, swelling in popliteal fossa, knee effusion
- **Bone**:
  - deformity or asymmetry
  - pelvic tilt
  - posterior subluxation of the tibia on the femur
  - varus/valgus deformities of the knee
  - flexion deformity or recurvatum

Physical Examination for Surgeons, ed. Petrut Gogalniceanu, James Pegrum and William Lynn. Published by Cambridge University Press. © Cambridge University Press 2015.

Feel
- **Skin**: temperature, tenderness
- **Soft tissues**:
    - knee effusion and 'bulge' test
    - patellar tap test
    - popliteal fossa: Baker's cyst, popliteal artery aneurysm
    - tendons: quadriceps tendon, patella tendon, pes anserinus, collateral ligaments and menisci, iliotibial band
    - pulses, capillary refill, neurology
- **Bone**:
    - tibial tuberosity and patella
    - femur, tibia and joint line
    - origin and insertion of collateral ligaments

Move
- **Active**:
    - straight leg raise
    - flexion and assess for crepitus
    - extension against gravity
- **Passive**:
    - flexion
    - hyperextension
- **Resisted**:
    - flexion

Special tests (* = essential tests)
- Patella: patella apprehension test,* patella tracking test, Clarke's test
- Collateral ligaments: valgus/varus pressure* (knee flexed at 30° flexion and extension)
- Menisci: McMurray's test*
- Cruciate ligaments: posterior sag test,* anterior & posterior drawer test,* Lachman's test,* pivot shift test, dial test

To complete the examination...
- Examine the joint above (hip joint) and the joint below (ankle joint).
- Check full neurovascular status of the lower limb.
- Order appropriate radiographs and further imaging.

Examination notes

How do you measure quadriceps diameter in order to assess wasting?
- Locate the tibial tuberosity. This is found on the proximal anterior tibia and demarcates the insertion of the patella tendon.
- Mark a point 20 cm proximal to this landmark, which is mid-thigh. (A longer measurement may be required in very tall individuals.)
- Measure the circumference of the thigh at this level and compare to the contralateral side.

How is the patella palpated?
- The patient is sitting on the edge of the couch.
- The examiner's hand is placed over the knee joint to feel the temperature (skin) or tenderness.
- The patella is held between index finger and thumb and patella tracking is assessed during active flexion and extension of the knee.
- Deviation the patella in the last 30° of knee extension equates to a 'J-sign' and indicates maltracking of the patella. This suggests that there is a shallow trochlea or poor soft tissues (medial quadriceps strength or disruption of medial patellofemoral ligament), which allows the patella to deviate laterally on flexion.
- The engaging of the patella in the trochlea in the last few degrees of knee extension causes the patella to suddenly straighten up, and this creates an appearance of an upside-down 'J'.

How are the tendons and muscles of the knee palpated?
- Palpate the insertion of the quadriceps tendon on the proximal pole of the patella, and the patella tendon distal to the patella. Discomfort in these areas may indicate a tendinopathy. A palpable gap with inability to extend lower leg against gravity indicates an extensor mechanism rupture.
- Palpate the pes anserinus, which is located three to four fingers distal to the anteromedial joint line. This marks the insertion of the sartorius, gracilis and semitendinosus tendons. These tendons also cause tendinopathy and are used in anterior cruciate ligament reconstruction, indicated by the presence of a scar with arthroscopic portals.

How are masses in the popliteal fossa differentiated?
A popliteal artery aneurysm can be pulsatile, whilst a Baker's cyst is not. Other possible diagnoses include skin masses, or more rarely tibial nerve neuroma and osteochondroma.

How are the ligaments and menisci of the knee assessed?

The knee is flexed to 90° to assess the medial and lateral joint line. Palpation tenderness suggests either meniscal or collateral ligament pathology. The origin and insertion of the collateral ligaments can also be felt, proximal and distal to the joint line. The other soft tissue structures that need to be palpated include the iliotibial band and its distal insertion on Gerdy's tubercle on the anterolateral tibia.

How do you assess and grade knee effusions?

A loss of normal patella contour indicates the presence of a knee effusion. In these cases, the patella is felt to float when it is compressed. A small knee effusion is detected by the 'bulge test', in which fluid is milked into the suprapatellar pouch from the medial gutter, with a vertical and upwards sweeping motion of one hand; the lateral side of the knee is then stroked from distal to proximal whilst assessing for a subtle bulge on the medial side.

Grades of knee effusion

Grade 1	Shows refilling of the medial gutter after it has been emptied
Grade 2	Gross fluctuation with no patellar tap test
Grade 3	Gross fluctuation with a positive tap test (although sometimes the effusion can be so large that a tap test is not possible)

Tip

The presence of an effusion after a twisting knee injury or valgus/varus stress is an important observation and warrants a careful history, examination and further investigation with an MRI scan.

How is movement of the knee joint assessed?

- The patient is asked to actively extend the knee against gravity. Evaluate range of flexion, noting any underlying discomfort. Palpate for crepitus during flexion.
- Active extension of the knee joint against gravity assesses competence of the extensor mechanism. The ability to perform a straight leg raise can be achieved with an intact retinaculum and iliotibial band, despite the extensor mechanism being ruptured. A loss to the terminal part of active extension signifies either an extensor lag or fixed flexion deformity.

> **Tip**
>
> Holding onto the heels will correct an extensor lag from muscle weakness but will not correct a fixed flexion deformity from osteoarthritis.

> **Tip**
>
> Excessive hyperextension (when compared to the contralateral side) indicates a significant ligamentous injury.

How is fixed flexion deformity of the knee joint assessed?

Holding onto the heels will correct an extensor lag from muscle weakness but will not correct a fixed flexion deformity from osteoarthritis. Excessive hyperextension (when compared to the contralateral side) indicates a significant ligamentous injury.

What is the patella apprehension test?*

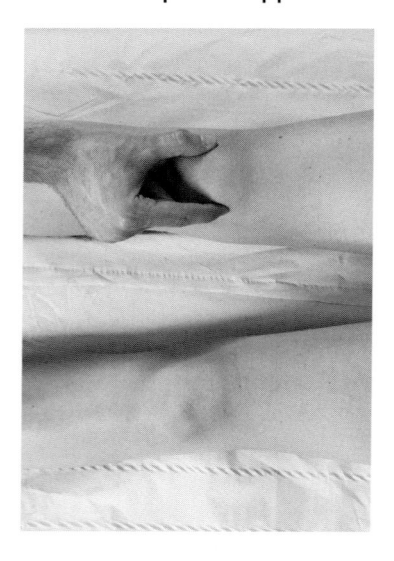

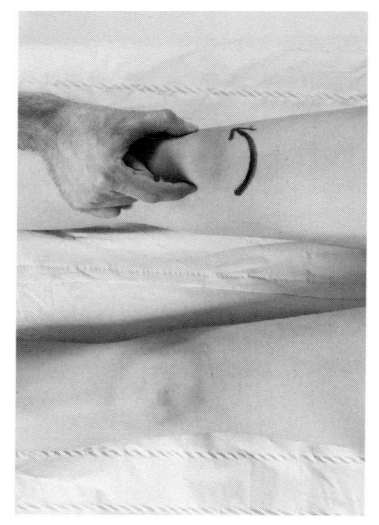

Rationale: Excessive lateral translation of the patella, compared to the contralateral side, may suggest previous dislocation and injury to the medial patellofemoral ligament and retinaculum.

Technique: The patient is supine and the knee is in extension. The examiner holds the medial and lateral patella edges and gently displaces the patella laterally, whilst carefully assessing change in the patient's facial expressions.

Positive test: Patient apprehension and asymmetrical lateral subluxation of the patella compared with the contralateral side. A useful grading system describes the amount of lateral movement as a percentage of the patella width – i.e. 25%, 50%, 75% or 100% lateral translation.

How is patella tracking assessed?*

Rationale: Maltracking patella is a cause of recurrent dislocations and can cause anterior knee pain.

Technique: Assess the linear movement of the patella during active knee flexion and extension with the patient sitting. Medial movement of the patella during the first 30° of knee flexion is found when the patella engages within the trochlea of the distal femur.

Positive test: A positive medial movement of the patella is referred to as a 'J-sign' and indicates patella maltracking.

What is Clarke's test?

Rationale: This tests helps isolate the cause of anterior knee pain.

Technique: The test involves compressing the patella against the trochlea during quadriceps muscle contraction to illicit patellofemoral pain. With the patient supine, place pressure over the patella and ask the patient to contract the quadriceps by extending the straight leg – 'pushing down' into the examination couch.

Positive test: Reproduction of the patient's discomfort. Comparison to the contralateral side is essential, as the test can be uncomfortable in a normal knee.

How are the collateral ligaments of the knee assessed?*

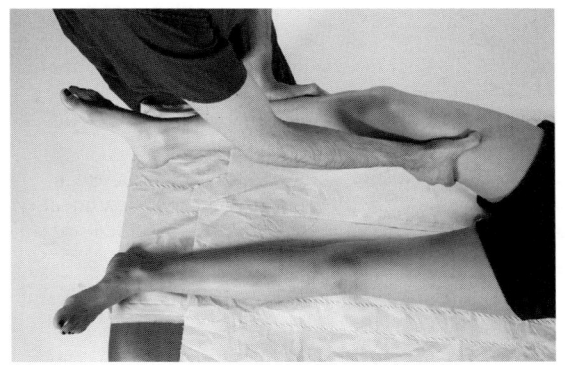

(A)

Varus pressure tests the lateral collateral ligament.

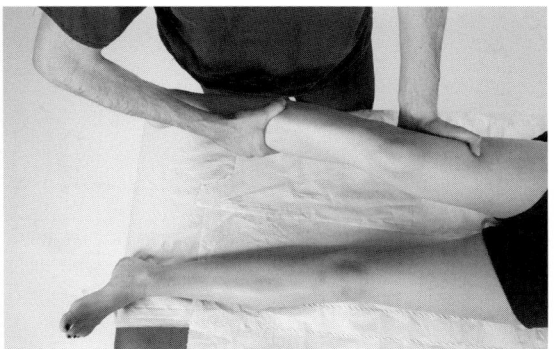

(B)

Valgus pressure tests the medial collateral ligament.

Rationale: Assesses the integrity of the collateral ligaments.

Technique: Varus stress is applied with the knee in extension and 30° of flexion; opening up the lateral joint line when compared to the contralateral knee indicates injury to the lateral collateral ligament and/or posterior lateral corner. Valgus stress in knee extension and 30° of flexion examines the medial collateral ligament and posteromedial capsule.

Positive test: Asymmetrical joint line gapping with no resistance or 'end point' to the examination indicates a complete rupture. Partial gapping with some resistance and (often significant) discomfort felt by the patient indicates a partial collateral ligament injury.

How are meniscal tests performed?*

Rationale: There are numerous available in the literature. They all have poor sensitivity and specificity but all aim to reproduce pain or catching from rotatory movements of the tibia.

Technique: The two commonly used tests are the McMurray's and Thessaly tests.

- McMurray's starts with the knee flexed and stresses the medial joint line with a varus and external rotation force to reproduce clicking or catching during knee extension. This movement is reversed for the lateral meniscus.
- The Thessaly test involves a twisting movement with the patient standing on the symptomatic leg with 20° of knee flexion. Reproduction of pain is reported to have a 95% diagnostic accuracy for meniscal tears.[16]

Positive test: Reproduction of the patient's discomfort, with catching and clicking felt by the patient.

---

[16] Karachalios T, Hantes M, Zibis AH, *et al*. Diagnostic accuracy of a new clinical test (the Thessaly test) for early detection of meniscal tears. *J Bone Joint Surg Am* 2005; **87**: 955–62.

How are the anterior and posterior drawer tests performed?*

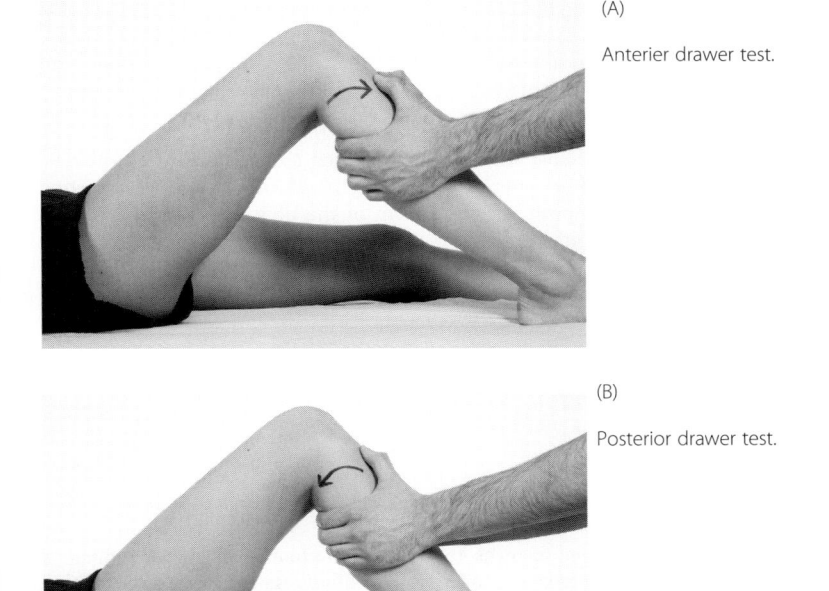

(A)

Anterier drawer test.

(B)

Posterior drawer test.

Rationale: Assess the integrity of the anterior and posterior cruciate ligaments, respectively.
Technique: The knee is flexed to 90° and the feet are placed flat on the couch.

- Assessment for a posterior sag of the tibia in the sagittal plane with both knees flexed to 90° is essential to correctly interpret an anterior drawer. The patient is supine with both knees flexed. Observe from the side for posterior displacement ('sag') of the tibia. A positive sag of the tibia signifies a posterior cruciate ligament injury. In this situation the anterior drawer will be incorrectly interpreted as positive, when in fact the anterior

translation of the tibia only brings the tibia back to a neutral position. This is an important cause of a false positive anterior drawer.
- Once a posterior sag has been excluded the examiner warns the patient that he/she is going to sit on the patient's toes. The examiner places both thumbs on the anterior joint line, either side of the patella tendon, and uses the index fingers of both hands to feel for hamstring laxity behind the knee.

Positive test: Excessive anterior drawer when compared to the contralateral knee indicates an anterior cruciate ligament injury. Analogous testing and asymmetrical posterior translation of the tibia is found in posterior cruciate ligament injuries.

Grades of anterior cruciate ligament deficiency

Grade 1	0–5 mm
Grade 2	6–10 mm
Grade 3	> 10 mm

Tip

A non-contact twisting injury to the knee with a 'pop', inability to continue participation and acute knee swelling within an hour is classical for an anterior cruciate ligament (ACL) injury.

What is Lachman's test*?

Rationale: Lachman's test has a high positive predictive value for detecting ACL rupture, and supplements the anterior drawer test.[17]

Technique: The knee is assessed in 30° of flexion. The femur is stabilised with one hand whilst the tibia is anteriorly translated perpendicular to the line of the tibia. This test has the highest positive predictive value of any of the ACL tests.

Positive test: A firm end point confirms the integrity of the ligament, whilst a boggy soft end point or excessive translation compared with the contralateral side indicates a rupture of the ACL.

---

[17] Solomon DH, Simel DL, Bates DW, Katz JN, Schaffer JL. The rational clinical examination. Does this patient have a torn meniscus or ligament of the knee? Value of the physical examination. *JAMA* 2001; **286**: 1610–20.

The pivot shift test

Rationale: Confirms complete ACL tear. Based on very early flexion causing anterior subluxation of the tibia that is reduced with further flexion (20–40°) due to the posterior pull of the iliotibial tract.

Technique: This is performed with the patient supine. With the knee extended the examiner grasps and internally rotates the tibia, whilst applying a valgus stress across the knee joint; the knee joint is then flexed.

Positive test: A positive test yields a palpable clunk in the knee at approximately 30° of flexion, when the lateral tibial plateau is reduced onto the lateral femoral condyle. Relocation event graded as 0 (absent), 1+ (pivot glide), 2+ (pivot shift), 3+ (momentary locking).[18]

The dial test

Rationale: This assesses the integrity of the posterolateral corner. The posterolateral corner is a combination of structures which include the popliteus muscle, joint capsule, arcuate ligament, lateral collateral ligament, biceps femoris muscle. The posterolateral corner can be injured alongside PCL and LCL injuries and needs to be assessed in any patients with these suspected injuries.

Technique: With the patient in the prone position, both knees are flexed to 30° and then to 90° with the knees and heels together. The feet and ankles are then externally rotated, likes the hands of a clock.

Positive test: Greater than 10° of rotational asymmetry is considered significant. Isolated rotational asymmetry at 30° and not 90° suggests an isolated posterolateral corner injury. Asymmetry at both 30° and 90° indicates combined posterior cruciate and posterolateral corner ligamentous injuries.

> **Tip**
>
> Hip pain can be referred to the inner aspect of the knee due to shared sensory innervation of both areas by the obturator nerve. L3 or L4 radicular symptoms may cause referred pain from the back.

---

[18] Galway HR, Beaupré A, MacIntosh DL. Pivot shift: a clinical sign of symptomatic anterior cruciate insufficiency. *J Bone Joint Surg Br* 1972; **54-B**: 763–4.

> **Tip**
>
> A history of an acute knee effusion (typically within an hour) after a twisting injury indicates an anterior cruciate ligament injury until proven otherwise, and warrants careful examination and further imaging with an MRI scan.

Differential diagnoses
What are the causes of knee pain?

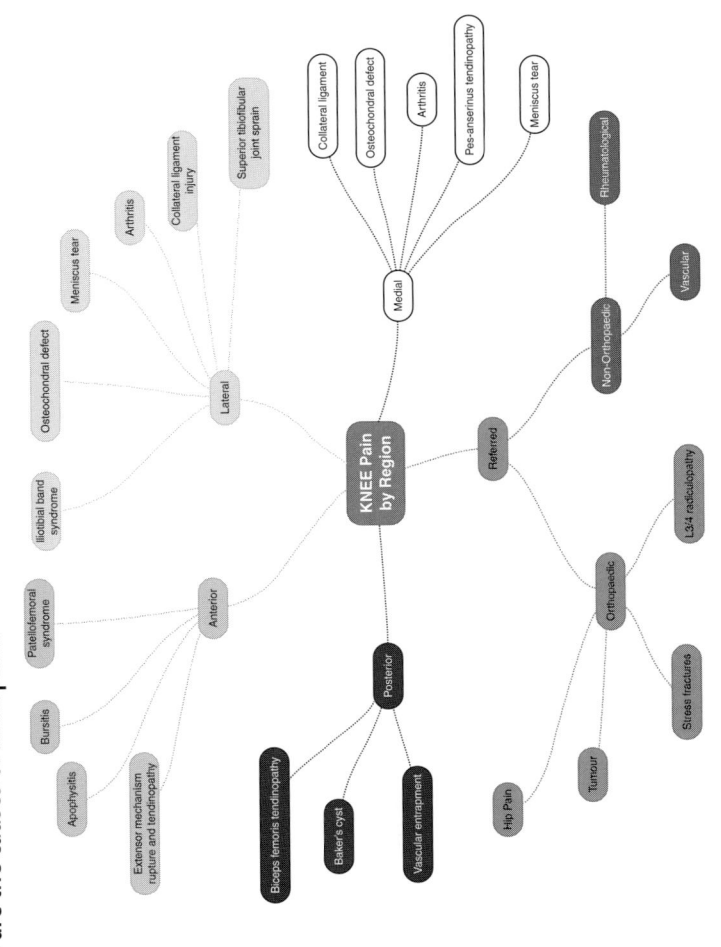

KNEE Pain by Region

- **Anterior**
  - Patellofemoral syndrome
  - Bursitis
  - Apophysitis
  - Extensor mechanism rupture and tendinopathy

- **Lateral**
  - Osteochondral defect
  - Meniscus tear
  - Arthritis
  - Collateral ligament injury
  - Superior tibiofibular joint sprain
  - Iliotibial band syndrome

- **Medial**
  - Collateral ligament
  - Osteochondral defect
  - Arthritis
  - Pes-anserinus tendinopathy
  - Meniscus tear

- **Posterior**
  - Biceps femoris tendinopathy
  - Baker's cyst
  - Vascular entrapment

- **Referred**
  - Orthopaedic
    - Hip Pain
    - Tumour
    - Stress fractures
    - L3/4 radiculopathy
  - Non-Orthopaedic
    - Vascular
    - Rheumatological

187

What causes reduced range of motion in the knee?

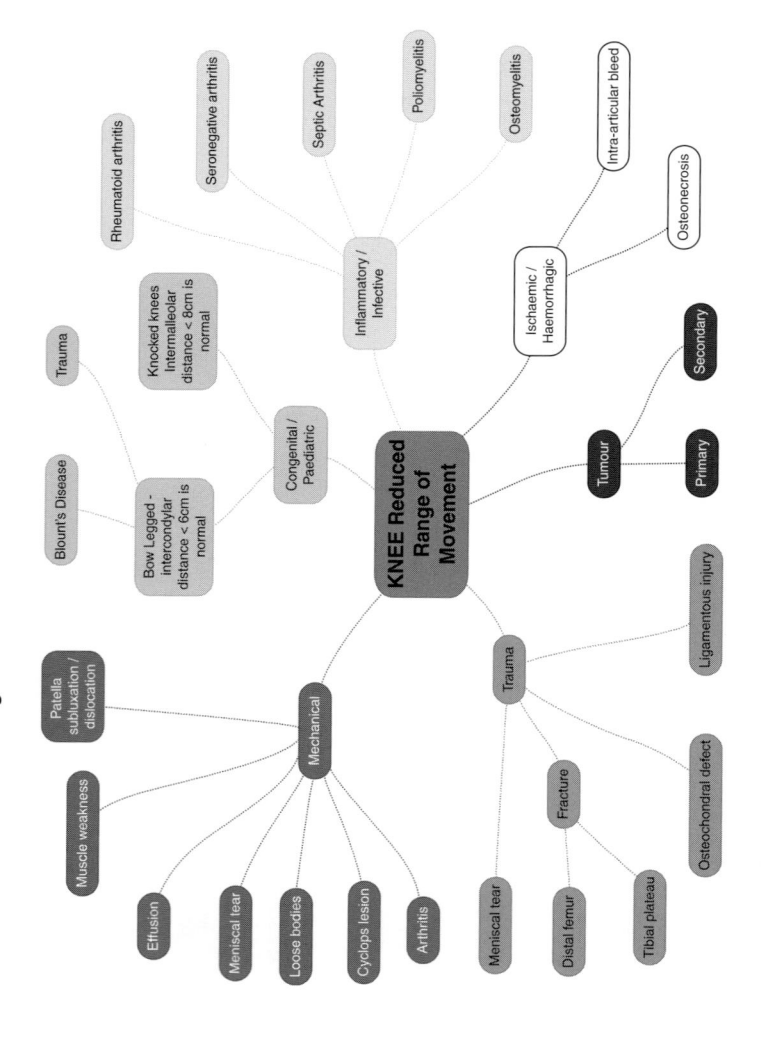

KNEE Reduced Range of Movement

- **Congenital / Paediatric**
  - Bow Legged - intercondylar distance < 6cm is normal
    - Blount's Disease
    - Trauma
  - Knocked knees Intermalleolar distance < 8cm is normal
- **Inflammatory / Infective**
  - Rheumatoid arthritis
  - Seronegative arthritis
  - Septic Arthritis
  - Poliomyelitis
  - Osteomyelitis
- **Ischaemic / Haemorrhagic**
  - Intra-articular bleed
  - Osteonecrosis
- **Tumour**
  - Primary
  - Secondary
- **Trauma**
  - Ligamentous injury
  - Fracture
    - Distal femur
    - Tibial plateau
  - Osteochondral defect
  - Meniscal tear
- **Mechanical**
  - Effusion
  - Meniscal tear
  - Loose bodies
  - Cyclops lesion
  - Arthritis
  - Muscle weakness
  - Patella subluxation / dislocation

188

What are the causes of a knee effusion?

- **Knee Effusion**
  - **Trauma**
    - Fracture
    - Osteochondral lesion
    - ACL / PCL
    - Meniscal tear
  - **Coagulopathy**
    - Acquired
      - Warfarin
    - Congenital
      - von Willebrand Disease
      - Factor deficiency
  - **Degenerative**
    - Osteoarthritis
  - **Inflammatory / Infective**
    - Sexually Acquired Reactive Arthritis
      - Gonorrhoea
    - Gout / Pseudogout
    - Iatrogenic
    - Polyarthritis
      - Rheumatoid arthritis
      - Reiter's Syndrome
      - Juvenile RA
  - **Tumour**
    - Malignant
    - Benign

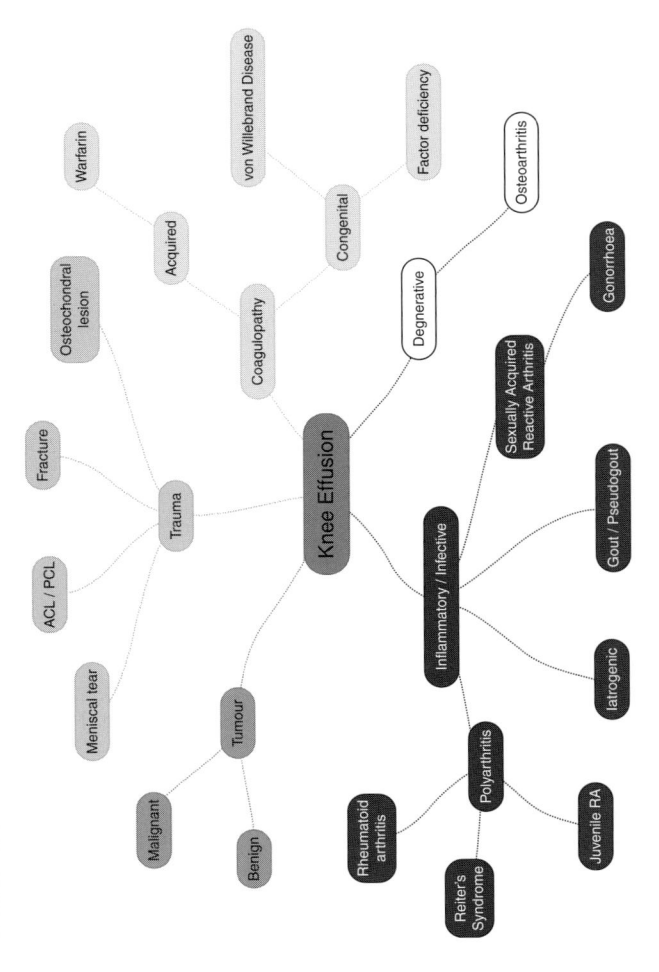

Section 5 Orthopaedic surgery

Chapter 23

Examination of the ankle

James Pegrum and Chris Lavy

Checklist

WIPER

- Patient standing in shorts or underwear; ankles and feet exposed with shoes and socks removed.
- Access is required to the spine, hip and knees to carry out a full biomechanical assessment.

Physiological parameters

Gait

- Antalgic gait
- Walking aids or orthotics
- Observation of footwear

Look

- **Skin**: scars, erythema, corns and callosities, skin or toe nail changes
- **Soft tissues**: swelling, proximal disuse muscle atrophy
- **Bone**:
  - foot: deformity, asymmetry, pes cavus, pes planus, equinus ankle, everted foot
  - heel: calcaneal valgus/varus
  - toes: toes number and alignment, overriding toes, hammer toes, hallux valgus, bunions

---

Physical Examination for Surgeons, ed. Petrut Gogalniceanu, James Pegrum and William Lynn. Published by Cambridge University Press. © Cambridge University Press 2015.

Feel
- **Skin**: temperature, tenderness, sensation
- **Soft tissues**:
    - anterior: extensor tendons, pulses, capillary refill time
    - sides: lateral and medial tendons and ligaments; sinus tarsi
    - posterior: Achilles tendon
    - plantar aspect: plantar fascia
- **Bone**:
    - bone and joint contours: proximal fibular head and neck; talus and calcaneum
    - Ottawa ankle rules for suspected ankle fractures

Move
- **Active**:
    - plantarflexion/dorsiflexion
    - eversion/inversion
- **Passive**:
    - plantarflexion/dorsiflexion
    - eversion/inversion
- **Resisted**:
    - ankle plantarflexion/ankle dorsiflexion
    - big toe flexion/big toe dorsiflexion
    - inversion/eversion

Special tests (* = essential tests)
- Coleman block test*
- Anterior drawer test*
- Talar tilt – medial and lateral tilt of talus while holding the heel (test medial and lateral ligaments)*
- Neuroma squeeze test (for Morton's neuroma)*
- Tinel's sign
- Simmonds–Thompson test

To complete the examination...
- Examine the joint above (knee) and the joint below (mid and forefoot).
- Check full neurovascular status of the lower limb.
- Order appropriate radiographs and further imaging.

Examination notes

What changes are inspected in the skin?

The quality of the skin around the foot and the presence and site of any ulcers will point the examiner towards underlying neuropathic, venous or arterial pathology.

- Scars from previous ankle open reduction and internal fixation will be sited over their respective malleoli.
- Anterior ankle approaches are used in trauma surgery, ankle replacement or fusion operations.
- Corns are skin thickening occurring to the dorsum or side of toes, whilst callosities are hardening of skin found in the heel and ball weight-bearing plantar surfaces of the foot.
- Atrophy of the toes or nails is a sign of vascular insufficiency, as are ulcers or gangrene.

What bone changes should be inspected?

- From the front: the foot should rest flat on the floor; failure to do so suggests a leg length discrepancy or equinus foot position.
- The great toe is assessed for:
  - valgus deformity (hallux valgus)
  - the presence of over-riding toes
  - hammer toe or claw toes
- From the side: the medial plantar arch is assessed for flattening, known as pes planus, or excessive arching, called pes cavus.
- From posterior inspection the angle of the calcaneum with the floor is noted and the number of lateral toes is counted. More than two toes seen laterally, known as the 'too many toes' sign, suggests an everted foot.

Causes of pes planus and pes cavus

Foot deformity	Cause
Pes planus	Normal variation (especially Afro-Caribbean patients), tibialis tendon dysfunction, inflammatory arthritis, tarsal coalition, arthritis, neuromuscular
Pes cavus	Muscle imbalances, idiopathic, neuromuscular disease, club foot, post compartment syndrome

How should sensation in the foot be examined?

Assessment of altered sensation must differentiate between:
- A glove and stocking distribution from diabetic peripheral neuropathy
- A dermatomal pattern secondary to spinal nerve root compression
- A mononeuropathy caused by nerve compression or iatrogenic transection

The foot sensation to touch or pain can also be altered due to underlying pathology.

Altered perception of pain

Sensation	Clinical features	Causes
Allodynia	Pain from innocuous stimulus, e.g. touch	Complex regional pain syndrome, fibromyalgia, diabetes, multiple sclerosis, vitamin B_{12} deficiency, neuroma, alcoholic neuropathy, Guillain–Barré syndrome
Dysaesthesia	Unpleasant sensation	
Hyperaesthesia	Increased sensitivity to touch	
Hyperalgesia	Increased pain from painful stimuli	

What soft tissue structures are palpable medially?

Soft tissues palpated posterior to the medial malleolus include the deltoid ligament, tibialis posterior, flexor hallucis longus and flexor digitorum longus tendon.

What soft tissue structures are palpable laterally?

- Soft tissues palpated behind lateral malleolus: the peroneal tendons.
- Soft tissues palpated distal to fibula: the lateral ligaments.
- The anterior talofibular ligament is commonly sprained in acute ankle inversion injuries. It is palpated between the tip of the distal fibula and the anterolateral talus at its insertion.
- Sinus tarsi or talocalcaneal sulcus is a tunnel between the talus and calcaneus. It is felt as a soft spot located distal and anterior to the tip of the fibula. Sinus tarsi pain can be found:
  - in everted feet causing soft tissue neural compression
  - in interosseous ligament sprains found in inversion injuries

What soft tissue structures are palpable anteriorly?
Tibialis anterior and the digital extensor tendons can be felt during resisted dorsiflexion of the toes and ankle anteriorly. The dorsalis pedis artery is found lateral to extensor hallucis longus.

What soft tissue structures are palpable posteriorly?
The Achilles tendon is palpated for:
- Defects suggesting acute tears
- Tenderness indicating tendinopathy
- Insertional pain consistent with Haglund's deformity, painful bony enlargement with associated bursitis or calcaneal apophysitis from Sever's disease in children

What soft tissue structures are palpated in the plantar aspect of the foot?
The plantar aspect of the foot is palpated just anterior to the calcaneum for characteristic plantar fascial pain.

How is the Ottawa ankle rule applied?
Rationale: The Ottawa ankle rule is a clinical assessment algorithm that guides clinicians as to whether patients with ankle sprains require radiological imaging in order to rule out bony injuries.

Technique: The inability to weight bear independently, or palpation pain found in these four bony prominences, warrants an ankle radiograph:
- the posterior distal 6 cm of the lateral and medial malleoli
- the navicular medially
- the 5th metatarsal base laterally

Positive test: The Ottawa ankle rule has high sensitivity but only modest specificity in adults and children.[19]

---

[19] Boutis K, Komar L, Jaramillo D, *et al*. Sensitivity of a clinical examination to predict need for radiography in children with ankle injuries: a prospective study. *Lancet* 2001; **358**: 2118–21; Derksen RJ, Bakker FC, Geervliet PC, *et al*. Diagnostic accuracy and reproducibility in the interpretation of Ottawa ankle and foot rules by specialized emergency nurses. *Am J Emerg Med* 2005; **23**: 725–9; Wang X, Chang SM, Yu GR, Rao ZT. Clinical value of the Ottawa ankle rules for diagnosis of fractures in acute ankle injuries. *PLoS One* 2013; **8**(4).

Why should the proximal fibula be palpated?

The proximal fibular head and neck need to be palpated in order not to miss a Maisonneuve fracture. A Maisonneuve injury will present with soft tissue medial ankle pain with a normal radiograph. This injury is a fracture of the proximal fibula and represents an unstable ankle injury. It requires a knee radiograph.

How do the ankle joints impact on movement?

- The ankle joint contains three separate joints which move in two planes.
- The joint between the tibia and talus, known as the talocrural joint, allows dorsiflexion and plantarflexion.
- The subtalar joint is the articulation between the inferior aspect of the talus and the calcaneum, and it includes an anterior articulation between the talus and the navicular bone. The subtalar joint controls and allows ankle inversion and eversion.
- The inferior tibiofibular joint or syndesmosis is formed by a convex recess on the lateral side of the tibia where the fibula is held in position by an interosseous membrane, anterior and posterior tibiofibular ligaments.

How is movement of the ankle joint assessed?

- Active movement is carried out with the patient sitting, noting the range of movement in dorsiflexion, plantarflexion, inversion (pointing the toes inwards) and eversion (pointing the toes outwards). The table below shows the typical range of movement expected, but more importantly there is a huge variation in the population, and thus contralateral ankle assessment is more important.
- The hand of the examiner is used to cup the heel, with the forearm against the under surface of the foot, which easily allows passive control of the ankle. The ankle is assessed for quality, ease and range of movement in the sagittal and coronal planes.
- Resisted muscle action aims to test the main foot and ankle muscle and tendinous function. The assessment of tibialis posterior tendon function is essential in patients with pes planus, as this is an acquired cause of flat foot deformity. Correction of the pes planus with tiptoeing or dorsiflexion of the hallux confirms that the deformity is flexible. The inability to complete 10 heel rises suggest tibialis posterior tendon dysfunction.

Range of movement of the ankle joint

Ankle movement	Typical range of movement
Dorsiflexion	20–30°
Plantarflexion	30–45°
Inversion	30°
Eversion	15°

Muscle function

Resisted movement	Muscle assessed
Ankle dorsiflexion (also L4 myotome)	Tibialis anterior
Great toe dorsiflexion (also L5 myotome)	Extensor hallucis longus
Lesser toe dorsiflexion	Extensor digitorum longus
Inversion and plantarflexion	Tibialis posterior
Eversion	Peroneal longus and brevis
Great toe plantarflexion	Flexor hallucis longus
Lesser toe plantarflexion	Flexor digitorum longus

> **Tips**
>
> Note that inversion and eversion are actually triplanar movements and include the movements in the transverse, sagittal and coronal planes.
>
> Inversion is a combination of plantarflexion, adduction and supination.
>
> Eversion is a combination of dorsiflexion, abduction and pronation.

The Coleman block test*

Rationale: This test aims to see if the varus hind foot position is correctable and caused by a fixed flexion deformity of the great toe.

Technique: With the patient standing, the lateral heel and foot border are placed on a block of wood 2.5–4 cm thick (or a suitably thick book). Correction of the hindfoot position confirms that the subtalar joint is flexible and the cause is in the forefoot.

Positive test: If the hindfoot does not correct, then the subtalar joint is not flexible, and surgery is aimed at both the forefoot and hindfoot.

The anterior drawer test of the ankle*

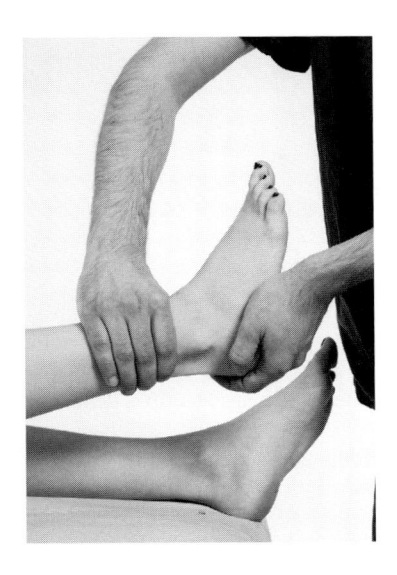

Rationale: This examination assesses the integrity of the anterior talofibular ligament (ATFL).

Technique: With the patient sitting and 10° of plantarflexion, stabilise the tibia, with one hand and cup the heel with the other, apply an anterior force to the foot.

Positive test: As with the anterior drawer test in the knee, asymmetrical anterior movement of the hindfoot in relation to the tibia confirms an ATFL injury.

The talar tilt test*

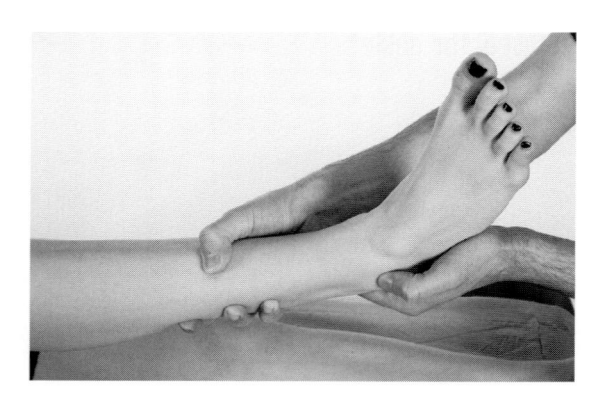

Rationale: this is a lateral ligament stress test and helps identify a deltoid or calcaneofibular ligament injury.

Technique: With the patient sitting with the knee flexed to 90°, a valgus or varus force is applied across the ankle joint, with one hand cupping the heel and the other the tibia.

Positive test:

- Asymmetrical opening up in valgus stress indicates a deltoid or medial ligament injury.
- Asymmetrical opening up in varus stress indicates a calcaneofibular ligament injury.

Examination for Morton's neuroma*

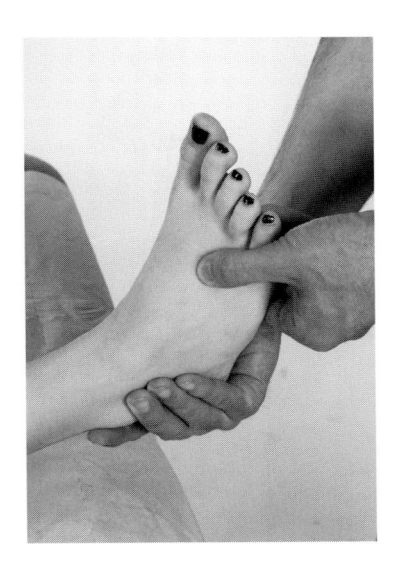

Rationale: A painful nerve neuroma is commonly found between the 3rd and 4th metatarsal heads.

Technique: A palpable or audible click, known as a Mulder's click, felt during compression of the forefoot. Importantly, neuromas are rarely found in the 4th metatarsal space, and are virtually unknown in the first metatarsal space. In these cases careful consideration of differentials is essential.

Positive test: A palpable click, typically felt between the 3rd and 4th metatarsal heads.

Tinel's tap test

Rationale: A neuropathic test assessing compression of the posterior tibial nerve.

Technique: The typical place for nerve compression is found within the tarsal tunnel, where the posterior tibial nerve is found.

Positive test: Tapping behind the medial malleolus reproducing the patient's symptoms indicates a positive test.

Simmonds–Thompson test

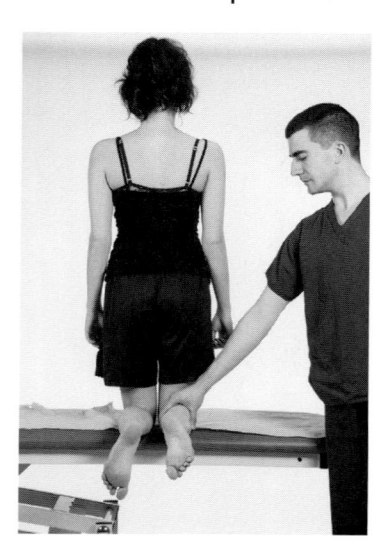

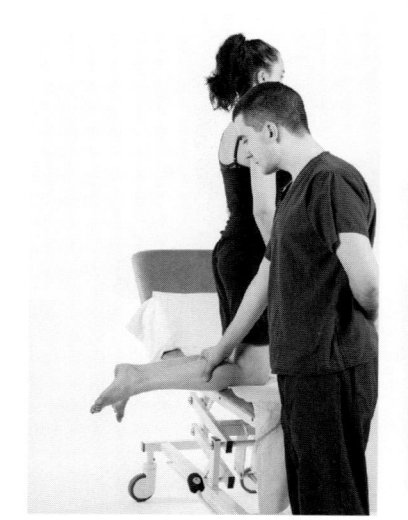

Rationale: Assesses for evidence of an Achilles tendon rupture.

Technique: The patient is examined either prone or with one leg kneeling on a chair with the knee flexed to 90°. The calf of the leg is squeezed.

Positive test: Reduced ankle plantarflexion compared with the contralateral side on squeezing the calf. The presence of this positive test with decreased resting tone and a palpable defect has 100% sensitivity.[20]

> **Tips**
>
> Foot and ankle pain can be referred from the knee and spine.
>
> Careful consideration of systemic pathology is warranted to avoid missing non-orthopaedic-related foot problems.

---

[20] Garras DN, Raikin SM, Bhat SB, Taweel N, Karanjia H. MRI is unnecessary for diagnosing acute Achilles tendon ruptures: clinical diagnostic criteria. *Clin Orthop Relat Res* 2012; **470**: 2268–73.

Differential diagnoses

What are the causes of ankle pain?

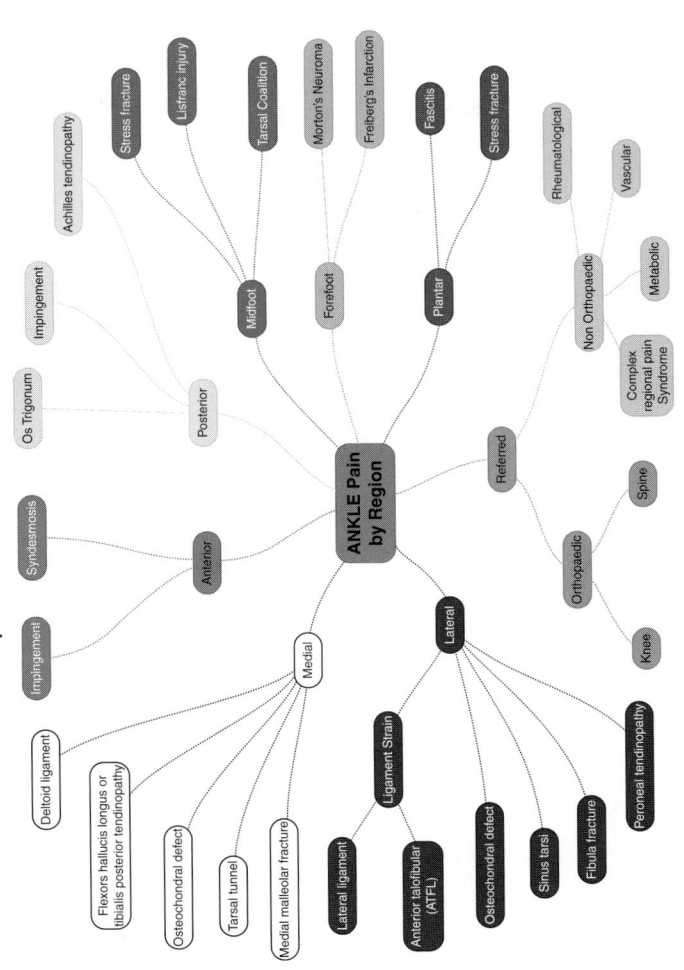

ANKLE Pain by Region

- **Anterior**
  - Impingement
  - Syndesmosis
- **Posterior**
  - Os Trigonum
  - Impingement
  - Achilles tendinopathy
- **Midfoot**
  - Stress fracture
  - Lisfranc injury
  - Tarsal Coalition
- **Forefoot**
  - Morton's Neuroma
  - Freiberg's Infarction
- **Plantar**
  - Fasciitis
  - Stress fracture
- **Referred**
  - Non Orthopaedic
    - Rheumatological
    - Vascular
    - Metabolic
    - Complex regional pain Syndrome
  - Orthopaedic
    - Spine
    - Knee
- **Lateral**
  - Ligament Strain
    - Lateral ligament
    - Anterior talofibular (ATFL)
  - Osteochondral defect
  - Sinus tarsi
  - Fibula fracture
  - Peroneal tendinopathy
- **Medial**
  - Deltoid ligament
  - Flexors hallucis longus or tibialis posterior tendinopathy
  - Osteochondral defect
  - Tarsal tunnel
  - Medial malleolar fracture

What are the causes of reduced range of motion of the ankle joint?

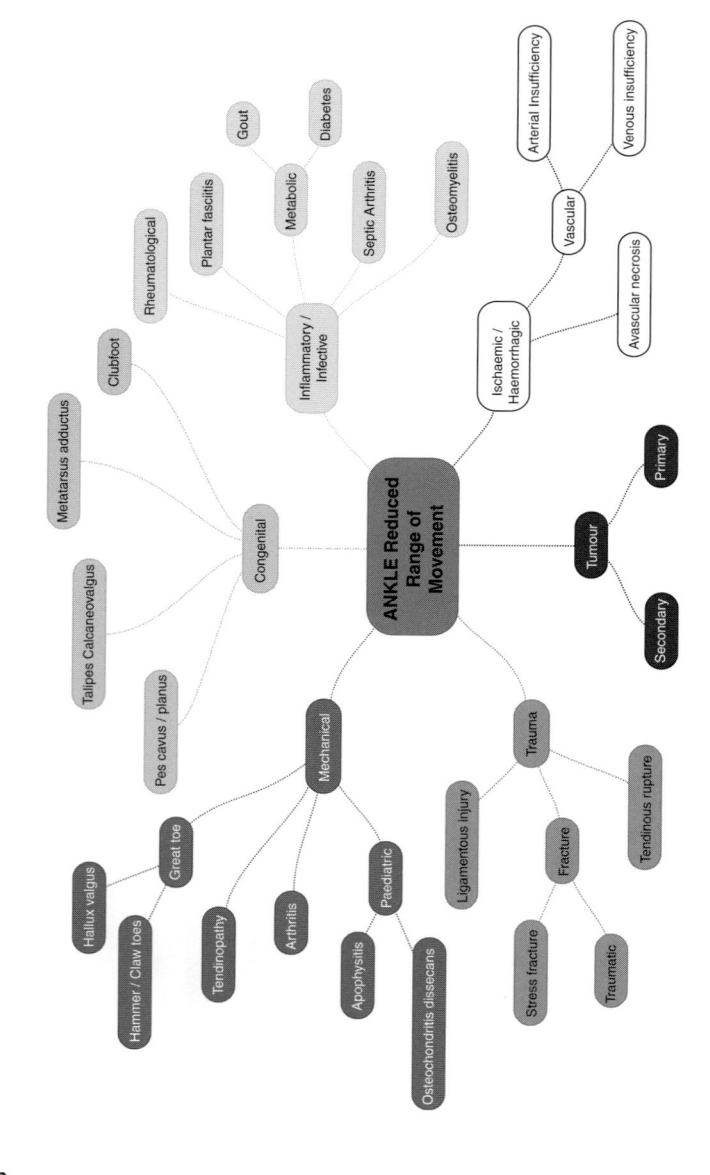

- **ANKLE Reduced Range of Movement**
  - **Inflammatory / Infective**
    - Clubfoot
    - Rheumatological
      - Plantar fasciitis
      - Metabolic
        - Gout
        - Diabetes
    - Septic Arthritis
    - Osteomyelitis
  - **Ischaemic / Haemorrhagic**
    - Vascular
      - Arterial Insufficiency
      - Venous insufficiency
    - Avascular necrosis
  - **Tumour**
    - Primary
    - Secondary
  - **Congenital**
    - Metatarsus adductus
    - Talipes Calcaneovalgus
    - Pes cavus / planus
  - **Mechanical**
    - Great toe
      - Hallux valgus
      - Hammer / Claw toes
    - Tendinopathy
    - Arthritis
    - Paediatric
      - Apophysitis
      - Osteochondritis dissecans
    - Trauma
      - Ligamentous injury
      - Fracture
        - Stress fracture
        - Traumatic
      - Tendinous rupture

Section editor: Petrut Gogalniceanu
Senior author: Vijay M. Gadhvi

Section 6: Vascular surgery

Chapter 24: Examination of the carotid artery
Petrut Gogalniceanu and Vijay M. Gadhvi

Checklist

WIPER
- Patient sitting in chair with neck, shoulders and upper chest exposed.

Physiological parameters

Inspection
- Scars from previous carotid endarterectomy
- Thoracic scars: midline sternotomy scar for CABG
- Scars from other head and neck surgery (hostile neck)
- Radiotherapy marks (hostile neck)
- Masses in anterior triangle or deep to SCM (carotid body tumours or aneurysms)
- Neurology: arm or leg weakness; facial asymmetry; speech disturbance

Palpation
- Radial pulse for AF
- Pulsatile neck masses (carotid body tumours or aneurysm)
- Carotid pulse
- Carotid thrill (arteriovenous fistula)

Physical Examination for Surgeons, ed. Petrut Gogalniceanu, James Pegrum and William Lynn. Published by Cambridge University Press. © Cambridge University Press 2015.

Move
- Neck mobility (to assess suitability for CEA)

Auscultation
- Carotid artery bruit
- Heart sounds

To complete the examination...
- Perform a full neurological and cardiovascular exam.
- Examine upper limb pulses to exclude steal syndrome.
- Check ECG: AF and ischaemic changes.
- Perform a fundoscopy of the retinal arteries to exclude embolism.

Examination notes

What aspects of carotid artery disease must be established?
- Establish presence of any neurological deficits: asymptomatic, transient ischaemic attacks, cerebrovascular accident.
- Establish the nature of neurological deficit: amaurosis fugax, speech impairment, facial asymmetry, focal neurological defect.
- Establish time since neurological event, recovery from stroke and residual functional deficit.

Where should the carotid bifurcation be palpated?
The carotid bifurcation is found at the level of the thyroid cartilage. Palpate this medially then slide fingers laterally to the anterior aspect of the sternocleidomastoid muscle. The presence of a carotid pulse does not exclude a stenosis of the internal carotid artery distal or proximal to it.

Where should one auscultate for carotid bruits?
Carotid bruits are best heard at the angle of the mandible. The absence of a bruit does not exclude carotid artery disease.

What are the different carotid endarterectomy scars?
- Longitudinal incision parallel and anterior to the anterior edge of the sternocleidomastoid muscle.
- Transverse incision across sternocleidomastoid at the level of the upper thyroid cartilage.

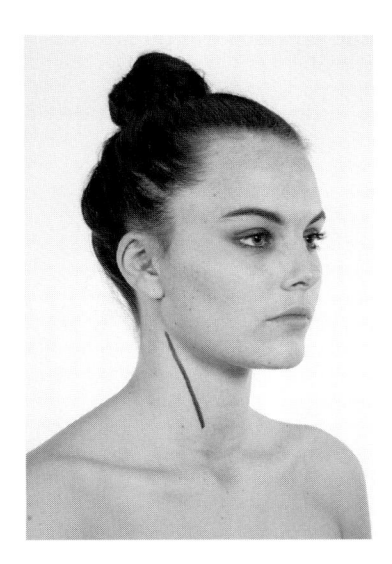

A longitudinal carotid endarterectomy scar is placed on the anterior aspect of the sternocleidomastoid muscle. The middle of the incision is situated at the level of the carotid bifurcation, which corresponds in most cases to the upper border of the thyroid cartilage.

What investigations are needed in the context of carotid artery stenosis and neurological deficits?

- Rule out cardiac embolic causes of neurological deficit: troponin (if indicated), check ECG (AF, ischaemia) and cardiac echocardiography (mural thrombi).
- Establish degree of carotid stenosis and patency of vertebral arteries using US Doppler, MRA or CTA.
- CT or MRI brain to rule out haemorrhage or space-occupying lesion; assess vascular territory affected; establish patency of circle of Willis and degree of collateralisation.

Why should patients with neck scars consistent with CEA have their chests examined?

Check for previous cardiac surgery/sternotomy. Carotid endarterectomy (CEA) is sometimes performed prior to on-pump CABG. This is done in order to avoid stroke in patients with significant internal carotid artery disease.

Does the absence of a CEA scar exclude previous carotid artery intervention?

No. Carotid artery stenting for occlusive disease may be used in selected groups of patients.

Differential diagnoses

What are the causes of carotid bruits?

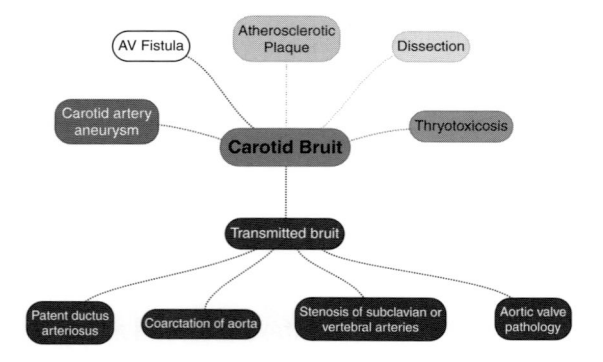

- Carotid Bruit
  - AV Fistula
  - Atherosclerotic Plaque
  - Dissection
  - Thyrotoxicosis
  - Carotid artery aneurysm
  - Transmitted bruit
    - Patent ductus arteriosus
    - Coarctation of aorta
    - Stenosis of subclavian or vertebral arteries
    - Aortic valve pathology

What are the causes of vascular neurological deficits?

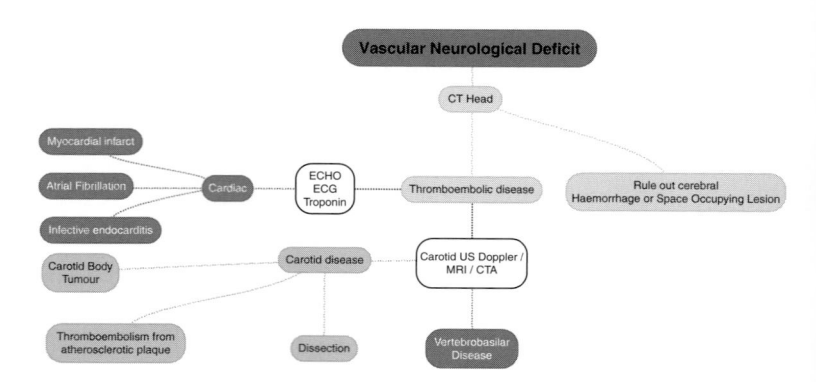

- Vascular Neurological Deficit
  - CT Head
  - Cardiac (ECHO / ECG / Troponin)
    - Myocardial infarct
    - Atrial Fibrillation
    - Infective endocarditis
  - Thromboembolic disease
  - Rule out cerebral Haemorrhage or Space Occupying Lesion
  - Carotid disease (Carotid US Doppler / MRI / CTA)
    - Carotid Body Tumour
    - Thromboembolism from atherosclerotic plaque
    - Dissection
    - Vertebrobasilar Disease

What are the causes of a pulsatile neck mass?

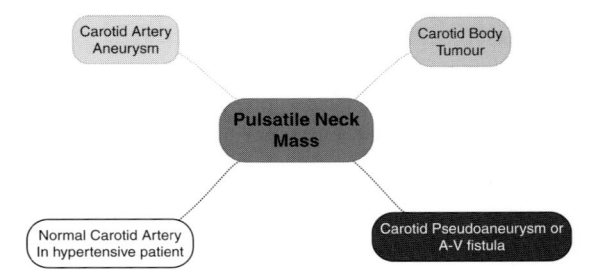

- Carotid Artery Aneurysm
- Carotid Body Tumour
- Normal Carotid Artery In hypertensive patient
- Carotid Pseudoaneurysm or A-V fistula

(Pulsatile Neck Mass)

Section 6: Vascular surgery

Chapter 25: Examination of an abdominal aortic aneurysm

Petrut Gogalniceanu and Vijay M. Gadhvi

Checklist

WIPER
- Patient lying flat; abdomen, chest and legs exposed
- Groin covered but accessible

Physiological parameters

General
- Pallor suggestive of anaemia
- Altered mental state
- Evidence of GI bleeding (aortoenteric fistula)

Inspection
- Scars: midline laparotomy, groin cut-down scars
- Visible pulsations
- Flank or periumbilical bruising (retroperitoneal haemorrhage)
- Feet: ischaemia or trash foot

Palpation
- Pulsatile +/- tender midline mass in abdomen: AAA
- Pulsatile +/- tender iliac fossa masses: iliac aneurysms
- Chest wall anteriorly and laterally: axillofemoral or bifemoral bypass grafts
- Femoral pulses

Physical Examination for Surgeons, ed. Petrut Gogalniceanu, James Pegrum and William Lynn. Published by Cambridge University Press. © Cambridge University Press 2015.

- Suprapubic soft tissues: femoro-femoral crossover graft
- Popliteal arteries: popliteal aneurysms
- Foot pulses

Auscultation
- Aortic bruits

To complete the examination...
- Perform full vascular and abdominal examinations.
- Perform a bedside US scan of the aorta.

Examination notes

What is the essential history that needs to be obtained?
The patient's baseline function and comorbidities need to be established, as open aortic surgery is associated with a considerable risk of death.

Where should the aorta be palpated?
Above the umbilicus. The identification of a pulsatile aorta warrants palpation of the right and left iliac fossae to identify aneurysmal changes in the iliac segment.

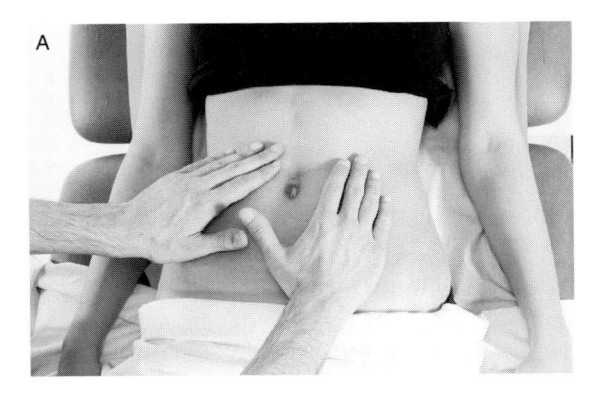

The aorta is always palpated with two hands, above the umbilicus and to the left of the midline (A). It is usually palpated with the tips of the fingers (B), but palpation between the thumbs has also been described (C).

(cont.)

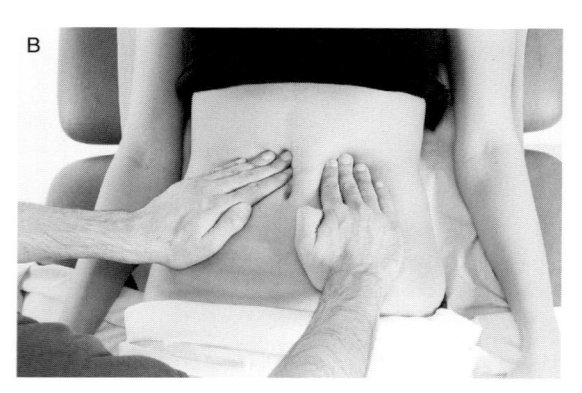

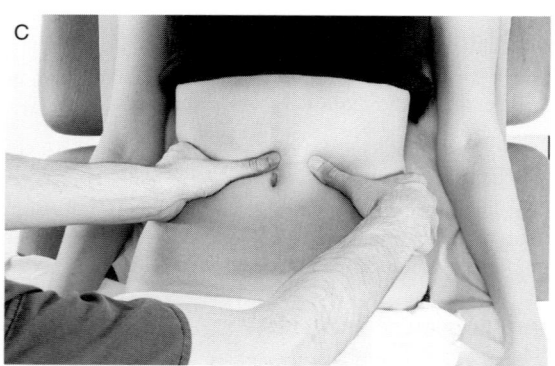

What are the differences between a normal palpable aorta and an aneurysmal aorta?

A normal aorta is pulsatile (displaces palpating hands vertically), whilst an aneurysmal aorta is expansile (displaces hands obliquely). In clinical practice this is not a definitive method of differentiation, and formal imaging should be arranged if there is clinical concern.

What is the relevance of an axillobifemoral or axillounifemoral bypass?

In the context of a midline laparotomy this may suggest that the aorta has been previously ligated or a previous aortic graft has been occluded or has failed.

Why should the femoral pulses be palpable?

Patients undergoing EVAR require good-calibre femoral and iliac vessels for insertion of endoprostheses (stents).

What is the relevance of femoral cut-down scars?

These may indicate previous EVAR, femoro-femoral bypass grafting (if bilateral) or common femoral artery endarterectomy (if unilateral).

Does the absence of groin cut-down scars exclude the possibility of a previous EVAR?

No. EVAR can be performed percutaneously (PEVAR) through 1 cm cuts in the groin.

Why should the popliteal arteries be palpated?

AAAs are associated with popliteal artery aneurysms.

How should the abdominal aorta be imaged?

- Diagnosis of AAA, screening and surveillance: ultrasound scan.
- Diagnosis of ruptured AAA and EVAR planning: CT angiogram of abdominal aorta, iliac and common femoral arteries.

Section 6 **Vascular surgery**

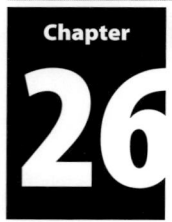

Chapter 26

Arterial examination of the upper limbs

Petrut Gogalniceanu and Vijay M. Gadhvi

Checklist

WIPER

Physiological parameters

Inspection
- Fingers: colour, cyanosis, finger-tip infarcts, Raynaud's syndrome
- Hand: atrophy of intrinsic muscles
- Arm: swelling, lymphoedema, arteriovenous fistulas

Palpation
- Digital tip tenderness
- Capillary refill time
- Hand temperature
- Pulses: radial, ulnar, brachial, axillary, subclavian arteries
- Sensation: dermatomal (C5 to T2) and nerve distribution (radial, ulnar, median, axillary nerves)
- Movement: fingers, wrist, elbow, shoulder
- Flexor and extensor compartments: tense or tender (compartment syndrome)
- Neck: cervical rib, first rib resection (treatment of TOS), carotid–subclavian bypass or carotid–carotid–subclavian bypass

Auscultation
- Bruits

Physical Examination for Surgeons, ed. Petrut Gogalniceanu, James Pegrum and William Lynn. Published by Cambridge University Press. © Cambridge University Press 2015.

Provocation tests in thoracic outlet syndrome (TOS)
- Adson's test
- Roos' stress test

Other tests
- Allen's test

Examination notes

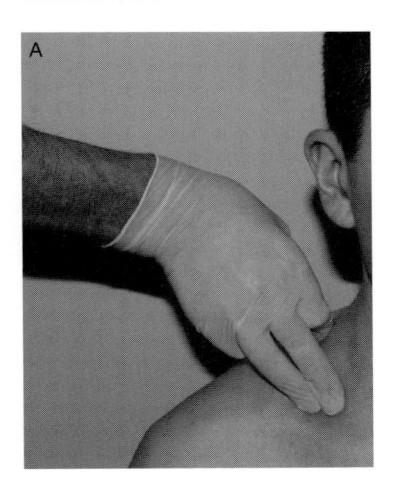

Palpation of upper limb arteries: (A) subclavian pulse (superior and posterior to clavicle), (B) axillary pulse (between humerus and biceps).

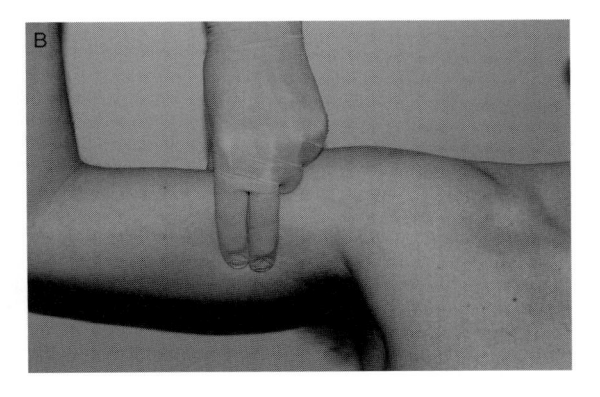

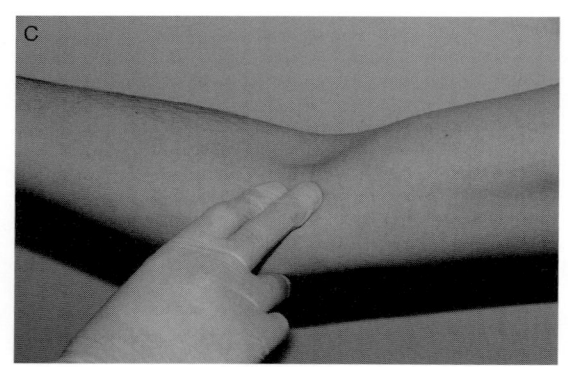

Palpation of upper limb arteries: (*cont.*) (C) brachial pulse (medial to biceps tendon), (D) radial pulse (proximal to wrist, over the radial bone).

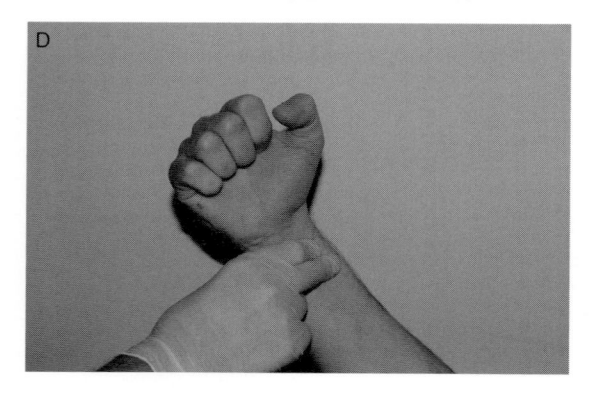

How is Allen's test interpreted?

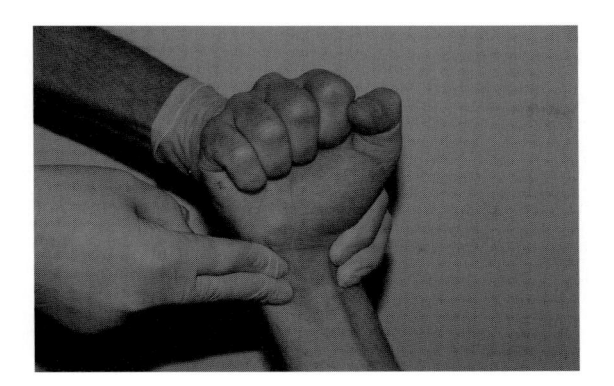

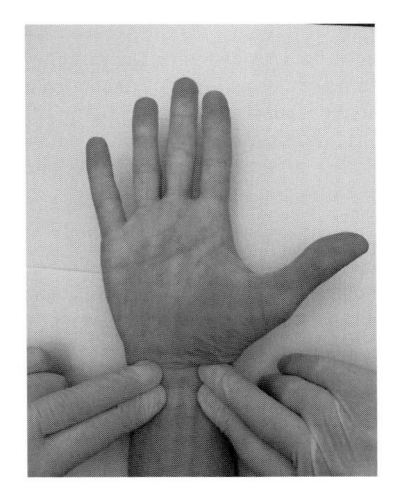

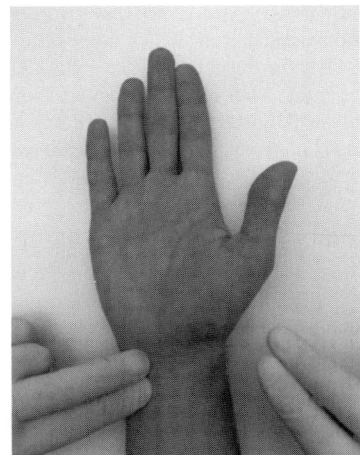

Allen's test: determining whether the hand can be perfused by a single artery.

Rationale: Determines whether the hand can be perfused from the ulnar artery alone. This needs to be assessed before performing an arterial puncture (blood gas sampling or arterial line placement) or prior to the formation of an upper limb arteriovenous fistula for haemodialysis.

Technique:

- Compress both ulnar and radial arteries until hand becomes pale.
- Maintain compression of radial artery.
- Release pressure on ulnar artery.
- Observe reperfusion of hand.

Positive test: If the hand becomes warm and pink whilst the radial artery is compressed, the test indicates that flow through the ulnar artery is sufficient to maintain independent perfusion of the hand.

When is a carotid–subclavian bypass performed?

Patients with thoracic aortic arch aneurysms that involve the origin of the left subclavian artery (LSA) may undergo endovascular stenting covering the origin of the LSA. If left arm ischaemia develops, a carotid–subclavian bypass may be performed.

When is a carotid–carotid–subclavian bypass performed?

Patients with more proximal thoracic aortic arch aneurysms may require an endovascular stent which covers the origin of the LSA as well as the origin of the left common carotid artery (LCCA). In these cases a bypass is made from the right to left carotid artery and subsequently from the left carotid to the left subclavian artery. In these circumstances the right carotid supplies the entire anterior circulation of the brain as well that of the left upper limb. The carotid–carotid bypass is palpable anterior to the trachea.

What is thoracic outlet syndrome (TOS)?

Thoracic outlet syndrome refers to neurological or vascular symptoms in the upper limb caused by compression of the brachial plexus, subclavian artery or subclavian vein on their course from the neck to the upper limb.

How does TOS present?

- Arterial TOS: thromboembolic events in hand
- Venous TOS: arm swelling, cyanosis or subclavian vein thrombosis
- Neurogenic TOS: muscle fatigue or wasting, paraesthesia and vasospasm

What is the relation of the subclavian artery and vein to the anterior scalene muscle?

The subclavian vein is anterior and the subclavian artery is posterior to the anterior scalene muscle.

Where are the possible areas of compression in TOS?
- Interscalene triangle: space between the first rib, anterior and middle scalene muscles in the neck. The subclavian vein lies outside the triangle and is therefore less commonly affected.
- Costoclavicular space: between clavicle and first rib (costoclavicular syndrome).
- Subcoracoid space: between coracoid process and pectoralis minor tendon.

What are the other causes of TOS?
Pregnancy, fibrous bands, Pancoast's tumour, fractured clavicle, repetitive strain injury, compression by cervical rib (cervical rib syndrome), enlargement of scalenus anterior muscle.

What is the commonest manifestation of TOS?
Neurogenic: usually in ulnar nerve distribution (C8, T1).

How is Adson's test interpreted?

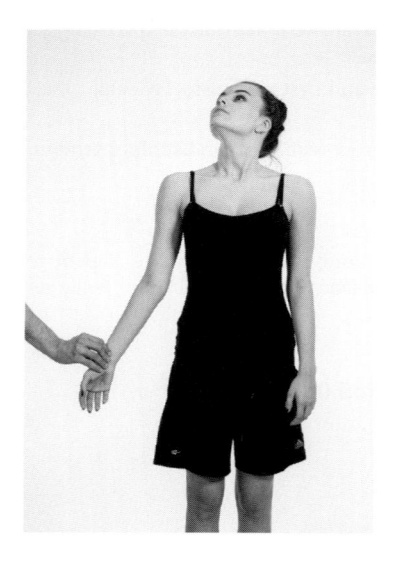

Adson's test for thoracic outlet syndrome.

Rationale: Test used in TOS.[21]

Technique:

- Ask the patient to extend the neck ('tilt your head backwards')
- Ask the patient to turn the head towards the symptomatic side
- Ask the patient to take a deep breath in and hold it
- On inspiration, the radial pulse is reduced, or paraesthetic symptoms are reproduced, in the presence of TOS
- Repeat the manoeuvre with the head turned away from the symptomatic side.

Positive test:

- With head turned towards the symptomatic side suggests possible cervical rib aetiology
- With head turned away from the symptomatic side suggests possible enlarged scalenus anterior aetiology.

---

[21] Bhattacharya V, Stansby G. *Postgraduate Vascular Surgery: the Candidate's Guide to the FRCS.* Cambridge: Cambridge University Press, 2010.

How is Roos' test interpreted?

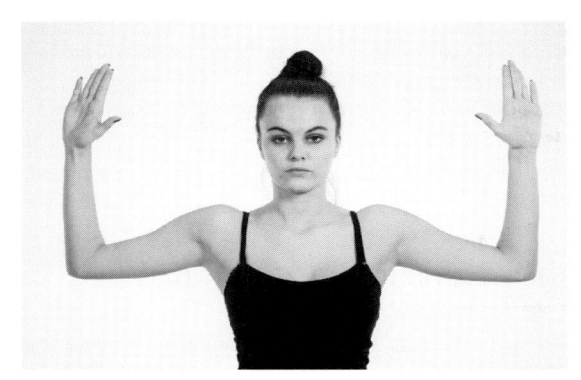

Roos' test for thoracic outlet syndrome.
(A) Hands up with elbows bent.

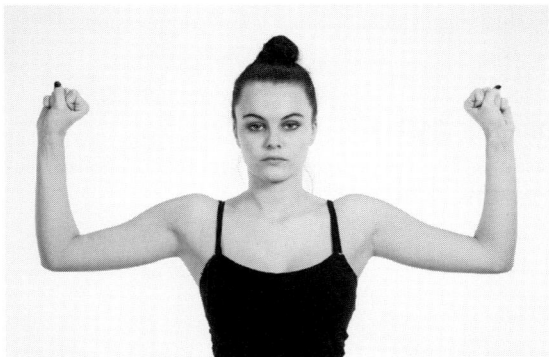

(B) Open and close hands for 1–3 minutes.

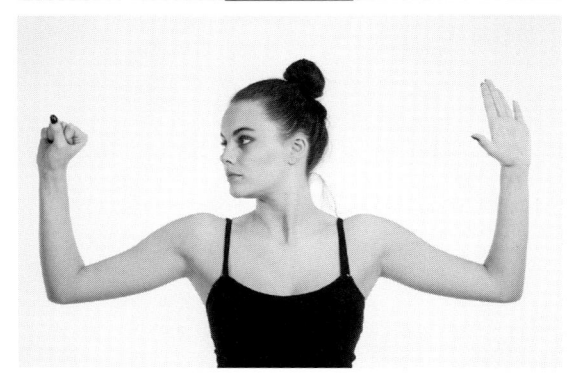

(C) Identify tingling, pain or fatigue in the affected hand or arm.

Rationale: Test used in TOS.[22] Also known as the elevated arm stress test (EAST).

Technique:

- Shoulders abducted (90°) and externally rotated (90°); elbows flexed (90°) (the 'put your hands up' position).
- Opening and closing of hands for several minutes reproduces symptoms.

Positive test: The affected hand/arm becomes cool, pale, tender or fatigued.

What imaging modalities can be used to diagnose TOS?

- X-ray neck: to rule out cervical rib.
- Duplex scanning: arterial and venous flow disturbance during provocation testing.
- MRI: to rule out brachial plexus or subclavian vessel compression.
- Nerve conduction studies.

What is Paget–Schroetter disease?

Paget–Schroetter disease refers to upper limb deep venous thrombosis secondary to venous compression in the context of TOS.

---

[22] Bhattacharya & Stansby, 2010.

Differential diagnoses
What are the causes of a 'blue' or cyanotic limb?

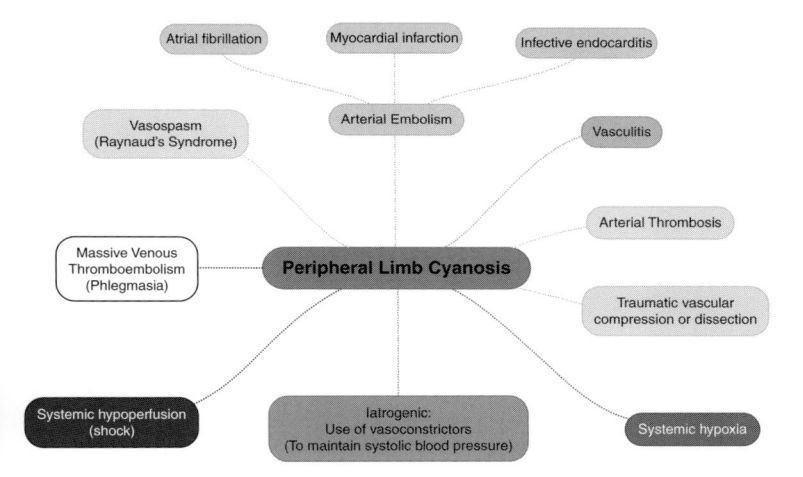

- Atrial fibrillation
- Myocardial infarction
- Infective endocarditis
- Arterial Embolism
- Vasospasm (Raynaud's Syndrome)
- Vasculitis
- Arterial Thrombosis
- Massive Venous Thromboembolism (Phlegmasia)
- Traumatic vascular compression or dissection
- Systemic hypoperfusion (shock)
- Iatrogenic: Use of vasoconstrictors (To maintain systolic blood pressure)
- Systemic hypoxia

Peripheral Limb Cyanosis

What are the causes of an oedematous limb?

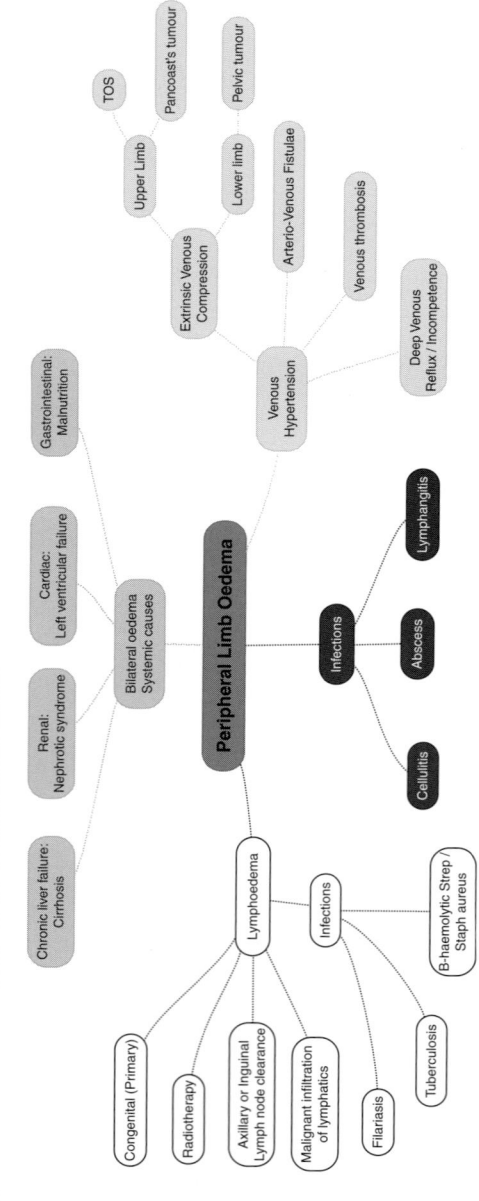

Peripheral Limb Oedema

- **Bilateral oedema: Systemic causes**
  - Chronic liver failure: Cirrhosis
  - Renal: Nephrotic syndrome
  - Cardiac: Left ventricular failure
  - Gastrointestinal: Malnutrition

- **Venous Hypertension**
  - Extrinsic Venous Compression
    - Upper Limb
      - TOS
      - Pancoast's tumour
    - Lower limb
      - Pelvic tumour
  - Arterio-Venous Fistulae
  - Venous thrombosis
  - Deep Venous Reflux / Incompetence

- **Infections**
  - Cellulitis
  - Abscess
  - Lymphangitis

- **Lymphoedema**
  - Congenital (Primary)
  - Radiotherapy
  - Axillary or Inguinal Lymph node clearance
  - Malignant infiltration of lymphatics
  - Filariasis
  - Tuberculosis
  - Infections
    - B-haemolytic Strep / Staph aureus

222

Section 6: Vascular surgery

Chapter 27: Arterial examination of the lower limbs

Petrut Gogalniceanu and Vijay M. Gadhvi

Checklist

WIPER
- Patient supine, legs and abdomen exposed
- Groin covered but accessible

Physiological parameters

General
- Bedside: GTN spray, cigarettes, lighter
- Hands: tar stains, finger pricks for glucose measurement (diabetes)
- Radial pulse: heart rate and rhythm (rule out AF)
- Eyes: xanthelasmas (hyperlipidaemia)
- Neck: carotid endarterectomy scar
- Chest: sternotomy or thoracotomy scars
- Abdomen: laparotomy scars, pulsating abdominal aortic aneurysm

Inspection
- **Skin:**
  - scars: laparotomy, femoral cut-down, crossover grafts, bypass grafts, vein harvest (upper and lower limbs)
  - sinuses or purulent discharge

Physical Examination for Surgeons, ed. Petrut Gogalniceanu, James Pegrum and William Lynn. Published by Cambridge University Press. © Cambridge University Press 2015.

- colour changes:
  - pallor/duskiness/cyanosis (ischaemia, thrombosis, phlegmasia)
  - erythema/cellulitis (infection)
- tissue loss: ulcers, gangrene (wet or dry)
- **Soft tissues**:
  - trophic changes: skin, hair, nails, toe-tip infarcts
  - calf swelling: DVT, lymphoedema
  - calf wasting
- **Bone**:
  - amputations

Palpation
- **Skin**: temperature
- **Soft tissues**: calf muscles and foot:
  - tender (ischaemic or infected)
  - tense (compartment syndrome)
  - fluctuant (abscess)
- **Vascular**:
  - capillary refill time (<3 sec)
  - pulses: aorta, femoral, popliteal, tibialis posterior (TP), dorsalis pedis (DP)
  - pulses: bypass grafts
- **Neurology**: short neurological exam (touch sensation and movement, L3, L4, L5, S1)

Auscultation
- Bruits: common femoral and superficial femoral arteries, grafts or arteriovenous fistulas (not routinely done)

Special tests
- Buerger's angle: cadaveric pallor and venous guttering on leg elevation
- Buerger's test: reactive hyperaemia/rubor in the dependent leg following elevation

To complete the examination...
- Ankle–brachial pressure index (ABPI)
- Venous, lymphatic and neurological examination of the lower limbs
- Complete abdominal and cardiovascular examinations

Examination notes

What are the symptoms of peripheral arterial disease?
- Intermittent claudication: pain on walking a fixed distance which is relieved by rest.
- Rest pain.
- Ulceration.
- Gangrene.
- Cellulitis or osteomyelitis can complicate ulceration and gangrene.

How can arterial and neurogenic claudication be differentiated?
- Arterial claudication presents with a muscular pain (**back** of calf, thigh or buttock) which is described as an ache, cramp or stiffness. It is brought on by exercise over a fixed and reproducible distance (claudication distance) and relieved by rest. The claudication distance can be shorter if walking uphill, in cold weather or at a faster pace.
- Spinal or neurogenic claudication is a sharp, shooting pain that is brought on by various movements at variable distances. The pain may be in the distribution of the sciatic nerve ('shooting pain in the back of the leg radiating to the **front** of the leg'). It may occur on standing or moving one's back and is relieved by lying or sitting down. Patients may have associated back pain or reduced range of spinal motion. Straight leg raise may be impaired or it can exacerbate symptoms.

How are the carotid and upper limb pulses collectively known?
Supra-aortic pulses.

How are the lower limb pulses collectively known?
Infrainguinal pulses.

Section 6: Vascular surgery

What is the basic anatomy of the lower limb arteries?

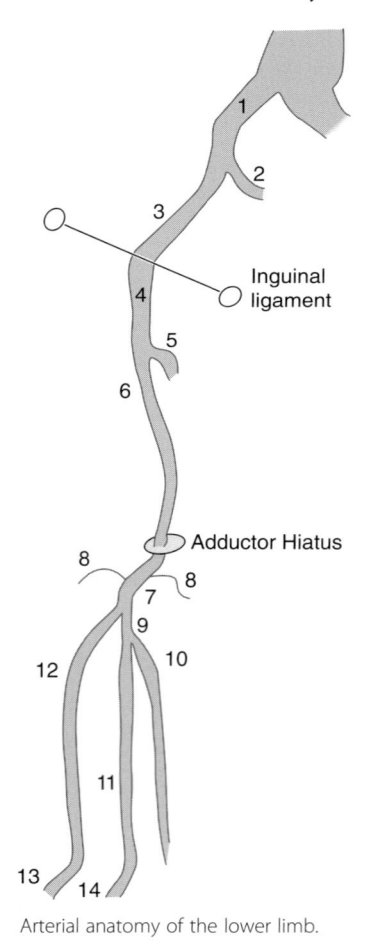

1. Common iliac artery (CIA)
2. Internal iliac artery (IIA)
3. External iliac artery (EIA)
4. Common femoral artery (Femoral pulse) (CFA)
5. Profunda femoris artery (PFA)
6. Superficial femoral artery (SFA)
7. Popliteal artery
8. Genicular arteries
9. Tibio-peroneal trunk
10. Peroneal artery
11. Posterior tibial artery (PT)
12. Anterior tibial artery (AT)
13. Dorsalis pedis pulse (DP)
14. Tibialis posterior pulse (TP)

Arterial anatomy of the lower limb.

What are the anatomical landmarks of the peripheral pulses in the lower limbs?

- Femoral pulse: just inferior to the midinguinal point (halfway between anterior superior iliac spine and pubic symphysis).

- Popliteal pulse: bimanual examination; knee slightly flexed, thumbs on tibial tuberosity anteriorly; index fingers palpate pulse deep in the popliteal fossa.
- Anterior tibial pulse: anterior to ankle joint, midway between the malleoli.
- Dorsalis pedis pulse: between first and second metatarsal bones, lateral to the tendon of the extensor hallucis longus.
- Tibialis posterior (or posterior tibial) pulse: medial foot, halfway between medial malleolus and Achilles tendon.

How are pulses graded?

- **3+** aneurysmal
- **2+** normal
- **1+** present but reduced
- **0** absent

How are lower limb pulses noted?

The example in the diagram shows a patient with an abdominal aortic aneurysm who has sustained an embolic event in his right SFA leading to loss of pulses in the right lower limb below the common femoral artery. Note that he has a full complement of pulses in his left lower limb, which may suggest this is an acute embolic event in the light of the fact that there is no evidence of atherosclerotic disease in the contralateral (left) limb.

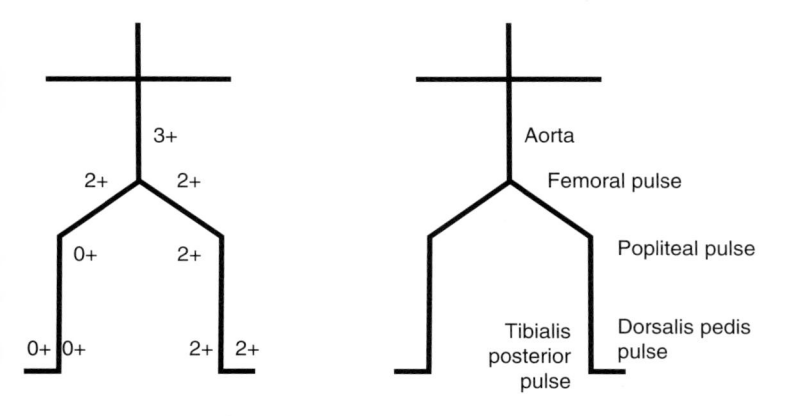

What is the most proximal pulse that should be palpated in the arterial examination of the lower limbs?

The aortic pulsation (not the femoral pulse).

How can the diseased arterial segment be deduced by the bypass graft identified?

- Axillofemoral or bifemoral bypass: aortic or bilateral common iliac disease.
- Femoro-femoral crossover bypass: iliac disease; aorto-iliac aortic endoprosthesis in EVAR.
- Femoro-popliteal (above or below knee): superficial femoral or popliteal arterial disease.
- Femoro-distal: SFA, popliteal and/or crural arterial disease.

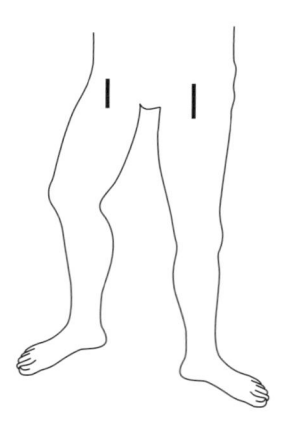

Lower limb arterial scars: bilateral groin cut-down scars are used to expose the common femoral arteries. These can be vertical or oblique.
Causes:
1. EVAR
2. Bilateral femoral endarterectomy
3. Femoral–femoral crossover graft

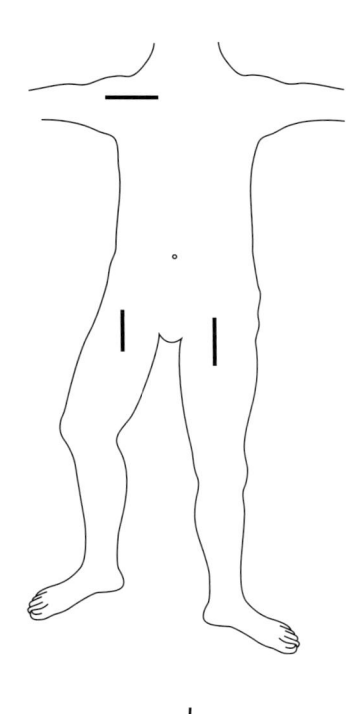

Chapter 27: Arterial examination of the lower limbs | 229

Lower limb revascularisation scars: axillo-bifemoral bypass.

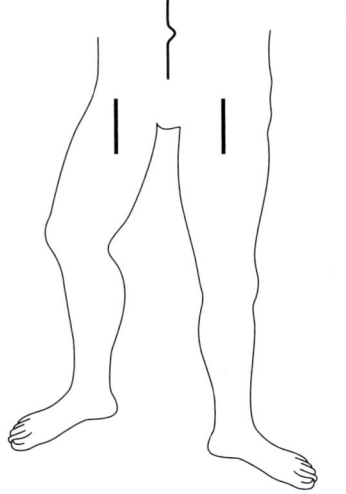

Lower limb revascularisation scars: aorto-bifemoral bypass.

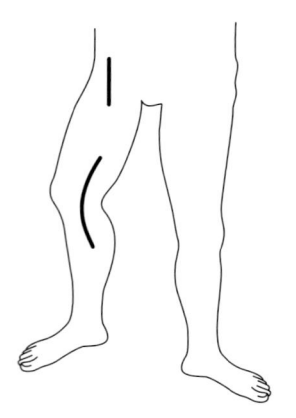

Section 6: Vascular surgery

Lower limb revascularisation scars: femoro-popliteal bypass.

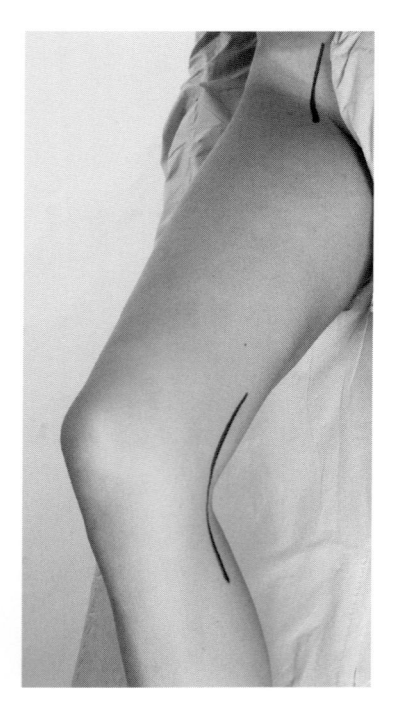

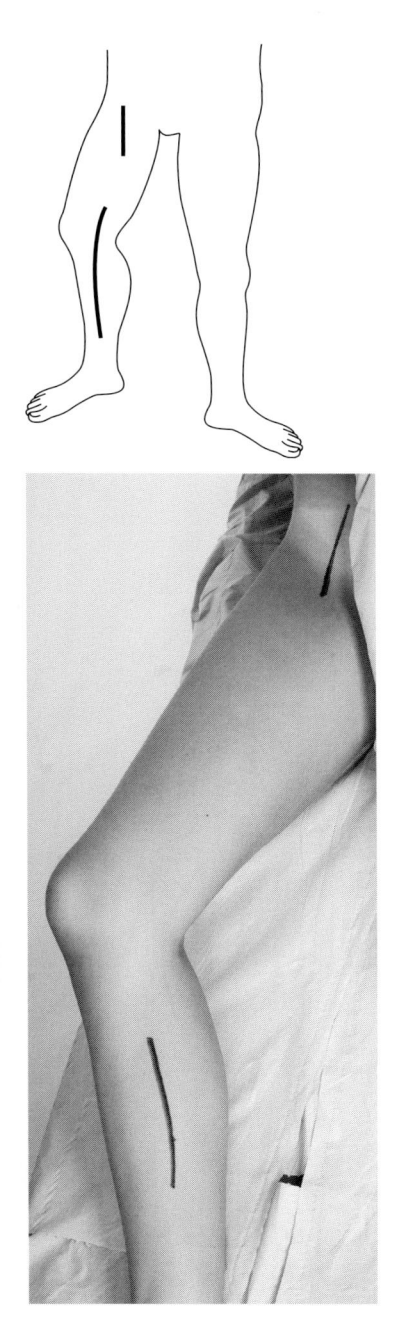

Lower limb revascularisation scars: femoro-distal bypass. Note this can be done using one long medial incision or through smaller 'skip' incisions reaching below the knee.

Can bypass grafts be palpated?

Grafts tunnelled subcutaneously may be palpable. Grafts tunnelled deeply may not be palpable, but the presence of pulses distal to them may suggest that they are patent. Bedside Doppler examination should be used to determine the patency of any graft.

What questions must be asked in the arterial examination of a limb?

1. What is the vascular anatomy?
2. What is the end-organ perfusion (tissue loss, function and viability)?
3. Is there infection?
4. Is the limb still viable?

What are Buerger's angle and test?

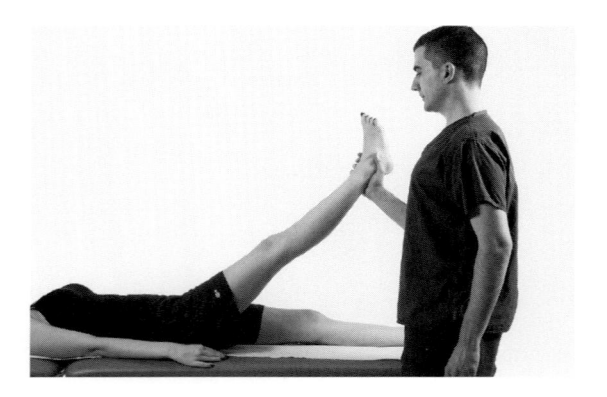

(A) Buerger's angle

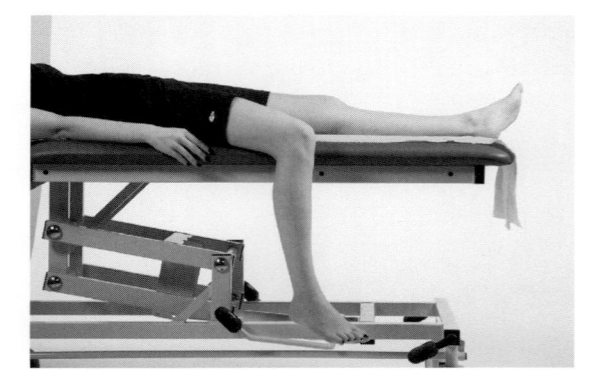

(B) Buerger's test.

Rationale: Identification of severe peripheral arterial disease.

Technique:
- Buerger's test involves straight leg elevation > 30° with the limb supported by the examiner
- Poor limb perfusion due to peripheral arterial disease will lead to impaired blood flow against the effect of gravity. This results in palor, venous guttering (due to absence of arterial inflow) and relative ischaemia of the affected limb.

Positive test:
- The angle at which the limb becomes pale is called Buerger's angle. The lower the angle, the greater the degree of ischaemia. In clinical practice this may be difficult to quantify.
- Once the limb has been elevated sufficiently, the patient is asked to stand or put legs in a dependent position. This causes a reactive hyperaemia (red discolouration) in the ischaemic leg due to reperfusion.
- Buerger's test is positive if a leg that was pale or dusky on elevation becomes hyperaemic on being placed in a dependent position.

Where are vascular bruits auscultated?

Note that this is not an accurate diagnostic method.

- Abdominal aorta (aneurysm): midline of abdomen above umbilicus.
- Renal arteries (renal artery stenosis): midclavicular line of the abdomen, above the umbilicus.
- Common femoral artery (stenosis): just below the midpoint of the inguinal ligament in the groin.
- Superficial femoral arteries (stenosis): in the subsartorial canal of the thigh (medial thigh, adductor compartment).

What are the crural vessels?

The term *crural vessels* describes the calf branches of the popliteal artery. The popliteal artery divides into the anterior tibial artery (ATA) and the tibioperoneal (TP) trunk. The tibioperoneal trunk further divides into the posterior tibial artery (PTA) and the peroneal artery (PA).

How are the crural vessels examined?

- Overall: capillary refill time.
- Specifically:
  - anterior tibial artery: dorsalis pedis pulse
  - posterior tibial artery: tibialis posterior pulse
  - peroneal artery: not readily palpable

How do you perform a brief neurological examination in the vascular examination?

- Sensory (touch sensation on foot): medial malleolus (L4), 1st metatarsal head (L5) and 5th metatarsal head (S1).
- Motor: ankle dorsiflexion (L4), toe dorsiflexion (L5), toe plantarflexion (S1–2).

How can suspected arterial disease be further investigated?

Bedside:

- ABPI: ankle–brachial pressure index (TBPI/toe–brachial pressure index in diabetes sufferers)
- PVR: pulse volume recording
- Doppler signal: triphasic, biphasic or monophasic waveforms

Specialist tests:

- Duplex ultrasound
- Angiography: computed tomography (CTA), magnetic resonance (MRA) or percutaneous diagnostic angiography
- Patients with renal failure or allergic to intravenous contrast can have CO_2 angiography

What clinical findings can be predicted from ABPI values?

> 0.95	normal
0.5–0.95	intermittent claudication
0.3–0.5	rest pain/critical ischaemia
< 0.2	ulcers and gangrene

What measurements can be performed in patients with diabetes and non-compressible vessels?

- Toe–brachial pressure index (TBPI).

What is PVR (pulse volume recording)?

PVR is a form of plethysmography which gives a graphical representation (waveforms) of blood flow through arteries.

How can the severity of acute ischaemia be determined?

Limb status	Sensory loss	Muscle weakness	Treatment
Viable	None	None	Treat as chronic limb ischaemia
Moderately threatened limb	Toes only	None	Angiography +/− thrombectomy or thrombolysis
Severely threatened limb	Proximal to toes/rest pain	Mild	Embolectomy/bypass
Irreversible	Paraesthesia	Paralysis	Amputation

Differential diagnoses

What are the causes of lower limb pain?

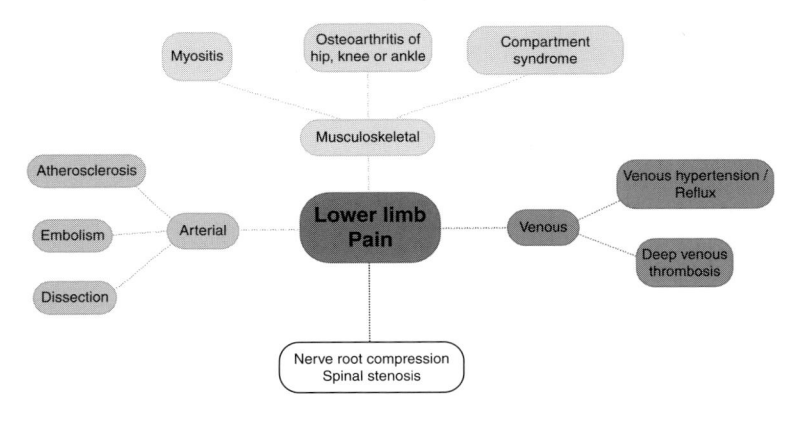

Lower limb Pain

- Musculoskeletal
  - Myositis
  - Osteoarthritis of hip, knee or ankle
  - Compartment syndrome
- Arterial
  - Atherosclerosis
  - Embolism
  - Dissection
- Venous
  - Venous hypertension / Reflux
  - Deep venous thrombosis
- Nerve root compression / Spinal stenosis

What are the causes of lower limb ischaemia?

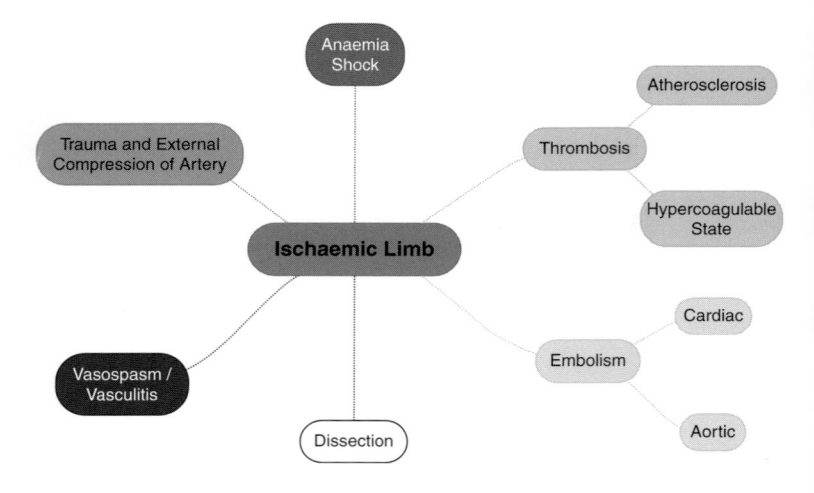

- **Ischaemic Limb**
  - Anaemia / Shock
  - Trauma and External Compression of Artery
  - Thrombosis
    - Atherosclerosis
    - Hypercoagulable State
  - Embolism
    - Cardiac
    - Aortic
  - Dissection
  - Vasospasm / Vasculitis

Section 6 **Vascular surgery**

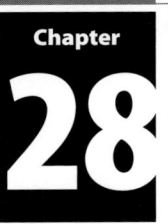

Chapter 28

Examination of the lower limb venous system

Petrut Gogalniceanu, William Lynn and Vijay M. Gadhvi

Checklist

WIPER
- Patient standing, legs and groins exposed

Physiological parameters

Inspection
- Limb girth/swelling/ankle oedema
- Scars:
  - groin: SFJ ligation
  - thigh: LSV stripping/endovenous ablation
  - calf: Stab phlebectomies
- Anatomical distribution of varicose veins:
  - long saphenous vein (LSV)
  - short saphenous vein (SSV)
  - anterior circumflex vein
  - intersaphenous vein
  - pudendal vein
- Skin complications of chronic venous hypertension (gaiter area/malleoli):
  - spider veins/venous telangiectasia
  - venous eczema
  - haemosiderin deposition

Physical Examination for Surgeons, ed. Petrut Gogalniceanu, James Pegrum and William Lynn. Published by Cambridge University Press. © Cambridge University Press 2015.

- lipodermatosclerosis
- venous ulcers
- scars from healed ulcers (atrophie blanche)

Palpation and percussion

- Groin: mass with a cough impulse suggestive of saphena varix
- Thigh: tap test (Chevrier's test)
- Calf and popliteal fossa: tenderness for DVT
- Ankle: pitting oedema
- Foot: dorsalis pedis pulse (check for adequate arterial perfusion)

Special tests

- Trendelenburg's test: SFJ/perforator incompetence
- Tourniquet test: SFJ/perforator incompetence
- Perthe's test: deep venous patency; tourniquet on calf then stand on toes
- ABPI

Auscultation

- Bruit at SFJ for arteriovenous fistula

To complete the examination…

- Abdominal exam: to rule out pregnancy or pelvic masses
- Doppler test: to identify superficial venous reflux
- Duplex ultrasound: to identify deep or superficial venous reflux, venous thrombosis and perforator incompetence

Examination notes
What is the anatomy of the superficial veins of the lower limb?

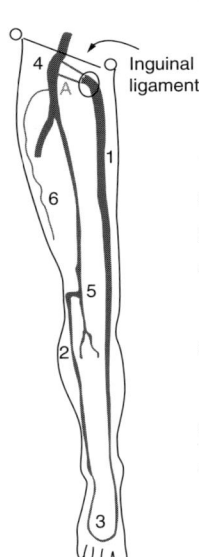

Lower limb venous anatomy.

1. Great or long saphenous vein
2. Lesser or short saphenous vein
3. Dorsal venous arch of the foot
4. Common femoral vein (receiving profunda femoris vein and superficial femoral vein)
5. Popliteal vein (Receiving anterior and posterior tibial veins)
6. Anterior thigh vein

A Sapheno-femoral junction (SFJ)

What are the symptoms of chronic venous disease?
- Leg ache, heaviness, tightness or bursting pain associated with prolonged periods of standing
- Skin irritation or itchiness
- Leg swelling

What is the CEAP classification?
The CEAP classification is a global method of describing the burden of venous disease, based on:
- **C**linical presentation (e.g. reticular veins, oedema, ulcers)
- **A**etiology (e.g. primary vs. secondary)
- **A**natomy (e.g. superfical, perforator, deep venous involvement)
- **P**athophysiology (e.g. reflux vs. obstruction)

What are the main disease processes that need to be identified?

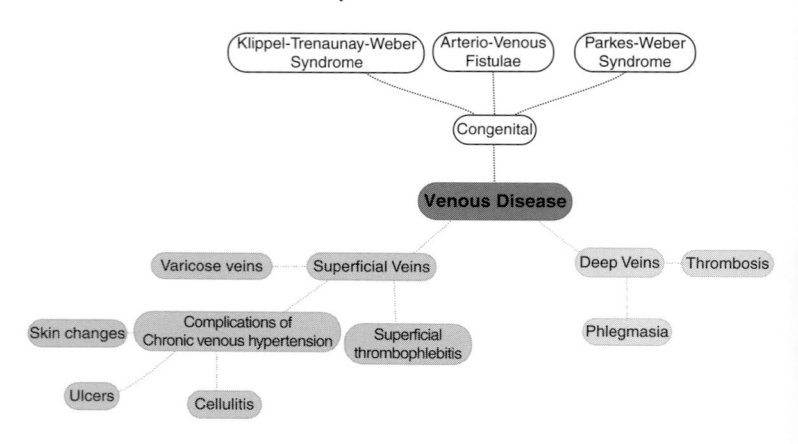

- Venous Disease
  - Congenital
    - Klippel-Trenaunay-Weber Syndrome
    - Arterio-Venous Fistulae
    - Parkes-Weber Syndrome
  - Superficial Veins
    - Varicose veins
      - Complications of Chronic venous hypertension
        - Skin changes
        - Ulcers
        - Cellulitis
    - Superficial thrombophlebitis
  - Deep Veins
    - Thrombosis
    - Phlegmasia

What are the main perforator/communicating veins called?
- Thigh – Dodd
- Gastrocnemius – Boyd
- Calf – Cockett
- Ankle – Kuster or May

Why should the arterial system be assessed in patients with varicose veins?
- Compression therapy for varicose veins can only be used in patients without peripheral arterial disease.
- Any planned surgery for varicose veins in the lower limb cannot be performed in the presence of significant arterial disease, because of the risk of wound non-healing.
- Always check foot pulses and ABPI.

What is phlegmasia caerulea dolens?
Phlegmasia caerulea dolens is a tender, blue discolouration of the entire limb. This is caused by acute massive venous thrombosis and obstruction of the entire venous system of the limb. It may extend proximally into the iliofemoral

veins. In the short term it can lead to limb-threatening venous gangrene (ischaemia) and life-threatening pulmonary embolism. In the long term it can cause post-thrombotic limb syndrome due to venous valve damage and deep venous incompetence.

What nerve travels with the long saphenous vein?
The saphenous nerve.

What nerve travels with the short saphenous vein?
The sural nerve.

How do you inspect for varicose veins?
The patient must always be standing, preferably on an examination stool/step. The inspection has four main end points:

- Has there been previous surgery for varicose veins? SFJ ligation is often performed through a groin-crease incision, which can be easily missed. Ensure you expose the groin adequately and stretch the groin-crease skin open with two fingers.
- Are there any varicose veins? Determine their anatomical distribution and the vein from which they arise. Inspect all aspects of the leg by asking the patient to turn 360°.
- Are there any skin changes caused by chronic venous hypertension?
- Is there any evidence of deep venous hypertension (thrombosis or reflux)?

Where is the saphenofemoral junction (SFJ) located?
Palpate the pubic tubercle. The SFJ is found 2–4 cm (2 fingers' breadths) inferior and 2–4 cm lateral to the pubic tubercle.

How do you perform a cough test?
Rationale: The aim is to identify incompetence of the SFJ valve.

Technique: Palpation is done just distal to the SFJ in the proximal long saphenous vein. The patient is asked to cough.

Positive test: In the presence of an incompetent SFJ, a cough impulse will be palpated in the vein upstream from the SFJ (lower in the leg).

How do you perform Chevrier's test (also described as Schwartz/tap/percussion test)?

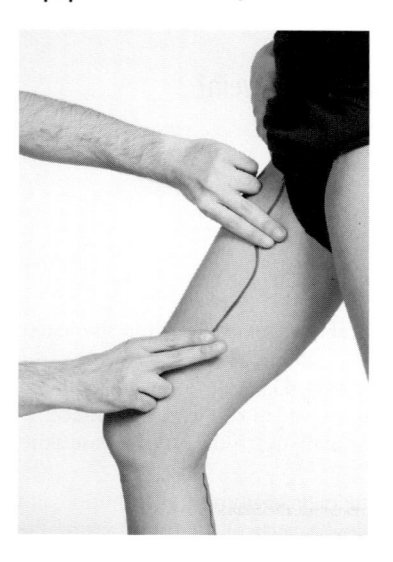

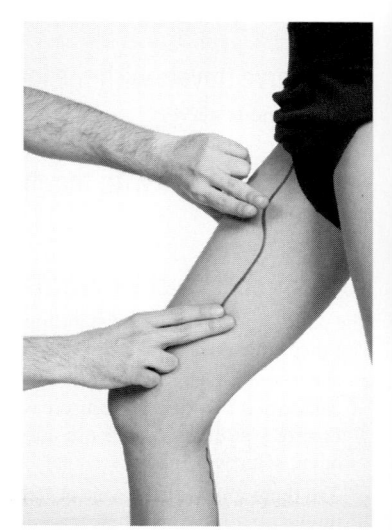

Rationale: Chevrier's test determines whether the superficial venous valves are incompetent or not. Venous blood should flow from the foot upwards towards the groin. Retrograde flow (from groin towards foot) suggests incompetence of veins.

Technique: The patient is standing. The right hand of the examiner taps dilated veins in the proximal thigh. The left hand feels for a transmitted (retrograde) impulse in the veins of the lower leg.

Positive test: A detectable impulse in the lower leg suggests that the venous valves in the vein between the examiner's hands are incompetent.

How do you perform Trendelenburg's test (vascular)?

Rationale: The test aims to identify the level at which incompetent perforators are found in the leg.

Technique:

- The patient is supine. The leg is elevated and the veins are massaged in order to drain blood from them.

- The SFJ is manually compressed. Pressure is maintained on the SFJ and the patient is asked to stand.

Positive test: If the varicose veins fail to refill whilst pressure is maintained, this suggests that venous incompetence occurs at the level of the SFJ (pressure on the vein simulates a competent valve).

How do you perform the tourniquet test?

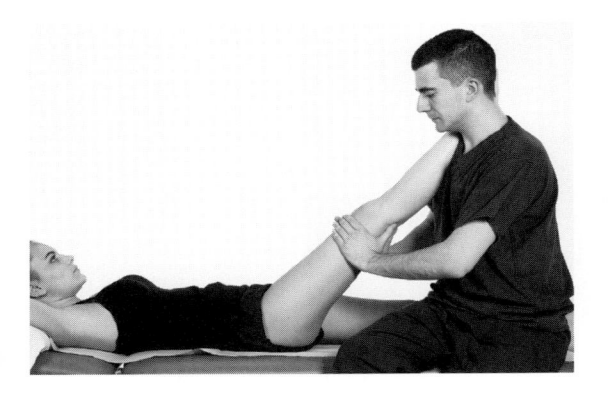

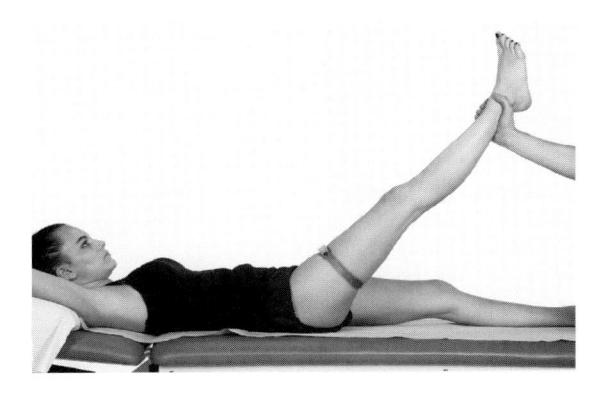

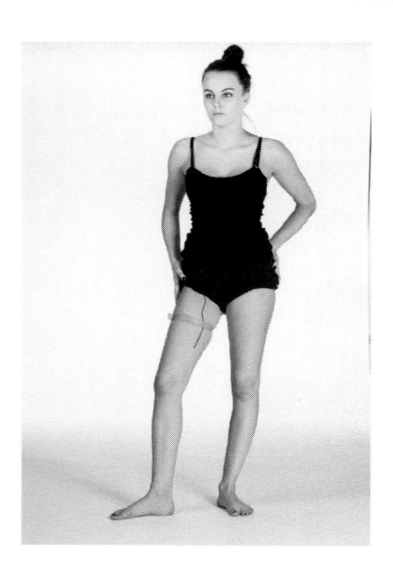

Rationale: The test aims to identify the level at which incompetent perforators are found in the leg. It is similar to Trendelenburg's test, but differs in that a tourniquet is used to apply pressure at various levels in the leg.

Technique:

- The patient is supine. The leg is elevated and the veins are massaged in order to drain blood from them.
- A tourniquet is applied in the upper thigh. The patient is asked to stand with the tourniquet on.

Positive test:

- If the varicose veins fail to refill whilst the tourniquet is on, it suggests that venous incompetence occurs at or above the level of the tourniquet (the tourniquet simulates a competent valve).
- If the varicose veins refill, the test is repeated with the tourniquet being applied at the level of the next distal perforator in the thigh. The test is repeated at subsequent perforator levels until the tourniquet controls venous refilling.

How do you perform Perthe's test?

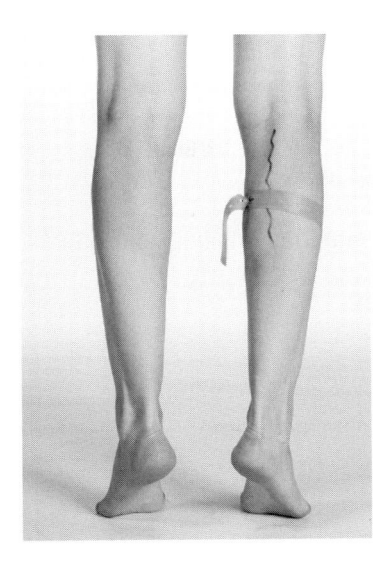

Rationale: In thrombosis of the deep venous system, the superficial veins provide the only venous return from the lower limb. Consequently, varicose veins develop due to increased venous pressure. Ablation of superficial varicose veins in the context of complete thrombosis of the deep venous system is contraindicated, as it eliminates the principal method of draining the lower limb. Perthe's test aims to determine whether the deep venous system is patent or not, and therefore whether it is safe to ablate superficial varicosities. Its aim is to simulate destruction of the superficial veins in order to determine whether the deep veins are patent.

Technique: The patient is standing, with the varicose veins distended. A tourniquet is placed around the upper calf to obstruct flow through the superficial veins. The patient is asked to exercise the calf muscles by repeatedly standing on the tips of the toes.

Positive test:
- Venous drainage should occur preferentially through the deep veins.
- If these are thrombosed the patient develops pain in the leg, indicating that ablation of the superficial veins should not be undertaken.

- If the deep and communicating veins are patent, the varicose veins below the tourniquet will empty into the deep system and reduce in size.

How do you assess for an arteriovenous fistula?
- The affected limb may be enlarged or warmer than the unaffected limb.
- Palpate for a thrill over the varicosities.
- Manual occlusion of the feeding artery leads to a reflex bradycardia.
- Auscultate for a machine-like bruit over the SFJ.

What are the features of Klippel–Trénaunay–Weber syndrome?
- Varicose veins
- Port wine stains
- Poorly developed lymphatics
- Lower limb bone and soft tissue hypertrophy

What are the features of Parkes–Weber syndrome?
- Limb hypertrophy
- Multiple arteriovenous fistulas

What is Homans' sign?
- In patients with deep vein thrombosis, dorsiflexion of the foot causes pain in the calf due to tension on the posterior tibial vein. This test is currently not used, because of the potential risk of dislodging the thrombus and causing a PE.

Section 6 | Vascular surgery

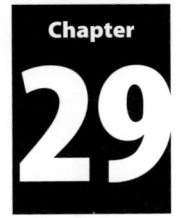

Chapter 29

Examination of ulcers

Petrut Gogalniceanu, William Lynn and Vijay M. Gadhvi

Checklist

WIPER

Physiological parameters

System
- **S-E-I-S** (Site, External, Internal, Surroundings)

Site
- Location and distribution: arterial/venous/pressure area

External
- Number of lesions
- Size
- Shape/contour/margin
- Depth
- Colour
- Discharge

Internal
- Edge: sloping, punched out, undermined, rolled, everted
- Base: healthy, sloughy, necrotic, avascular
- Floor: bone, tendon, muscle
- Sensation: sensate or insensate

Physical Examination for Surgeons, ed. Petrut Gogalniceanu, James Pegrum and William Lynn. Published by Cambridge University Press. © Cambridge University Press 2015.

Surroundings
- Identify cellulitis, abscesses or excoriation.
- Look for chronic venous changes.
- Look for signs of peripheral arterial disease.
- Palpate pulses and capillary refill time (CRT) to rule our peripheral arterial disease.
- Palpate regional lymph nodes for lymphadenopathy.
- Check sensation to rule out neuropathy.

To complete the examination...
- Examine contralateral side.
- Perform an ABPI to rule out peripheral arterial disease.
- Perform a venous Duplex scan to identify venous reflux.
- Check blood and urine glucose levels to rule out diabetes.

Examination notes

What are the common ulcers in a surgical examination?
- Arterial
- Venous
- Neuropathic/diabetic
- Malignant

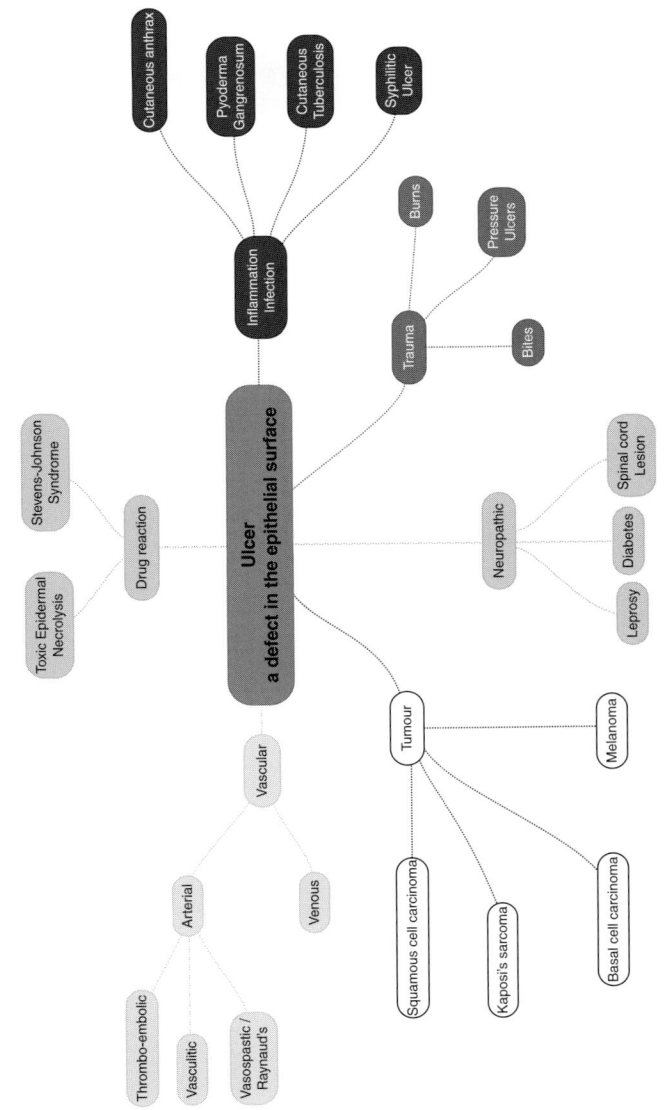

What are the causes of ulcers?

Ulcer — a defect in the epithelial surface

- **Inflammation / Infection**
  - Cutaneous anthrax
  - Pyoderma Gangrenosum
  - Cutaneous Tuberculosis
  - Syphilitic Ulcer
- **Trauma**
  - Burns
  - Pressure Ulcers
  - Bites
- **Neuropathic**
  - Leprosy
  - Diabetes
  - Spinal cord Lesion
- **Tumour**
  - Squamous cell carcinoma
  - Kaposi's sarcoma
  - Basal cell carcinoma
  - Melanoma
- **Vascular**
  - Arterial
    - Thrombo-embolic
    - Vasculitic
    - Vasospastic / Raynaud's
  - Venous
- **Drug reaction**
  - Stevens–Johnson Syndrome
  - Toxic Epidermal Necrolysis

249

How can the aetiology of an ulcer be deduced from the examination findings?

	Arterial	Venous	Neuropathic	Diabetic	Malignant
Location	Distal areas: heels, tips of toes, metatarsal heads, dorsal and plantar aspects of foot	Gaiter area: medial and lateral malleoli and lower legs	Pressure areas: heels, metatarsal heads, toe tips	Variable	Variable
Edge	Punched out, deep	Sloping, shallow	Punched out, deep	Variable	Rolled, everted, irregular or pigmented
Base	Bloodless, pale or necrotic	Sloughy, pink or bleeding	Pink or bleeding	Sloughy, necrotic	Indurated, hard
Sensation	Painful	Painful	Insensate (stocking distribution)	May be insensate	Normal
Surroundings	Cold limb, reduced capillary refill time	Chronic venous changes	Foot deformity / Charcot's joint	Cellulitis	Satellite lesion, lymphadenopathy
Pulses	Absent	Present (unless mixed arteriovenous), foot well perfused	Variable	Variable	Present
ABPI	Low	Normal	Normal	High	Normal

Chapter 29: Examination of ulcers | 251

What can be deduced from the ulcer edge?

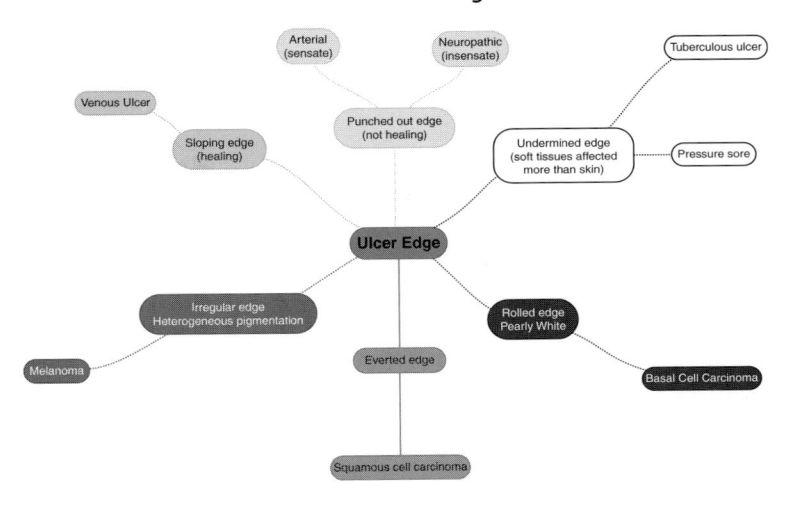

- **Ulcer Edge**
  - **Sloping edge (healing)** — Venous Ulcer
  - **Punched out edge (not healing)** — Arterial (sensate), Neuropathic (insensate)
  - **Undermined edge (soft tissues affected more than skin)** — Tuberculous ulcer, Pressure sore
  - **Rolled edge, Pearly White** — Basal Cell Carcinoma
  - **Everted edge** — Squamous cell carcinoma
  - **Irregular edge, Heterogeneous pigmentation** — Melanoma

What features of an ulcer base can lead to a diagnosis?

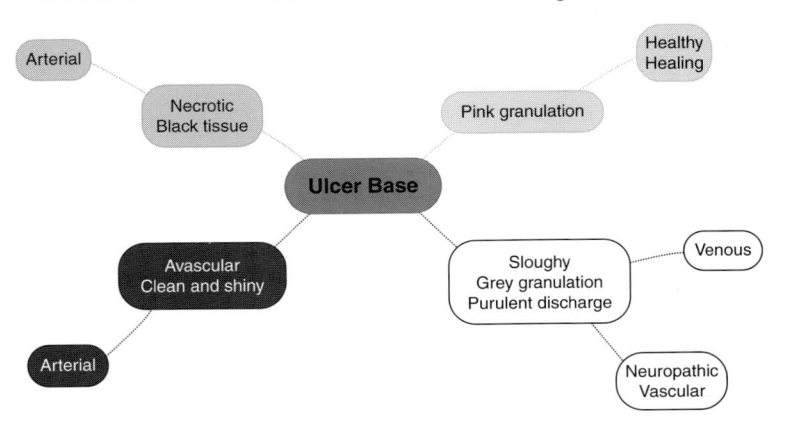

- **Ulcer Base**
  - **Necrotic Black tissue** — Arterial
  - **Pink granulation** — Healthy Healing
  - **Sloughy, Grey granulation, Purulent discharge** — Venous, Neuropathic Vascular
  - **Avascular, Clean and shiny** — Arterial

How is an ulcer diagnosed?

Ask three questions:

1. Where is the ulcer?
2. Is there evidence of ischaemia/absent pulses?
3. Is there loss of sensation?

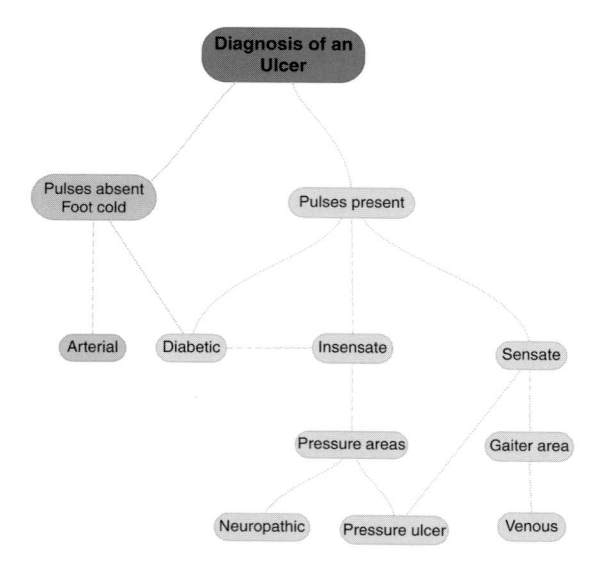

```
                    Diagnosis of an
                        Ulcer

     Pulses absent                Pulses present
       Foot cold

  Arterial    Diabetic     Insensate         Sensate

                          Pressure areas    Gaiter area

                  Neuropathic   Pressure ulcer   Venous
```

What are the causes of gangrene?

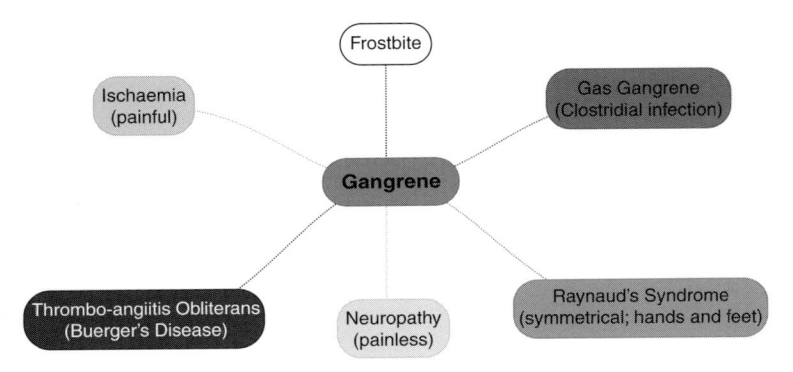

- Frostbite
- Ischaemia (painful)
- Gas Gangrene (Clostridial infection)
- Thrombo-angiitis Obliterans (Buerger's Disease)
- Neuropathy (painless)
- Raynaud's Syndrome (symmetrical; hands and feet)

What ulcers are most variable in their presentation?

Diabetic ulcers have the most variable sensation, arterial supply and concomitant infections on physical examination.

What is the difference between the base and the floor of an ulcer?

The base describes the pathological state of the ulcer's surface (e.g. slough). The floor describes the anatomical structures involved in the ulcer's base (e.g. bone or tendons).

What can be deduced from the ulcer floor?

The presence of tendons, bone or large vessels on the floor of an ulcer would suggest that skin grafting would not be recommended.

What signs of chronic venous hypertension should be assessed?

- Varicose veins in the long (great) and short (lesser) saphenous vein distribution
- Ankle oedema
- Flare veins, haemosiderin deposits, lipodermatosclerosis and venous eczema

What signs of peripheral arterial disease should be assessed?
The presence of peripheral arterial disease needs to be excluded in all ulcers, even if there is convincing evidence that the aetiology is primarily venous, neuropathic or diabetic.

- Assess all pulses.
- Check capillary refill time and limb warmth.
- Look for trophic changes in the nails and secondary hair loss.
- Perform ABPI in all patients.

How are arterial ulcers investigated?
- ABPI
- Duplex ultrasound
- CTA/MRA
- DSA

How are venous ulcers investigated?
- Doppler (bedside): identify venous reflux in LSV and SSV.
- Duplex US (vascular lab): identify patency and reflux in deep (iliac, femoral, popliteal and tibial) and superficial (LSV and SSV) veins.

Why is the ABPI often elevated in diabetic ulcers?
Calcium deposition within the wall of the artery renders it more difficult to compress, resulting in a higher ABPI, which may not accurately reflect the arterial inflow to the ulcerated area.

Section editor: Martin T. Yates
Senior author: Ian Hunt

Section 7: Heart and thorax

Chapter 30: Examination of the thorax and lungs

Martin T. Yates, Petrut Gogalniceanu and Ian Hunt

Checklist

WIPER
- Patient sitting on edge of examination couch with all clothing above the waist removed

Physiological parameters

General
- End of bed: shortness of breath, wheeze
- Bedside: sputum pot, bedside oxygen, cigarettes, inhalers
- Hands: nicotine staining and finger clubbing
- Face: Horner's syndrome (ptosis and meiosis) and venous engorgement of head and neck veins

Inspection
- Neck: lymphadenopathy, low transverse cervical scar for mediastinoscopy, tracheostomy scar, tuberculous abscesses
- Chest wall deformities: pectus excavatum (pushed in) or pectus carinatum (pushed out)
- Chest movement: asymmetry of expansion, contraction of one side of the chest wall, paradoxical movement (flail chest)

Physical Examination for Surgeons, ed. Petrut Gogalniceanu, James Pegrum and William Lynn. Published by Cambridge University Press. © Cambridge University Press 2015.

- Scars: midline sternotomy, lateral/posterior/posterolateral thoracotomy, small scars (video-assisted thoracoscopic surgery or chest drains)
- Radiotherapy tattoos
- Chest drains

Palpation
- Neck: lymphadenopathy, goitre, position of trachea
- Chest: sternal tenderness or instability, rib tenderness, asymmetry of expansion

Percussion
- Chest wall: resonant, dull or hyper-resonant

Auscultation
- Chest wall: breath sounds (vesicular, crackles, wheeze, reduced air entry)

To complete the examination...
- Bedside spirometry
- Chest x-ray

Examination notes

What are the basic thoracic and pulmonary symptoms?

The main symptoms of thoracic disease are shortness of breath, fatigue, wheeze, stridor, cough, sputum production, haemoptysis, chest pain and voice hoarseness.

How do you prepare for the examination of the thorax?

The patient needs to be sitting on the edge of the examination couch, exposed from the waist up.

What do you look for during inspection?

- Start the examination by inspecting the hands. Look for nicotine stains from cigarette smoking (risk factor for lung malignancy) and finger clubbing (a possible sign of malignancy or chronic lung disease).
- Move up to the face, looking at the eyes for evidence of ptosis (drooping of the eyelid) and meiosis (a constricted pupil), which are signs of Horner's syndrome. This may be caused by a Pancoast's tumour originating from the superior sulcus of the lung.

Chapter 30: Examination of the thorax and lungs | 257

- Distended neck veins may indicate obstruction of the superior vena cava (SVC).
- A low transverse scar just above the sternal notch may suggest previous mediastinoscopy performed for biopsy of suspicious lymph nodes in the mediastinum. This can be undertaken in patients with primary lung cancer, haematological malignancies or interstitial lung disease. It must not be confused with a tracheostomy scar, which is generally higher in the neck, over the trachea.
- On the chest wall look for scars from front, side and back, asking the patient to raise his or her arms to specifically look in the axilla.
- Look for tattoos from radiotherapy and chest drain scars.
- Increasingly, thoracic surgical procedures are performed as 'keyhole' operations, known as VATS (video-assisted thoracoscopic surgery). Several small incisions in the lateral part of the chest (mid-axillary line) may suggest this approach.
- A small pleural drain may be tunnelled under the skin into the pleural cavity for palliation of symptomatic pleural effusion.
- Ask the patient to take a deep breath in and out and look at the expansion of both sides of the chest. Compare for asymmetry.

What are the common scars in thoracic surgery?

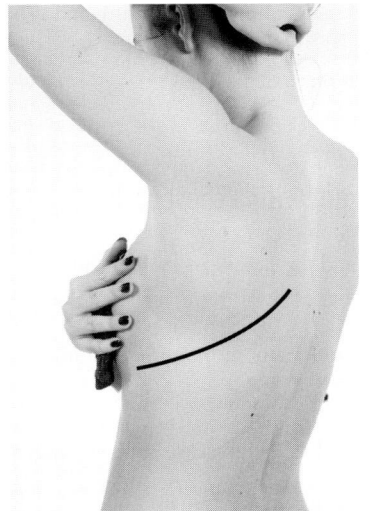

Left posterolateral thoracotomy.

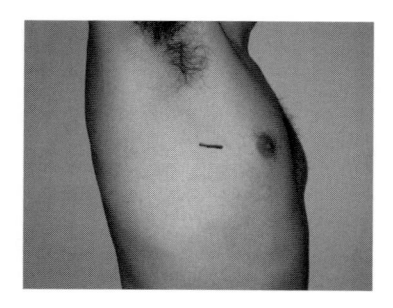

Right-sided chest drain scar in the 5th intercostal space, anterior to the mid-axillary line.

- Posterolateral thoracotomy (5th intercostal space) to access the lungs and pleura
- Anterolateral thoracotomy (5th intercostal space) to access heart and pleural cavity
- Clamshell (bilateral 5th intercostal spaces) for trauma or transplantation
- 2 cm transverse incision above sternal notch for mediastinoscopy for lung cancer staging
- Video-assisted thoracoscopic surgery (VATS):
  - 3 cm incision in 3rd intercostal spaces in the anterior axillary line with two or three other 1 cm incisions in 6th intercostal spaces
  - one to four ports are typically used, depending on procedure and pathology
- Chest drains (5th intercostal space anterior axillary line)
- Tattoos for radiotherapy

What are the basic checks for a patient with a chest drain?

1. **What is being drained?**
   Establish the need for chest drainage and the nature of the effluent:
   - air (pneumothorax) via a flutter valve or chest drain bottle with a water seal
   - fluid (effusion)/pus (empyema)/blood (haemothorax) into a stoma bag or chest drain bottle with a water seal

2. **Is the drain on suction?**
   Establish if the drain is on suction as well as the pressure applied (routine suction pressure −5 kPa).

3. **Is the drain 'swinging'?**
   Movement of fluid in the drain on inspiration/expiration suggests that the drain is in continuity with the thoracic cavity and is therefore working.
4. **Is there an air leak?**
   Establish if there is air bubbling during normal breathing, talking and coughing:
   a. on breathing suggests a large air leak
   b. on talking suggests a moderate air leak
   c. on coughing suggests a small air leak

There has been an increased use of devices that offer a digital readout of air-leak rate and suction applied.

What do you palpate when examining the thorax?

- Stand behind the patient, who is sitting upright.
- Palpate systematically for cervical lymphadenopathy, and specifically feel in the supraclavicular areas for masses. It is unusual for lung cancer to metastasise to cervical nodes, but they can be associated with other pathology in the thorax and neck such as TB, head and neck cancers or lymphoma. Lymphadenopathy in the supraclavicular area can be seen in patients presenting with an advanced stage of lung cancer (classically small-cell lung cancer), or lymphoma.
- Palpate for a thyroid goitre, which can extend into the mediastinum.
- Place your hands on the patient's back with your thumbs touching. Ask the patient to take a deep breath in and feel for expansion, looking for asymmetry.

What do you percuss when examining the thorax?

You should percuss both the front and back of the chest whilst the patient breathes normally. You should feel for dullness (effusion or consolidation) or hyper-resonance (pneumothorax), comparing one side to the other.

What do you auscultate on examining the thorax?

Listen both front and back, comparing sides. Auscultate bilaterally, assessing for reduced air entry of consolidation, pleural effusion, or collapse associated with central mass. A completely dull chest on one side associated with thoracotomy scar suggests a previous pneumonectomy.

Differential diagnoses

What are the causes of haemoptysis?

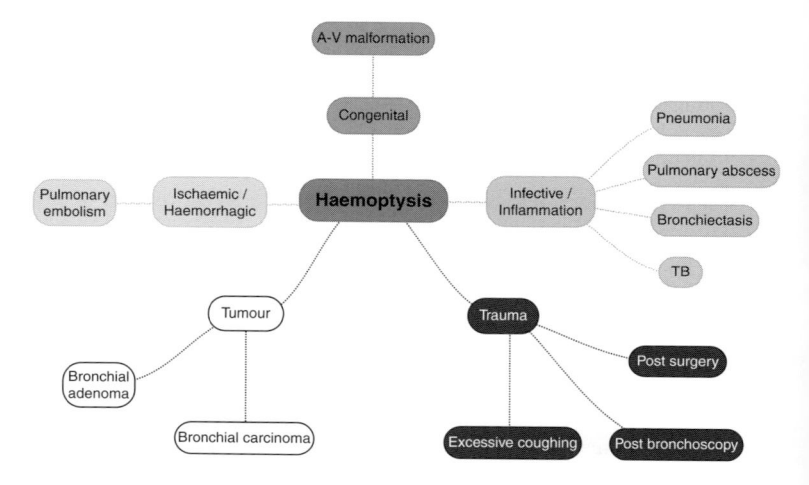

- **Haemoptysis**
  - Congenital
    - A-V malformation
  - Ischaemic / Haemorrhagic
    - Pulmonary embolism
  - Infective / Inflammation
    - Pneumonia
    - Pulmonary abscess
    - Bronchiectasis
    - TB
  - Tumour
    - Bronchial adenoma
    - Bronchial carcinoma
  - Trauma
    - Post surgery
    - Post bronchoscopy
    - Excessive coughing

What are the causes of a discharging chest wall sinus/lesion?

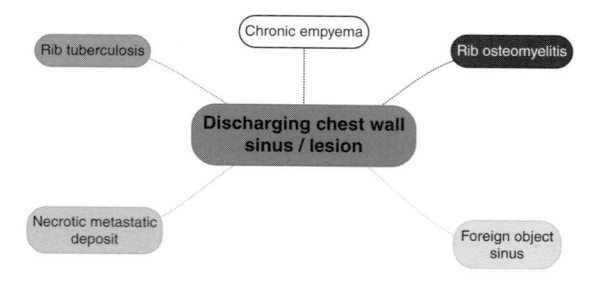

- **Discharging chest wall sinus / lesion**
  - Chronic empyema
  - Rib tuberculosis
  - Rib osteomyelitis
  - Necrotic metastatic deposit
  - Foreign object sinus

Chapter 30: Examination of the thorax and lungs

What are the causes of SVC obstruction?

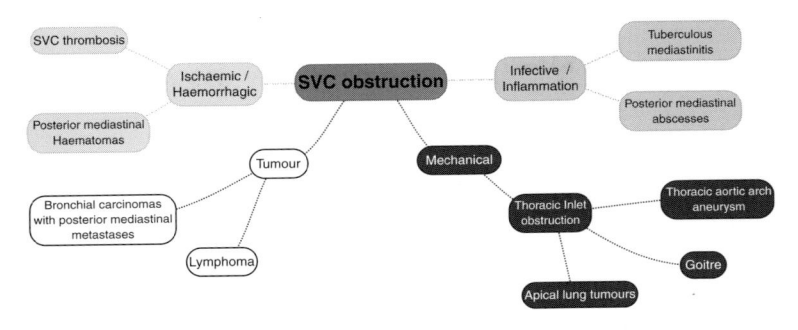

SVC obstruction

- **Ischaemic / Haemorrhagic**
  - SVC thrombosis
  - Posterior mediastinal Haematomas
- **Tumour**
  - Bronchial carcinomas with posterior mediastinal metastases
  - Lymphoma
- **Infective / Inflammation**
  - Tuberculous mediastinitis
  - Posterior mediastinal abscesses
- **Mechanical**
  - **Thoracic Inlet obstruction**
    - Thoracic aortic arch aneurysm
    - Goitre
    - Apical lung tumours

What is the differential diagnosis of SVC obstruction?
Cardiac tamponade and acute heart failure.

What are the causes of a haemothorax?

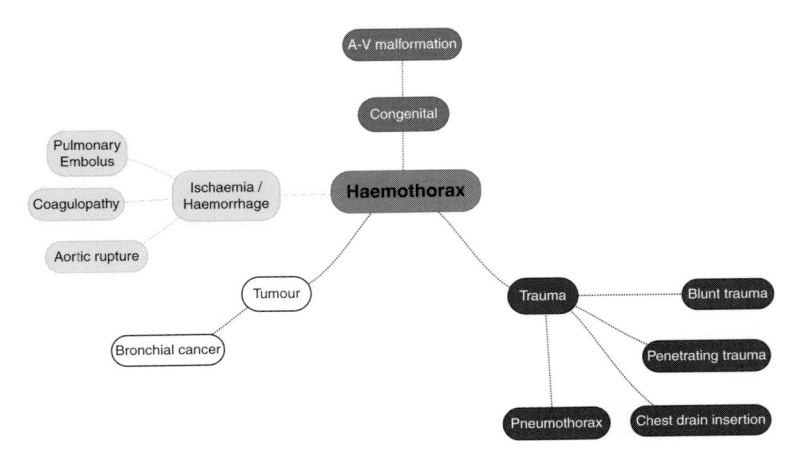

Haemothorax

- **Congenital**
  - A-V malformation
- **Ischaemia / Haemorrhage**
  - Pulmonary Embolus
  - Coagulopathy
  - Aortic rupture
- **Tumour**
  - Bronchial cancer
- **Trauma**
  - Blunt trauma
  - Penetrating trauma
  - Chest drain insertion
  - Pneumothorax

What are the causes of a pneumothorax?

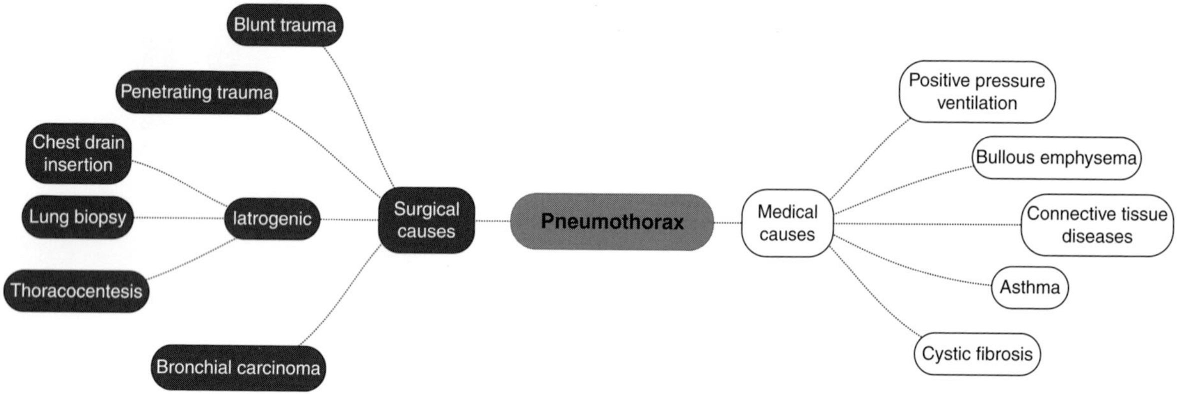

- **Pneumothorax**
  - **Medical causes**
    - Positive pressure ventilation
    - Bullous emphysema
    - Connective tissue diseases
    - Asthma
    - Cystic fibrosis
  - **Surgical causes**
    - Blunt trauma
    - Penetrating trauma
    - Iatrogenic
      - Chest drain insertion
      - Lung biopsy
      - Thoracocentesis
    - Bronchial carcinoma

Chapter 30: Examination of the thorax and lungs | 263

What are the causes of surgical emphysema?

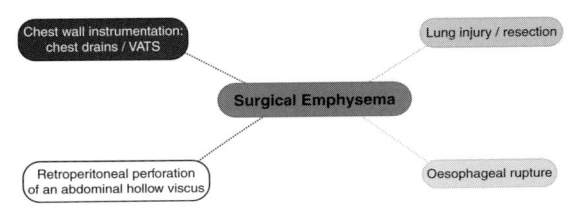

- **Surgical Emphysema**
  - Chest wall instrumentation: chest drains / VATS
  - Lung injury / resection
  - Oesophageal rupture
  - Retroperitoneal perforation of an abdominal hollow viscus

What are the causes of tracheal deviation?

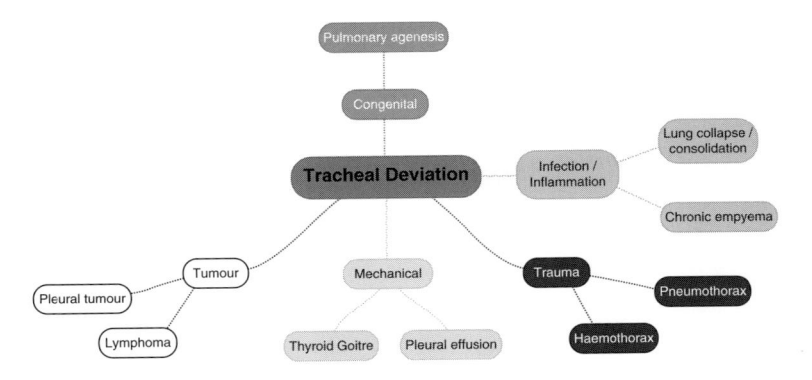

- **Tracheal Deviation**
  - Congenital
    - Pulmonary agenesis
  - Infection / Inflammation
    - Lung collapse / consolidation
    - Chronic empyema
  - Tumour
    - Pleural tumour
    - Lymphoma
  - Mechanical
    - Thyroid Goitre
    - Pleural effusion
  - Trauma
    - Pneumothorax
    - Haemothorax

Section 7: Heart and thorax

Chapter 31: Examination of the heart and great vessels

Martin T. Yates, Petrut Gogalniceanu and Ian Hunt

Checklist

WIPER
- Patient sitting on edge of examination couch with all clothing above the waist removed

Physiological parameters

General
- Bedside: GTN spray, cigarettes, oxygen
- Cachexia: severe mitral valve disease
- Morbidly obese: cor pulmonale

Inspection
- Hands: nicotine stains, radial artery harvest
- Neck: JVP
- Chest wall : scars of previous chest surgery (midline, lateral and posterior)
- Legs: groin incisions, varicose veins, scars from vein harvest

Palpation
- Hands: radial artery pulse: rate and rhythm
- Neck: carotid pulse, pulsatile trachea (aortic arch aneurysm), carotid–carotid or carotid–subclavian bypass, visible JVP
- Chest wall: apex beat, heaves, thrills, pacemaker, implantable defibrillator

---

Physical Examination for Surgeons, ed. Petrut Gogalniceanu, James Pegrum and William Lynn. Published by Cambridge University Press. © Cambridge University Press 2015.

- Sacrum: sacral oedema
- Legs : peripheral oedema, radio-femoral delay

Auscultation
- Carotid artery: bruit
- Precordium: heart sounds, murmurs, pericardial rub
- Lung bases: effusion, pulmonary oedema

To complete the examination. . .
- Chest x-ray
- ECG

Examination notes

What are the basic cardiac symptoms?

The main symptoms of cardiac disease are chest pain, shortness of breath, ankle swelling, orthopnoea, paroxysmal nocturnal dyspnoea, palpitations and syncope.

How do you prepare for the examination of the cardiac surgery patient?

The patient needs to be lying at 45° in underwear on the examination couch. The groins are covered but the legs are exposed.

What do you inspect in the examination of the heart?

- Jugular venous pressure (JVP). The patient is positioned at 45° with the head slightly turned to the contralateral side. Look for the JVP wave form and the height above the sternal notch. It should normally be seen 3 cm vertically above the sternal angle. A raised JVP is associated with congestive cardiac failure, pericardial tamponade or constrictive pericarditis.
  A collapsed JVP is caused by dehydration or shock.
- Identify scars from previous carotid endarterectomy.
- Inspect the chest for scars from previous cardiac or thoracic surgery.
- Inspect the legs for scars from previous saphenous vein harvest or varicose vein avulsions.
- The groins must be checked for evidence of previous vascular or endovascular surgery or percutaneous intervention.
- At the beginning or end of the examination the patient should be asked to stand, to look for varicose veins.

What do you palpate in the examination of the heart?

- Palpate the radial arteries bilaterally. Feel for rate and rhythm of the pulse. Identify a radio-radial delay. This signifies that there is a discrepancy in the blood flow between the right and left upper limbs. Possible causes include subclavian artery dissection, thrombosis or external compression, or aortic arch pathology such as coarctation of the aorta or aortic dissection. Aortic pathology distal to the origin of left subclavian artery will also cause a radio-femoral delay.

> **Tip**
>
> If assessing a radio-radial or radio-femoral delay, ensure that the distal arm pulses are present, in case you are palpating a locally damaged radial artery (e.g. following catheterisation).

- Palpate the carotid pulse and assess the character.
- In the thorax use your forefingers to palpate the apex beat of the heart. This is normally found in the 5th intercostal space in the mid-clavicular line. In cardiomegaly the apex beat moves laterally. If the apex beat is absent, feel for a right-sided apex beat in patients with dextrocardia.
- The palm of the hand is then placed on the left and right side of the sternum to feel for heaves or thrills.
- Palpate for pitting oedema in the pre-tibial region. If there is oedema, determine the level it extends to from the thigh, groin and back.
- The femoral artery should be palpated simultaneously with the right radial artery for a radio-femoral delay. A delay may be caused by aortic occlusion or dissection.

What do you auscultate in the examination of the heart?

- Auscultate the carotid arteries bilaterally for a bruit, followed by auscultation of the four areas of the precordium in the anterior chest wall. This assesses the four heart valves and pericardium. Remember that the auscultation areas do not coincide with the anatomical position of the valves but are the areas where the murmurs from these valves are best heard.

Valve	Site of auscultation
Aortic	2nd ICS, right sternal edge
Pulmonary	3rd ICS, left sternal edge
Tricuspid	4th ICS, left sternal edge
Mitral	5th ICS, left mid-clavicular line

- Complete the examination by auscultating the lung bases for signs of pulmonary oedema.

How do you differentiate murmurs?

- Palpate the carotid pulse whilst auscultating the heart sounds to determine if the murmur is systolic or diastolic.
- Systolic murmurs should then be differentiated into pan-systolic (mitral regurgitation, if left sided) and ejection systolic (aortic stenosis, if left sided).
- Diastolic murmurs are heard from blood flowing through a valve during diastole. On the left side of the heart these are due to either mitral stenosis or aortic regurgitation.

When might carotid–carotid or carotid–subclavian bypasses be used?

Revascularisation of the left subclavian (carotid–subclavian bypass) or left common carotid (carotid–carotid bypass) arteries is performed to allow endovascular management of proximal aortic arch aneurysms, which involves occlusion of the aortic arch vessels by an endoprosthesis.

What are the common scars in cardiac surgery?

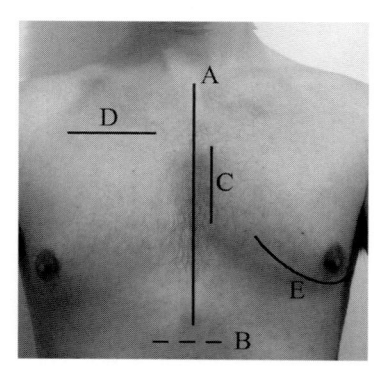

Common scars in cardiac surgery: (A) median sternotomy scar; (B) three chest drain scars associated with cardiac surgery (one draining the pericardial space and one in each pleural cavity); (C) mini sternotomy (aorta and aortic valve access); (D) 2nd intercostal space mini thoracotomy (atrial septal defect or aortic valve surgery); (E) 5th intercostal space mini thoracotomy (minimally invasive CABG).

- Median sternotomy: most common incision to access heart and great vessels.
- Mini sternotomy: smaller midline scar commonly used to access aorta and aortic valve.
- Right 2nd intercostal space mini thoracotomy: access to aortic valve or atrial septal defect (ASD).
- Left 5th intercostal space mini thoracotomy: minimally invasive CABG or transapical transcatheter aortic valve implantation.
- Subxiphisternal scars: three stab wound scars from three chest drains placed following CABG surgery.
- Anterior aspect of forearm: radial artery harvest.
- Medial aspect of leg: long saphenous vein harvest.
- Posterior calf: short saphenous vein harvest.
- Groin incisions: cannulation for cardiopulmonary bypass for minimally invasive surgery, re-do surgery, surgery on thoracic aorta or in patients with severe aortic calcification.

Differential diagnoses

What are the causes of heart failure?

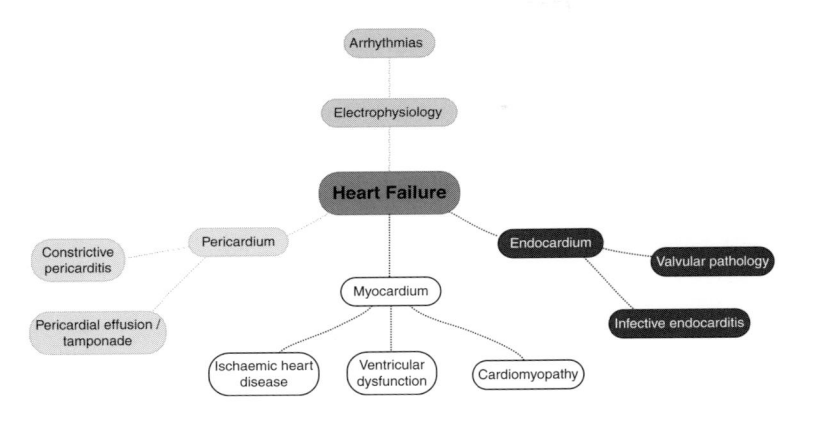

- **Heart Failure**
  - Arrhythmias
    - Electrophysiology
  - Pericardium
    - Constrictive pericarditis
    - Pericardial effusion / tamponade
  - Myocardium
    - Ischaemic heart disease
    - Ventricular dysfunction
    - Cardiomyopathy
  - Endocardium
    - Valvular pathology
    - Infective endocarditis

What are the causes of a pericardial rub?

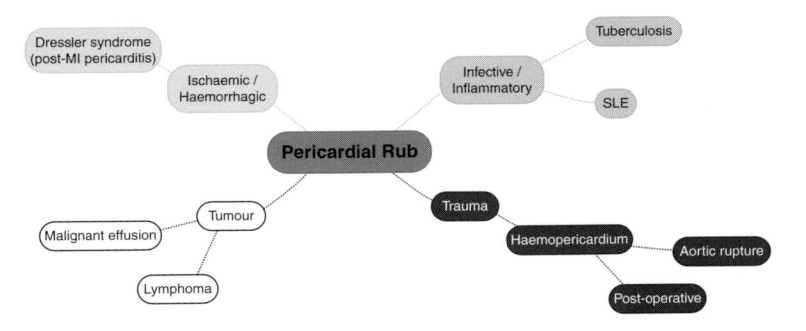

- **Pericardial Rub**
  - Ischaemic / Haemorrhagic
    - Dressler syndrome (post-MI pericarditis)
  - Infective / Inflammatory
    - Tuberculosis
    - SLE
  - Trauma
    - Haemopericardium
      - Aortic rupture
      - Post-operative
  - Tumour
    - Malignant effusion
    - Lymphoma

Section editors: William Lynn, Rajeev Mathew, Petrut Gogalniceanu
Senior authors: S. Alam Hannan, Parag M. Patel, Dan Gogalniceanu, John Lynn

Section 8 — Head and neck surgery

Chapter 32 — Examination of the ear

Rajeev Mathew, S. Alam Hannan and Parag M. Patel

Checklist

WIPER
- Perform with headlight and inspect from the front and the side.

Physiological parameters

Inspection
- Scars: tragal, endaural, postaural, retrosigmoid, middle cranial fossa
- Devices: hearing aid (aural or bone-anchored), cochlear implant in scalp
- Pinna: symmetry, prominence, microtia, accessory auricle, tophi, auricular pit/sinus, tumours, chondrodermatitis nodularis helicis, eczema, psoriasis

Otoscopy
- External auditory canal: wax, furuncle, exostosis/osteoma, papilloma, discharge, polyp, granulation, stenosis/canal atresia
- Mastoid cavity: type, state, facial ridge, meatoplasty
- Tympanic membrane: quadrants, colour, perforation, retraction, mobility (pneumatic), fistula test

Hearing
Ask: 'Which is your better hearing ear?'

Physical Examination for Surgeons, ed. Petrut Gogalniceanu, James Pegrum and William Lynn. Published by Cambridge University Press. © Cambridge University Press 2015.

- Free field hearing test
- Weber's test
- Rinne's test

To complete the examination...
- Cranial nerves, in particular the facial nerve.
- Inspect the postnasal space with nasendoscope (otitis media with effusion or referred otalgia).
- Regional lymphadenopathy (tumours).

Examination notes

How do you position the patient for examination of the ear?

The patient is seated with hair tied back (if applicable) and neck exposed. For an examination of the left ear, examiner and patient face each other, with knees together and legs to the right of each other. If you are using a head mirror, place the lamp at eye level over the patient's left shoulder.

What features of the patient should be noted on general examination?

- Down's syndrome is associated with low-set ears, narrow ear canals and otitis media with effusion. General features include stunted growth, epicanthic folds, flattened nose, short neck and macroglossia.
- Look for the scar of a cleft lip repair, which may be associated with a cleft palate. A history of cleft palate increases the risk of otitis media with effusion and can be associated with other craniofacial malformations resulting in microtia or aural atresia.
- Other signs in the head and neck associated with abnormalities of the ear/hearing are shown in the table:

Head and neck signs	Diagnoses	Notes
Small stature	Down's syndrome	*See above*
	Achondroplasia	Sensorineural hearing loss (SNHL),
	Turner's syndrome	SNHL, low hairline, webbed neck
Tall stature	Marfan's syndrome	Mixed hearing loss, arachnodactyly
Changes in skin		
– loss of pigmentation	Albinism	SNHL
– café-au-lait spots	Neurofibromatosis type 2	Bilateral acoustic neuromas/ SNHL
– depigmented patches	Vitiligo	SNHL
Eye signs		
– heterochromia	Waardenburg's syndrome	SNHL, white forelock of hair
– hazy cornea	Congenital syphilis	SNHL
– opacification of lens	Congenital rubella	SNHL
Goitre	Pendred's syndrome	SNHL
Branchial cyst/fistula	Branchio-oto-renal syndrome	Conductive hearing loss/ SNHL, microtia, auricular sinus

What abnormalities may be noted on examination of the pinna?

- Prominent ears/bat ears are usually due to deficiency of the antihelical folds and deep conchal bowls.
- A lop ear is a deformity where the superior edge of the helix is folded down.
- Preauricular sinuses usually occur at the root of the helix and are connected to the perichondrium of the auricular cartilage. They occur superior and lateral to the facial nerve. Where there is a sinus in an unusual position, look for another opening around the angle of the mandible, as this may represent a collaural fistula from 1st branchial groove duplication.
- Accessory auricles are small tags containing cartilage anterior to the ear.
- Hypoplasia of the external ear is called microtia. It may be an isolated finding or associated with craniofacial malformation.

- The pinna is one of the most common sites for basal and squamous cell carcinoma.
- Chondrodermatitis nodularis helicis presents as a painful scaly nodule on the helical or antihelical rim.

What is the technique for otoscopy?
- Ask the patient to turn his or her head contralaterally.
- The examination of the right ear is performed with the right hand, and the left ear with the left hand.
- Point the base of the otoscope 30–45° above the horizontal.
- Pull the ear canal posteriorly and superiorly in adults and posteriorly in children to straighten the auditory canal.
- Insert the otoscope under direct vision and inspect the canal and all four quadrants of the tympanic membrane (TM).
- A pneumatic otoscope has a squeezable air reservoir which can be used to pump air and generate positive pressure.
    - Lack of movement of an intact TM suggests middle ear fluid.
    - If the eyes deviate to the contralateral ear and there is ipsilateral nystagmus this is called a positive fistula test and implies a perilymphatic fistula or labyrinthine fistula.

How can you tell if a patient has a mastoid cavity?
This is a cavity in the mastoid bone which has been drilled to remove cholesteatoma or treat infection. There will be an associated postaural or endaural scar. The cavity will only be visible if the posterior canal wall has been removed at the time of surgery. The otoscope should be angled posteriorly, and comment should be made on the size and cleanliness of the cavity as well as the height of the facial ridge.

What signs should be noted on examination of the tympanic membrane?
Examine the whole TM – do not forget to examine the attic. Look for the following:
- Changes in colour
- Segmental changes:
    - white plaques on the TM: tympanosclerosis (scarring)
    - white pearly lesion behind TM: cholesteatoma

- red/purple lesions of the TM/behind the TM: glomus tumours; glomus jugulare tumours can have a 'rising sun' appearance
- hypervascularity of promontory (Schwartze's/flamingo pink sign): otosclerosis

- Global TM changes:
  - amber/gold with or without air bubbles: otitis media with effusion
  - blue discolouration: haemotympanum
  - red, bulging: acute otitis media

- Perforations – comment on:
  - position (anterior or posterior, pars tensa or pars flaccida)
  - size (as percentage of TM size) and whether it extends to the annulus (marginal perforation) or not (central perforation)
  - whether it is dry or wet
  - what middle ear structures can be seen through perforation and if they are normal (remember that a perforation of the attic may indicate underlying cholesteatoma)

- Retraction pockets – comment on:
  - position (pars tensa or pars flaccida)
  - classification:
    - **Pars tensa** (Sade, 1979)
      Stage 1 Mild retraction
      Stage 2 Retraction onto incudostapedial joint
      Stage 3 Retraction onto promontory
      Stage 4 Adhesion to medial wall cannot be lifted off
    - **Pars flaccida** (Tos and Poulsen, 1980)
      Type 1 Retraction towards neck of malleus but airspace visible
      Type 2 Retraction onto neck of malleus
      Type 3 Retraction extends beyond malleus full extent seen
      Type 4 Erosion of scutum
  - whether dry or wet
  - whether you can see the whole extent of retraction
  - any associated erosion of the ossicles or cholesteatoma

How do you perform a free field hearing test?

Ensure a quiet environment. When examining the right ear, sit on the right-hand side of the patient at 90° so that he or she cannot see you. Sit approximately 60 cm from the patient and mask the contralateral ear by rubbing the tragus (masking level of 50 dB) or with a Barany noise box (masking level up to 90 dB). Use random number–letter combinations and ask the patient to repeat these. If the patient is able to repeat > 50% of combinations correctly at a particular loudness of speech, the test can be stopped.

Start with a whisper; if the patient succeeds, this implies normal hearing. If the patient fails, use a conversational voice; success implies mild/moderate hearing loss. If the patient fails again, use a loud voice; a Barany noise box must be used to provide enough masking for the contralateral ear. Success with a loud voice implies moderate/severe hearing loss. Inability to hear anything with a loud voice is indicative of a dead ear.

What tuning fork should be used?

A 512 Hz tuning fork should be used to perform Weber's and Rinne's tests.

How do you perform Weber's test?

Strike the tuning fork on your patella and place the base on the patient's vertex, whilst supporting the back of the head with your other hand. Ask the patient 'Is the sound louder in the right ear or the left ear, or is it in the middle?'

If Weber's test localises to the better hearing ear, this implies SNHL, while if it localises to the poorer hearing ear this implies CHL. If it is in the middle, this usually implies symmetric hearing.

How do you perform Rinne's test?

Strike the tuning fork on your patella and place the base on the mastoid process to assess bone conduction. To assess air conduction, place the prongs of the tuning fork vertically 2 cm away from the ear, ensuring the acoustic axis is in line with the ear canal. At all times support the opposite side of the skull with your other hand. Ask the patient, 'Which is louder, number 1 [while testing bone conduction] or number 2 [while testing air conduction]?'

Louder air conduction implies normal hearing or sensorineural hearing loss (SNHL), while louder bone conduction implies a conductive hearing loss (CHL) or rarely a dead ear (as the contralateral ear picks up bone conduction). Rinne's test will detect a CHL of >30dB in 90% of cases.

The table below shows examples of how to interpret the tuning fork tests in combination.

	Weber's	Rinne's test right ear
CHL right ear	Localises to right	Bone conduction louder = negative Rinne's
SNHL right ear	Localises to left	Air conduction louder = positive Rinne's
Dead right ear	Localises to left	Bone conduction louder = false negative Rinne's

When should you perform flexible nasendoscopy as part of your ear examination?

- In an adult with otitis media with effusion, to look for a nasopharyngeal carcinoma or chronic rhinosinusitis.
- In patients with otalgia for which no cause can be found, to examine the upper aerodigestive tract for a malignancy which could be causing referred pain.

What additional tests would you perform in a patient with tinnitus?

Examine the cranial nerves, as a lesion of the cerebellopontine angle may give unilateral tinnitus. If a patient has pulsatile tinnitus, perform the following additional tests:

- Check blood pressure.
- Auscultate:
  - carotid arteries to check for a bruit or transmitted murmur.
  - heart for a murmur.
  - preauricular region/mastoid to check for objective pulsatile tinnitus (glomus tumour, arteriovenous malformation, venous hum).
- Consider oropharyngeal examination and nasendoscopy. Palatal myoclonus produces rhythmic contraction of the soft palate muscles, which can mimic tinnitus.

What additional tests would you perform in a patient with vertigo?

The dizzy patient requires full neuro-otological assessment. This includes assessment of gait, cranial nerves, cerebellar function and the peripheral nervous system. Some of the key tests of vestibular function are listed below.

a. **Nystagmus:**
   - Spontaneous: look for nystagmus while the patient looking straight ahead. This usually indicates central pathology, unless the patient is suffering from acute vertigo at the time of testing.
   - Gaze-evoked: tested by asking the patient to look at your finger as you move it to the right, left, up and down. Peripheral vestibular lesions cause jerk nystagmus, which has a slow phase generated by the vestibular system and a fast corrective phase in the opposite direction. The direction of nystagmus is described according to the fast phase. Peripheral vestibular lesions cause nystagmus which is horizontal with a minor rotatory component. The direction is contralesional where there is vestibular hypofunction and ipsilesional with vestibular irritation. Central nystagmus has a pendular waveform and can occur in all directions.
   - Head shaking: eliminate visual fixation by using video Frenzel goggles. Observe the eyes at rest and then turn the patient's head from side to side at 2 Hz for 20 cycles with around 30° excursion to either side. Stop the movement abruptly and observe for nystagmus. Peripheral vestibular hypofunction will result in horizontal jerk nystagmus which is contralesional.
   - Dix–Hallpike manoeuvre: warn the patient that you may induce vertigo with this test, and ask them to keep their eyes open. The patient is seated upright lengthwise on a couch with the head turned 45° to one side. Quickly move the patient into the supine position with the head hanging beneath the couch edge by 30°, with the head still turned. Keep the patient in this position for 20–30 seconds and observe the eyes. If there is nystagmus, wait for it to stop and then bring the patient back to the original position. If the head is turned to the right, this tests the right posterior semicircular canal. If benign paroxysmal positional vertigo (BPPV) is present the patient will experience vertigo and there will be rotatory (clockwise) up-beating nystagmus after a short latent period. A right Dix–Hallpike manoeuvre also tests the left anterior semicircular canal, but BPPV from this canal will result in down-beating nystagmus with a rotatory component. This is rare. Horizontal canal BPPV causes purely horizontal nystagmus. It is best tested by lying the patient supine with the head flexed 30° and turning the head fully in each direction. If for example there is right horizontal canal BPPV, there will be nystagmus on turning the head in both directions but it will be more pronounced on right turn.
   - Central pathologies can also cause positional nystagmus. Features of central pathology include lack of a latent period and persistent nystagmus in a particular position. Vertical nystagmus is usually central in origin.

b. **Head thrust test**. This is a test of the vestibulo-ocular reflex. Rule out any cervical spine pathology or neck pain. Sit opposite the patient and ask him or her to stare at your nose while you hold the head with both hands. Gently turn the head from side to side and ensure the patient is staring at your nose. Then briskly turn to the left and observe eye position. Repeat the test with a brisk movement to the right. If the patient fails to maintain fixation on right head turn this is indicative of a right peripheral vestibular lesion. You will see catch-up saccades as the eye tries to focus on the nose again.

c. **Unterberger's test**. The patient is asked to walk on the spot with eyes closed and hands stretched out for at least 30 seconds. A patient with vestibular hypofunction will turn to the ipsilesional side by > 30°.

Tips

1. Insert the otoscope under direct vision and this will avoid causing pain to the patient.
2. Remember that a hand-held otoscope provides a monocular view. The tympanic membrane should be examined with a microscope, which will provide depth of field. This is essential for examination of retraction pockets.
3. Tuning fork tests have limited sensitivity and specificity and should be supplemented with pure tone audiometry where possible.

Differential diagnoses

What are the causes of conductive hearing loss?

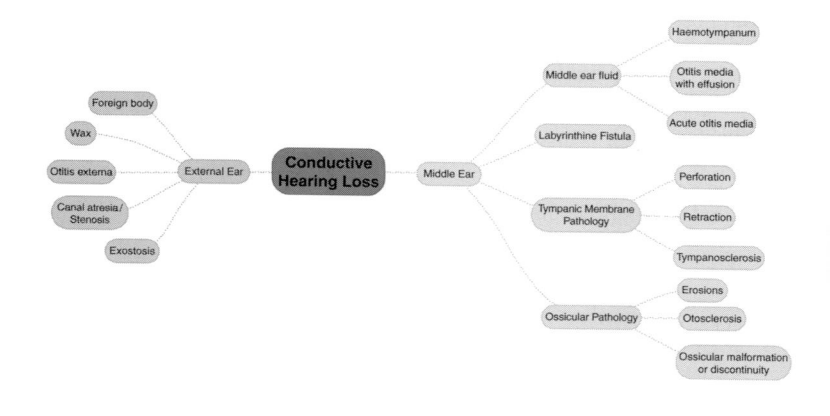

Conductive Hearing Loss

- External Ear
  - Foreign body
  - Wax
  - Otitis externa
  - Canal atresia/Stenosis
  - Exostosis
- Middle Ear
  - Middle ear fluid
    - Haemotympanum
    - Otitis media with effusion
    - Acute otitis media
  - Labyrinthine Fistula
  - Tympanic Membrane Pathology
    - Perforation
    - Retraction
    - Tympanosclerosis
  - Ossicular Pathology
    - Erosions
    - Otosclerosis
    - Ossicular malformation or discontinuity

What are the causes of sensorineural hearing loss?

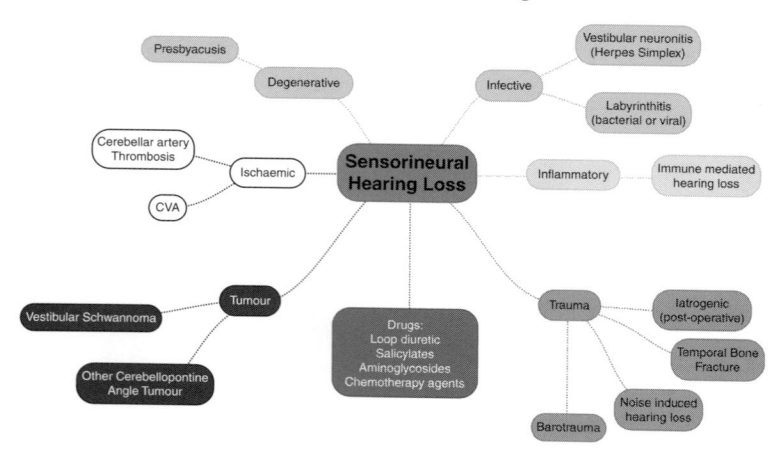

Sensorineural Hearing Loss

- Degenerative
  - Presbyacusis
- Infective
  - Vestibular neuronitis (Herpes Simplex)
  - Labyrinthitis (bacterial or viral)
- Inflammatory
  - Immune mediated hearing loss
- Ischaemic
  - Cerebellar artery Thrombosis
  - CVA
- Tumour
  - Vestibular Schwannoma
  - Other Cerebellopontine Angle Tumour
- Drugs:
  - Loop diuretic
  - Salicylates
  - Aminoglycosides
  - Chemotherapy agents
- Trauma
  - Iatrogenic (post-operative)
  - Temporal Bone Fracture
  - Noise induced hearing loss
  - Barotrauma

Section 8: Head and neck surgery

Chapter 33: Examination of the nose

Rajeev Mathew, S. Alam Hannan and Parag M. Patel

Checklist

WIPER
- Position and expose as for ear examination. Perform with headlight.

Physiological parameters

General inspection (from the front)
- Listen to the voice and breathing.
- Inspect face, eyes, lips and mouth.

External examination of the nose
Inspection:
- Front:
  - symmetry: height, width, bony deformity, septal deviation
  - scars: columella, lateral rhinotomy, Lynch–Howarth, bicoronal
  - skin: erythema, rash, swelling, ulcer
  - alar collapse
- Sides:
  - profile: dorsal hump, saddling, tip ptosis
- Below:
  - narrowing of external nasal valve
  - triangularity

Physical Examination for Surgeons, ed. Petrut Gogalniceanu, James Pegrum and William Lynn. Published by Cambridge University Press. © Cambridge University Press 2015.

Palpate:
- Skin: quality
- Nasal bones: steps, fractures
- Nasal tip support and recoil

Patency:
- Misting test/nostril occlusion
- Cottle's manoeuvre

Internal examination of the nose
- Elevate tip.
- Inspect position of the caudal septum: dislocation/deviation.
- Inspect the external nasal valve.
- Anterior rhinoscopy with Thudicum's speculum: nasal vestibule, septal deviation, septal perforation, mucosa (rhinitic), turbinates (congested), polyps, papillomas, granulomas, tumours, ulcers, crusting, Little's area (prominent vessels), telangiectasia.
- Rigid nasendoscopy.

Oral examination
- Inspect and percuss the upper teeth for dental disease.

To complete the examination...
- Regional lymphadenopathy.
- Cranial nerve examination and ear examination if evidence of postnasal space lesion.

Examination notes

What features should be noted on general inspection?

Full aesthetic assessment of the nose is beyond the scope of this chapter. Start by examining from the front.

- Patients with bilateral nasal congestion have a typical hyponasal voice – make a note of this at the start of the consultation.
- Listen to the patient's breathing – a whistling sound may indicate a septal perforation or crust inside the nose.
- Note if the patient is mouth breathing.
- A long face with an open mouth in children is referred to 'adenoid facies' and may indicate adenoidal hypertrophy.

- A 'frog face' is caused by gross nasal polyposis resulting in a broadened nasal bridge.
- Look at the lips for telangiectasia, which may indicate hereditary haemorrhagic telangiectasia in a patient with epistaxis.
- Proptosis of the eye may be caused by a sinonasal tumour.
- Look for the scar of a cleft lip; this is often associated with characteristic unilateral nasal deformity including shortened columella with deviation to the non-cleft side, collapse of the lower lateral cartilage, widened nares and broad nasal dorsum.

What skin changes should be examined?
Identify actinic keratosis, skin tumours, lupus pernio, acne rosacea/rhinophyma, and midline dermoid cysts.

What is the relevance of alar collapse?
Alar collapse is seen as the patient quietly inspires – this is a sign of a narrow nasal valve.

How is the nose divided anatomically?
Divide the nose into thirds (upper bony third and lower cartilaginous two-thirds) and note symmetry. Bony deformity and septal deviation can impact the nasal airway.

What are the features of saddling of the nose?
Nose saddling is characterised by loss of vertical height, dorsal concavity and reduced projection.

Why should the tip of the nose be palpated?
If the tip of the nose is soft this is a sign of loss of support, usually because of previous septal fracture or surgery.

How do you examine nasal patency?
Place a cold Lack tongue depressor under the patient's nostrils and compare the misting from each nostril during quiet respiration. An alternative method is to occlude the nostril from below with a gloved thumb and listen to nasal breathing. Occluding the nostril from the side can put pressure on the septum and artificially constrict the contralateral nostril. If airflow is reduced on one side, then perform Cottle's manoeuvre.

What is Cottle's manoeuvre?

Lateral traction is applied to the cheek on the side of reduced flow. If the patient reports improved breathing then this is suggestive of narrowing of the internal nasal valve.

How is the internal nasal examination performed?

Start by gently elevating the tip. Note the position of the septum: look for deviation of the septum and whether the caudal septum lies within the columella in the midline.

What is the internal nasal valve?

The boundaries of the internal nasal valve are the septum medially, caudal edge of the upper lateral cartilage superiorly and inferior turbinate laterally. This is the narrowest area in the nasal airway and therefore critical to flow.

How should the internal nasal valve be assessed?

The most accurate way of assessing the nasal valve is with an endoscope at the tip of the nose. Narrow nasal valve can be caused by septal deviation, thick septum, enlarged inferior turbinate, upper lateral cartilage abnormality (shape, position, weakness) or scar tissue. Note that the normal angle between the septum and upper lateral cartilage is 10–15° in Caucasians.

How should the Thudicum's speculum be used?

The Thudicum's speculum is placed in the non-dominant hand, suspended on the index finger, and the prongs are controlled between the middle and ring fingers. Systematically examine the vestibule, septum, middle turbinate, inferior turbinate and floor of the nose. With rhinitis, the mucosa is typically swollen and either pale or red. In sarcoid the mucosa has a 'strawberry skin' appearance with pale granulomas against an erythematous background.

How do you perform nasendoscopy?

- Explain the procedure to the patient.
- Apply topical co-phenylcaine spray to decongest and anaesthetise the nose. Multiple decongestions may be needed during the examination.
- A 4 mm 30° rigid endoscope is normally used. A 2.7 mm endoscope can be used in patients with narrow nasal airways.
- Hold the endoscope in the non-dominant hand between thumb and forefinger.
- Systematically examine the nose with three passes, avoiding trauma to the nasal mucosa.

What should be examined on nasendoscopy?

1. First pass along the floor of the nose. Note the size of the inferior turbinate, check for an old inferior meatal antrostomy and attempt to visualise the nasolacrimal duct, Eustachian tube and postnasal space. Note the position of mucous and pus: if it passes superior to the Eustachian tube it is likely to come from the posterior ethmoid or sphenoid sinus, while if it passes below the Eustachian tube it is likely to arise from the middle meatus.
2. Second pass between the inferior and middle turbinate. Examine the middle turbinate and middle meatus. Then pass the endoscope medial and superior to the middle turbinate to visualise the superior turbinate and sphenoethmoidal recess.
3. Third pass. This is usually done on the way out from the second pass. The endoscope is gently rolled under the middle turbinate, which allows a view of the uncinate process, ethmoid bulla and accessory ostia.

The technique for flexible nasendoscopy (flexible nasolaryngopharyngoscopy) is described in Chapter 34, *Examination of the throat*. The same landmarks described above should be examined.

What is the relevance of the dental assessment when examining the nose and sinuses?

The roots of the second premolar and first molar teeth underlie the floor of the maxillary sinus. Caries or pain on central percussion are signs of pulpitis. Gingival fullness, tooth mobility and pain on lateral percussion are signs of a periodontal abscess. Sublabial scars from previous surgery may be noted (Caldwell–Luc, midfacial degloving) or there may be an oroantral fistula (iatrogenic, trauma, tumour).

Tips

1. Assess the nasal airway during quiet breathing; forced inspiration will cause alar collapse in most people.
2. Pay attention to the internal nasal valve, and ideally assess this with an endoscope.
3. The appearance of a mild dorsal hump can be caused by saddling of the nose. It is important to be aware of such a pseudohump, as augmentation of the nasal septum is more appropriate than reduction of the hump in these cases.

Differential diagnoses

What are the causes of septal perforation?

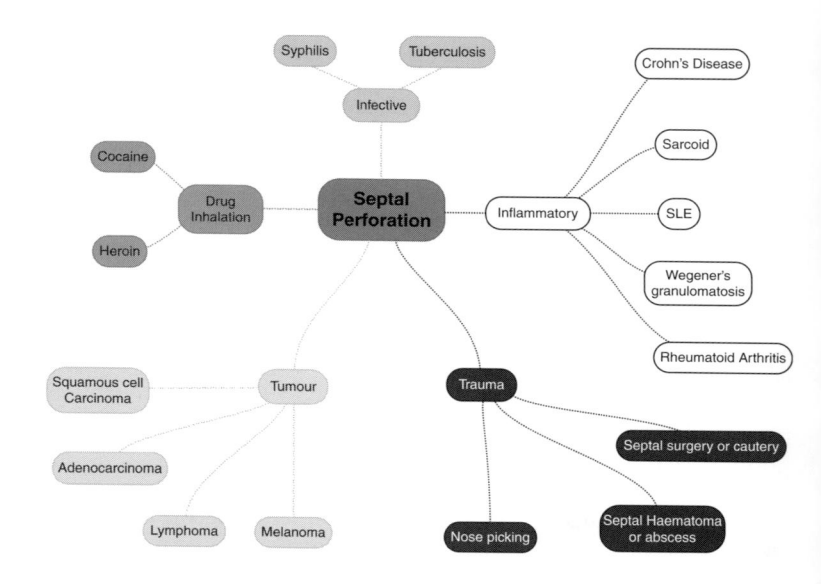

- **Septal Perforation**
  - Infective
    - Syphilis
    - Tuberculosis
  - Drug Inhalation
    - Cocaine
    - Heroin
  - Inflammatory
    - Crohn's Disease
    - Sarcoid
    - SLE
    - Wegener's granulomatosis
    - Rheumatoid Arthritis
  - Tumour
    - Squamous cell Carcinoma
    - Adenocarcinoma
    - Lymphoma
    - Melanoma
  - Trauma
    - Septal surgery or cautery
    - Septal Haematoma or abscess
    - Nose picking

Nasal Mass

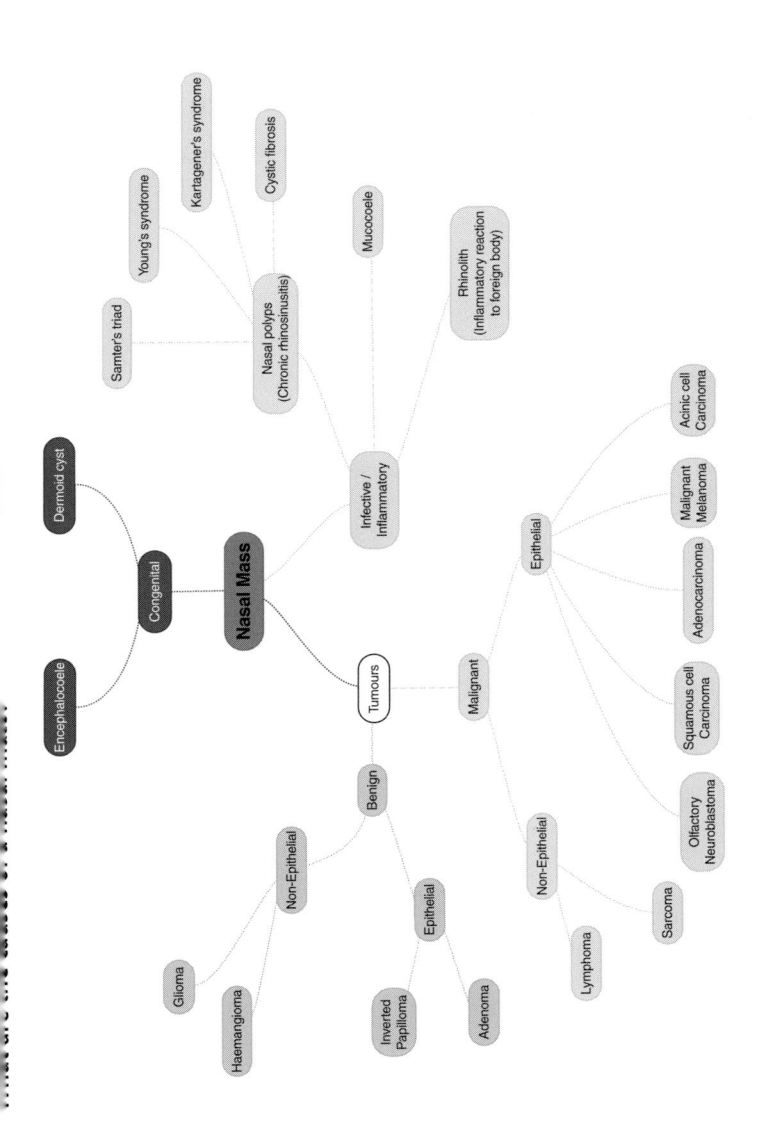

- **Congenital**
  - Encephalocoele
  - Dermoid cyst
- **Infective / Inflammatory**
  - Nasal polyps (Chronic rhinosinusitis)
    - Samter's triad
    - Young's syndrome
    - Kartagener's syndrome
    - Cystic fibrosis
  - Mucocoele
  - Rhinolith (Inflammatory reaction to foreign body)
- **Tumours**
  - **Benign**
    - Non-Epithelial
      - Glioma
      - Haemangioma
    - Epithelial
      - Inverted Papilloma
      - Adenoma
  - **Malignant**
    - Epithelial
      - Olfactory Neuroblastoma
      - Squamous cell Carcinoma
      - Adenocarcinoma
      - Malignant Melanoma
      - Acinic cell Carcinoma
    - Non-Epithelial
      - Sarcoma
      - Lymphoma

Section 8 Head and neck surgery

Chapter 34

Examination of the throat

Rajeev Mathew, S. Alam Hannan and Parag M. Patel

Checklist

WIPER

- Position and expose as for ear examination. Ensure dentures are removed. Inspect with a headlight.

Physiological parameters

Inspection

- Listen to the voice and breathing.
- Front and side: neck scars, stigmata of radiotherapy to the head and neck.
- Oral cavity/oropharyngeal inspection (see Chapter 35, *Oral and maxillofacial examination*):
  - 2 tongue depressors: lips, tongue, teeth, gingiva, parotid duct opening, floor of mouth, submandibular duct
  - 1 tongue depressor: hard palate, soft palate, tonsil, posterior pharyngeal wall, posterior tongue

Palpate

- Floor of mouth: submandibular salivary calculus, tumour
- Parotid duct: salivary calculus
- Tonsils and tongue for tumour

Laryngopharyngoscopy

- Flexible nasolaryngopharyngoscopy

Physical Examination for Surgeons, ed. Petrut Gogalniceanu, James Pegrum and William Lynn. Published by Cambridge University Press. © Cambridge University Press 2015.

> *To complete the examination...*
> - Examine the neck for regional lymphadenopathy (see Chapter 36, *Examination of the neck and thyroid*).

Examination notes
How do you perform flexible nasolaryngopharyngoscopy?
- Explain what you are going to do. In particular, warn that the eyes may water, that one may feel the need to sneeze and that the endoscope can cause discomfort.
- Spray co-phenylcaine into both nostrils and ideally allow it to work for 5–10 minutes.
- Warn the patient not to eat or drink for the next 30 minutes to avoid aspiration or burning the throat.
- Wear gloves and prepare the endoscope – connect the light source, if a sheath is available place it over the endoscope, lubricate the end with aqueous jelly and then either use anti-fog on the tip or warm the tip of the endoscope on the patient's tongue.
- The patient should be sitting with the head resting against a wall, so that the head cannot be drawn back.
- Pass the endoscope into the nasal vestibule on either side under direct vision. Once in the vestibule, if the examined side looks obviously narrowed then pass the endoscope through the contralateral side. In almost all patients the endoscope can be successfully passed between the middle and inferior turbinate. The alternative is to go along the floor of the nose. The key is to stay away from the septal mucosa, which is very sensitive; control the rotation and angulation of the endoscope in order to achieve this. Inspect the nasopharynx, looking at the Eustachian tube orifice, the fossa of Rosenmuller and the adenoid pad.
- Ask the patient to sniff or breathe through the nose. This will bring the soft palate forward, and the endoscope can be passed into the oropharynx.
- Keep the tip of the endoscope at the level of the soft palate and inspect the tongue base; ask the patient to protrude the tongue and look at the valecula and lingual surface of the epiglottis.
- With the tongue back in, systematically examine the larynx.
- Inspect the laryngeal surface of the epiglottis, arytenoids, false cords, ventricle and true cords.
- Assess vocal cord mobility by asking the patient to say a high-pitched 'eeee' and also ask him or her to count to five.

- Ask the patient to blow the cheeks out; this will open up the hypopharynx and allow inspection of the pyriform fossa. Then pass the endoscope behind the epiglottis to get a closer view of the vocal cords, subglottis and tracheal rings. Gently withdraw the endoscope under direct vision and then give the patient a tissue.

Tips

1. When depressing the tongue, ensure the patient does not protrude the tongue. For a patient who warns you that he or she has a strong gag reflex, anaesthetise the throat prior to examination.
2. Flexible nasolaryngopharyngoscopy is facilitated by the use of local anaesthetic, good explanation and reassurance during the examination.
3. It is important to feel the tonsils and tongue base if possible. If there is a submucosal lesion, this will not be evident on inspection.
4. Semon's law: In a progressive lesion of the recurrent laryngeal nerve, the abductors are paralysed before the adductors. Therefore, in an incomplete paralysis, the cord will be brought to the midline by the adductors, but in complete paralysis it falls away to the paramedian position.

Differential diagnoses

What are the causes of asymmetrical tonsils?

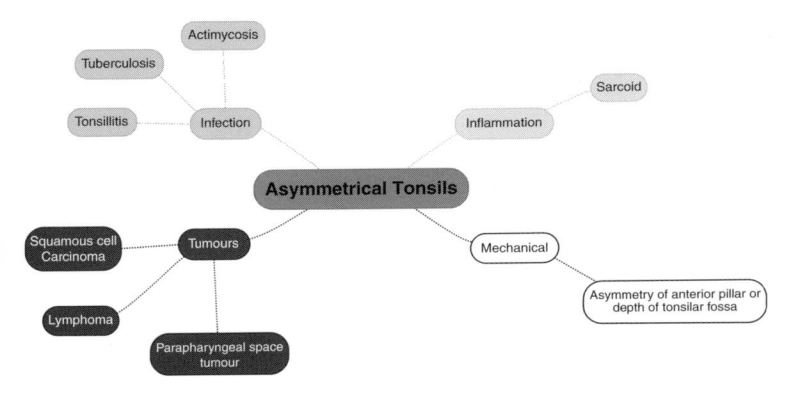

Asymmetrical Tonsils

- Infection
  - Tuberculosis
  - Actimycosis
  - Tonsillitis
- Inflammation
  - Sarcoid
- Mechanical
  - Asymmetry of anterior pillar or depth of tonsilar fossa
- Tumours
  - Squamous cell Carcinoma
  - Lymphoma
  - Parapharyngeal space tumour

What are the causes of vocal cord immobility?

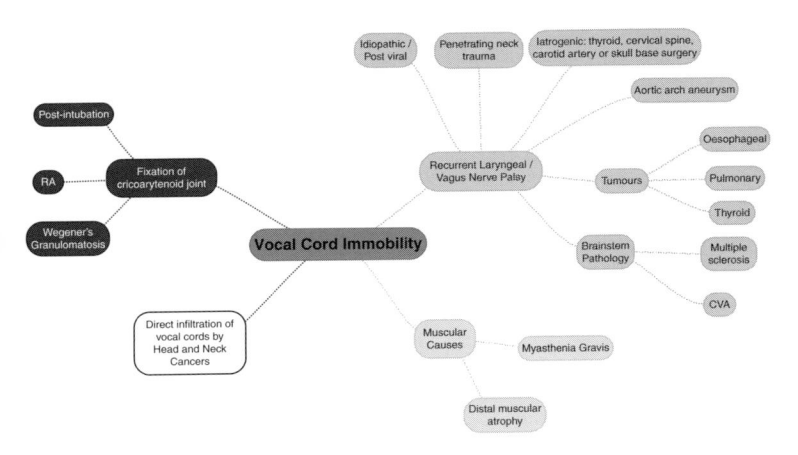

Vocal Cord Immobility

- Fixation of cricoarytenoid joint
  - Post-intubation
  - RA
  - Wegener's Granulomatosis
- Recurrent Laryngeal / Vagus Nerve Palsy
  - Idiopathic / Post viral
  - Penetrating neck trauma
  - Iatrogenic: thyroid, cervical spine, carotid artery or skull base surgery
  - Aortic arch aneurysm
  - Tumours
    - Oesophageal
    - Pulmonary
    - Thyroid
  - Brainstem Pathology
    - Multiple sclerosis
    - CVA
- Direct infiltration of vocal cords by Head and Neck Cancers
- Muscular Causes
  - Myasthenia Gravis
  - Distal muscular atrophy

Section 8 Head and neck surgery

Chapter 35

Oral and maxillofacial examination

David C. McAnerney, Petrut Gogalniceanu, Rajeev Mathew and Dan Gogalniceanu

Extra-oral examination of the face

Checklist

WIPER

- Good light source. The patient needs to be sitting with neck exposed to the clavicles. Necklaces and glasses must be removed.
- Examine the head from the front, from the sides and from above.
- Compare the left and right sides of the face.
- Look for deviation of midline structures.

Physiological parameters

General facial examination

- First, rule out:
    - airway compromise
    - cervical spine injuries
    - scalp, cranial or intracranial injuries
    - major haemorrhage
- Facial appearance: expression, symmetry, facial muscle palsy or congenital syndromes
- Nutritional status

Inspection

- Skin of all facial structures: scars, masses (tumours), defects (ulcers, lacerations, tissue loss), colour changes (cyanosis, ecchymoses, erythema, pallor)

Physical Examination for Surgeons, ed. Petrut Gogalniceanu, James Pegrum and William Lynn. Published by Cambridge University Press. © Cambridge University Press 2015.

- Scalp: lacerations, foreign bodies, haematomas, masses
- Ears:
    - mastoid bruising (Battle's sign) in skull base fractures
    - auricle: lacerations, haematomas or avulsions
    - external acoustic meatus: blood or CSF
- Eyes:
    - periorbital ecchymoses ('panda eyes') in skull base fractures
    - 'sunken' eye (enopthalmos) and diplopia in orbital floor fractures
    - swelling of the eyelids
    - symmetry of movement
    - subconjunctival haemorrhage
- Nose:
    - deformity or deviation from midline
    - CSF leak
    - bleeding
    - septal haematomas
- Lips:
    - lacerations, haematomas, masses, asymmetry of the mouth
- Parotid and submandibular glands:
    - swelling
- Hard tissues:
    - loss of bony contours or deformities of facial skeleton
    - malocclusion of teeth, prognathism or retrognathism

Palpation

- Skin: temperature, tenderness.
- Soft tissues: tenderness, fluctuance, surgical emphysema:
    - eyelids, nose, lips and cheeks
    - submandibular region: induration (rule out Ludwig's angina or abscesses)
- Hard tissues: step deformities, irregularities, mobility or tenderness:
    - supraorbital ridge and frontal bones
    - inferior orbital ridge and lateral orbital ridge
    - zygomatic arch
    - ramus, angle and body of mandible
    - nasal bone, midface, teeth
- Sensation:
    - numbness in distribution of infraorbital nerve (cheek and upper lip) in orbital blow-out fracture or zygoma fractures

- numbness in distribution of inferior alveolar nerve (chin and lower lip) in mandibular fractures
- Sinuses: tenderness
- Salivary glands: parotid, submandibular for enlargement and tenderness.
- Lymph nodes: pre- and post-auricular, occipital, submental, submandibular, cervical and supraclavicular nodes for enlargement, tenderness and mobility.
- Neck:
  - anterior and posterior triangles of the neck for masses
  - sternocleidomastoid muscle for induration
  - thyroid, larynx and trachea
  - carotid pulse

Movement
- Temporomandibular joint (TMJ): open and close the mouth while palpating the joint:
  - malocculsion
  - pain
  - interincisal distance (4–6.5 cm)
  - lateral deviation
  - symmetry of movement
  - joint clicking, locking or crepitus
- Mandibular condyle: place index fingers bilaterally in front of tragus to palpate condylar heads.

Auscultation
- Airway: stridor
- Speech: dysarthria
- Voice: hoarseness
- TMJ movement: clicking

To complete the examination...
- Perform a cranial nerves examination (see Chapter 38, *Focal neurological examination*). Special attention must be given to the hypoglossal nerve (tongue movement), trigeminal nerve (facial sensation) and facial nerve (facial movement).
- Perform a full neck and ENT examination.
- Perform an intra-oral examination.
- Imaging, as required:
  - Skull and facial radiographs
  - OPG (orthopantomogram)

- CT facial bones
- FNE (fine nasendoscopy)

Intra-oral examination

Checklist

WIPER
- Good light, examination gloves, suction apparatus, dental mirror or other retraction instruments. Inspection of teeth using a dental mirror.

Physiological parameters

Inspection
- General inspection: oral hygiene, hydration of mucosal surfaces
- Lips: masses, cyanosis, angular cheilitis, hydration (vermillion border and labial mucosa)
- Oral mucosa: lacerations, ulcers, sinuses, fistulas, neoplastic lesions, swellings or colour changes
  - labial frenulum, buccal (cheek) mucosa, opening of Stensen's (parotid) duct, vestibule and retromolar area

    Ask: 'Push your tongue to the top of your mouth and towards each cheek'

  - floor of mouth, inferior aspect of tongue, lingual frenulum, opening of Wharton's (submandibular) duct

    Ask: 'Stick your tongue out and to both sides'

  - dorsum and lateral surfaces of tongue: surface lesions, wasting, movement
- Anterior (hard) and posterior (soft) palates.
  'Say "Ahh".'
- Tonsils, fauces, uvula
- Tongue
- Gingiva: bleeding, regression, abscesses, trauma, hypertrophy and tumours
- Teeth:
  - chart presence or absence of teeth
  - tooth disease: colour changes, erosions, fractures, caries
  - occlusion
  - dental appliances and prostheses

Palpation
- Soft tissues: lips, cheeks, tongue, soft palate, floor of the mouth
- Hard tissues: hard palate, inner aspect of mandible
- Teeth: mobility and tenderness

To complete the examination...
As required:
- Skull and facial radiographs
- OPG (orthopantomogram)
- FNE (fine nasendoscopy)

Examination notes

Note that the intra-oral examination described here is a general screening examination of the oral cavity for the general surgeon in acute or trauma settings prior to referral to a specialist. Specific examination of teeth in the elective setting should be performed by a dental or oral & maxillofacial surgeon.

What symptoms should be sought?

- Facial, head, ear or tooth pain
- Pain or clicking in the jaw
- Masses, swellings, ulcers or other lesions in the mouth
- Loose or missing teeth
- Problems with mouth opening, chewing or swallowing
- Speech or breathing difficulties
- Background information on oral hygiene, dietary preferences, alcohol and tobacco use
- Past medical history on previous dental or oral surgery

What associated examination should be performed when examining the face?

Eyes:
- Eyelid movement, swelling or masses
- Eye position and symmetry
- Orbital alignment, exophthalmos, ocular movement
- Sclera and conjunctiva: injection
- Pupillary reflexes, visual acuity

Nose (See Chapter 33):
- Shape and midline deviation
- Tenderness
- Bilateral nostril patency: swelling, polyps, septal haematoma, oral respiration
- Discharge: bleeding, mucus, pus, CSF

Ears (See Chapter 32):
- External deformities or injuries
- Meatus: redness, discharge, masses, foreign objects
- Otoscopy
- Hearing tests: voice, Weber's and Rinne's tests

What signs should be sought in head and neck trauma?

All trauma patients should be managed according to the ATLS guidelines in order to diagnose and treat life-threatening injuries first. Note that the assessment of deformity can be difficult in the immediate post injury phase because of swelling.

Some considerations specific to head and neck trauma include:
- Airway compromise: stridor, foreign objects or fluids in mouth, tracheal deviation or posterior displacement of the tongue
- Cervical spine trauma requiring immediate in-line immobilisation
- Bleeding: external, mouth, nose or ears
- Glasgow Coma Scale ($n/15$)
- Scalp lacerations
- Skull vault fractures (step deformities)
- Basal skull fractures: raccoon or panda eyes (periorbital ecchymoses), Battle's sign (mastoid ecchymosis) in middle cranial fossa fractures and CSF leaks from the ears (otorrhoea) or nose (rhinorrhoea)
- Facial bone fractures (tenderness, deformity or instability)

What is bimanual examination?

A mass or lesion in the orofacial region should be examined in relation to surrounding structures and with a view to establishing its anatomic plane. Bimanual assessment is performed with simultaneous insertion of the gloved fingers of one hand in the oral cavity while the other hand palpates externally. Palpate:
- Submandibular, sublingual and parotid glands
- Base of tongue
- Floor of mouth
- Buccal region

How can the facial bones be palpated?

Sequence of palpation of facial bones:

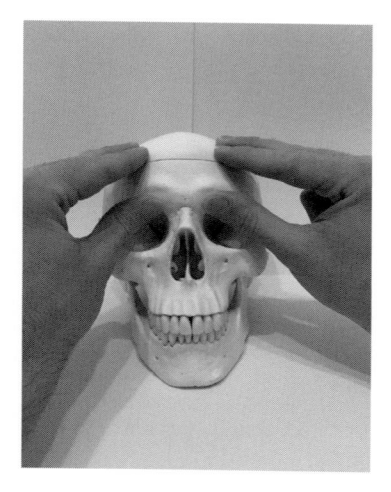

1. Palpation of supraorbital ridge and frontal bone.

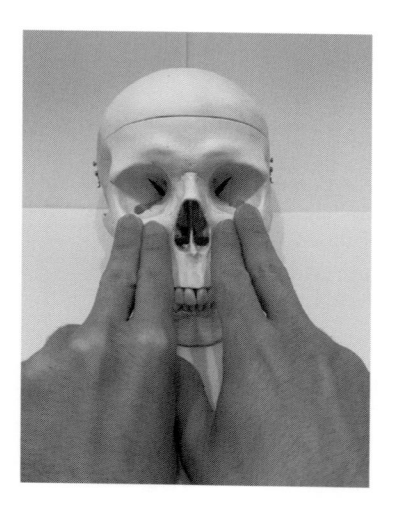

2. Palpation of infraorbital and lateral orbital ridges.

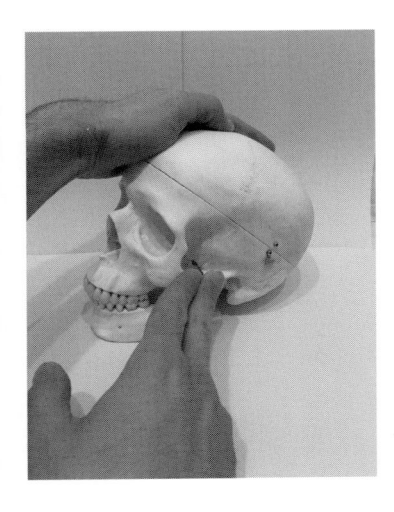

Chapter 35: Oral and maxillofacial examination | 299

3. Palpation of zygomatic arch.

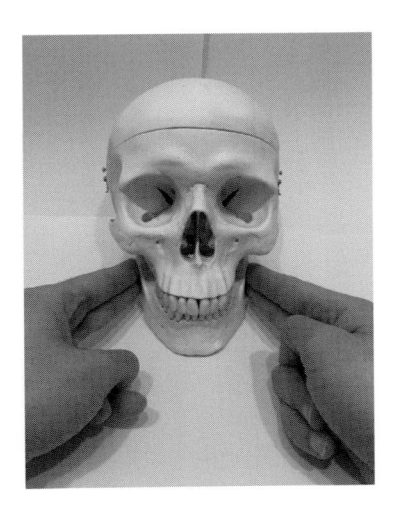

4. Palpation of mandibular ramus and angle.

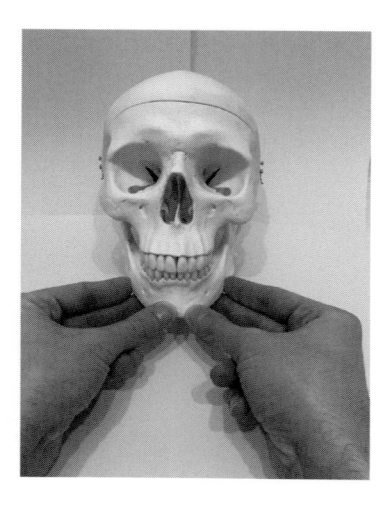

5. Palpation of mandibular body and mental protuberance.

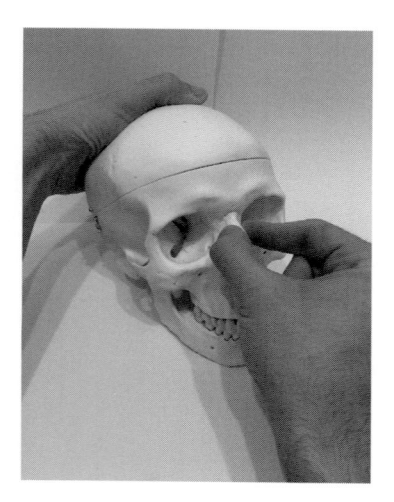

6. Palpation of nasal bones.

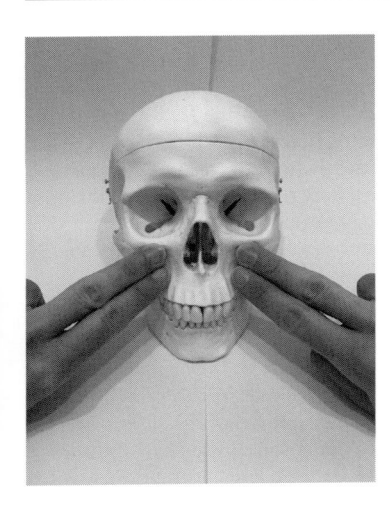

7. Palpation of malar/zygomatic bones.

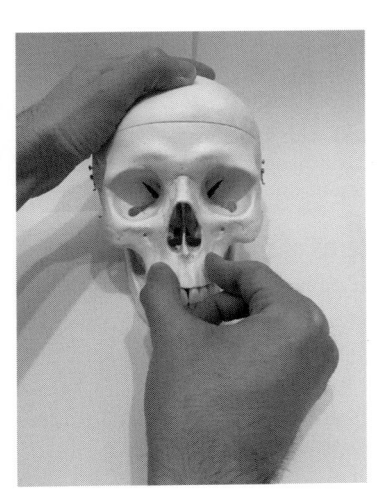

8. Palpation of maxilla/midface stability.

How is a nasal septal haematoma diagnosed?

A septal haematoma presents as an anterior blue-red septal swelling. This can be confused with septal deviation due to a fracture. Palpation with a Jobson–Horne probe or a gloved little finger will determine whether the swelling is soft and fluctuant (haematoma) or firm (deviated septum).

Are there specific tests for the maxilla?

Maxillary fractures are important, because they can cause both obstruction of the naso-/oropharynx and signify trauma to the base of the skull. The maxilla is held between the thumb and forefinger of one hand while the free hand examines for movement externally with gentle anterior–posterior pressure. The two points of reference are the sides (Le Fort I) and the bridge of the nose (Le Fort II/III). The maxilla should not be manipulated if there are signs of a base of skull fracture, in which case one should proceed straight to CT scanning.

What are the features of an orbital blow-out fracture?

Blow-out fractures are caused by direct blunt trauma to the orbit resulting in fracture of the orbital floor or medial wall. It is characterised by enophthalmos (depression of the eyeball in the orbit) and entrapment of the inferior rectus muscle, which does not allow the eye to look superiorly. Eye movement assessment is performed with a standard 'H' pattern, which can be augmented by including a central vertical movement up. This is particularly sensitive for entrapment secondary to an infraorbital fracture. Other features may include exophthalmos/proptosis due to a retrobulbar haematoma.

What are the features of a zygomatic arch fracture?

Zygomatic arch fractures may be associated with facial asymmetry due to a depressed cheekbone. Lateral subconjunctival haemorrhage in the eyes may indicate a potential fracture at the zygomaticofrontal suture.

What are the common fracture patterns of the midface?

These are described by the Le Fort classification:

- Le Fort I Bilateral detachment of the alveolar complex and palate or low-level subzygomatic fracture
- Le Fort II Pyramidal, subzygomatic fracture of the maxilla
- Le Fort III Craniofacial dislocation; high-level suprazygomatic fracture of the central and lateral parts of the face

It is important to appreciate that these are an approximation of potential injury, as high-energy facial traumas can lead to variable and often mixed injury patterns.

How do you differentiate clinically between Le Fort fractures?

Hold the upper teeth and maxilla in one hand and palpate the skeleton of the face with the other hand:

Le Fort I   The maxilla moves independently
Le Fort II The maxilla moves together with the bridge of the nose
Le Fort III The maxilla moves together with the cheekbones

What are the causes of cranial nerve deficits secondary to facial trauma?

CN I	Anterior fossa floor fracture disrupting cribiform plate
CN II	Compression usually due to fractures of the optic canal, orbit, extensions of skull base fractures or haematoma (retrobulbar haemorrhage)
CN III, IV, VI	Any fractures involving the superior orbital fissure or haematoma causing compression
CN V	Va – supraorbital fractures Vb – zygomatic or Le Fort II/III Vc – mandibular fracture
CN VII	Temporal bone fracture (although can be injured due to soft tissue trauma anywhere along its path)
CN VIII	Temporal bone fracture
CN IX, X, XI	Base of skull fracture

How should the neck be palpated?

- Stand behind the patient.
- Begin the examination below the chin and proceed posteriorly along the body of mandible towards its angle.
- Palpate the submental lymph nodes as well as the submandibular and parotid salivary glands.
- Palpate the preauricular, retroauricular and occipital lymph nodes.
- Palpate inferiorly along the sternocleidomastoid, feeling the cervical chain of lymph nodes.
- At the inferior end of the stenocleidomastoid palpate laterally in the supraclavicular fossa.
- Subsequently move medially to feel the trachea and thyroid.

- At the end of the examination palpate the anterior and posterior triangles of the neck (anterior and posterior to sternocleidomastoid muscles, respectively) including the carotid artery.

What special considerations are necessary in examining a mass arising from the parotid gland?

The parotid gland is intimately associated with the facial nerve (CN VII). Its function needs to be assessed (see Chapters 36 and 38).

What is Stensen's duct?

Stensen's duct or the parotid duct drains secretions from the parotid gland. It opens on the buccal mucosa in the region of the upper molars. It can be palpated externally over a contracted masseter muscle.

What is Wharton's duct?

Wharton's ducts drain the submandibular glands on either side of the lingual frenulum on the floor of the mouth. They can be palpated bimanually.

What preparation is necessary prior to examining the soft tissues?

It is important to remove any prostheses, as these can both impair examination and hide pathology.

Damage to which nerves causes vocal hoarseness?

Damage to the vagus nerve or recurrent laryngeal branch.

What areas of the oral cavity are difficult to inspect?

- **Lingual sulci**: the posterior parts of the lingual sulcus on either side of the tongue have been called 'coffin corners', as neoplastic lesions can grow undetected by clinician or patient. These regions should be gently palpated by slipping the index finger posteriorly and inferiorly to the back and base of the tongue (left index to left lingual sulci and right to right). This must be done gently, as a gagging reflex may be induced.
- **Tongue**: lateral borders.

How can teeth be charted?

Tooth notation in adults (permanent teeth) can be done by a variety of methods. The simplest is to divide the oral cavity into quadrants. Each tooth is then individually numbered 1–8 from medial (central incisor) to lateral (3rd molar). For example, the upper left first premolar would be notated simply as UL4.

Upper

Right　87654321 | 12345678　Left

　　　--

　　　87654321 | 12345678

Lower

> **Tip**
>
> As in radiographs, *left* and *right* refer to the patient's left and right rather than the examiner's.

How should teeth be examined?

Gentle movement or tapping of an infected or damaged tooth can cause pain or sensitivity. Adjacent oral mucosa must be assessed for evidence of ulceration, abscess formation or trauma. If dentures are present it is important to examine them both in and outside the mouth. Damaged/repaired or ill-fitting prostheses can cause irritation and trauma to the local tissues.

How is dental occlusion assessed?

- Ask patient: 'When biting teeth does it feel normal to you?'
- Ask the patient to bite together while exposing the front teeth, to reveal any gross step deformities.
- Biting on a tongue depressor can produce pain localised to a fracture site.

How should teeth be imaged?

An orthopantomogram (OPG) can give good general assessment of the entire dentition, although there are limitations. The anterior teeth may be hard to assess due to spinal contour overlap. An accurate assessment of individual teeth can be achieved with an intra-oral periapical radiograph.

Any soft tissue trauma to the lips in conjunction with lost or fractured teeth requires a soft tissue radiograph to ensure that no foreign bodies are embedded within.

What other investigations can be performed?

- **Ultrasound +/- fine needle biopsies** is a safe first-line investigation for neoplasms of the salivary glands.
- **CT/MRI** are used for diagnosing complex facial bony trauma and for the assessment of extent, invasion and potential metastases in patients with head and neck cancers.
- **Sialography** is a specialised radiological technique used to assess the salivary ductal system for integrity and obstruction (e.g. in Sjögren's syndrome and sialoliths). Stone retrieval can also be attempted during this investigation.
- **Mucosal pathology** can be further investigated using excisional or incisional biopsies to gain a tissue diagnosis, depending on access, size of lesion and suspected diagnosis.

Section 8: Head and neck surgery

Chapter 36: Examination of the neck and thyroid

William Lynn, Petrut Gogalniceanu and John Lynn

Neck examination

Checklist

WIPER
- Patient on chair, away from wall, both clavicles exposed.
- Examine from the front, sides and behind the neck.
- Glass of water available.

Physiological parameters

General
- Hoarse voice or stridor
- Position of the head: sternocleidomastoid tumour or torticollis
- Open mouth: thyroglossal cyst, lingual thyroid, ranula, cystic hygroma

Inspection
- Scars or radiotherapy tattoo
- Sinuses, fistulas or erythema
- Masses/swellings
- Distended neck veins: SVC obstruction or compression
- Protrusion of tongue: rule out mobile masses or hypoglossal/lingual nerve pathology
- Swallow water: rule out mobile masses (thyroglossal cyst), cough or dysphagia
- Blow nose: identify laryngocoele

Physical Examination for Surgeons, ed. Petrut Gogalniceanu, James Pegrum and William Lynn. Published by Cambridge University Press. © Cambridge University Press 2015.

Palpation

Ask: 'Do you have any pain?'

From behind:
- Temperature and tenderness
- Lumps:
  - during swallowing
  - whilst patient is protruding tongue
  - during coughing
- Submandibular and parotid glands
- Trachea: central or deviated
- Thyroid: goitre, discrete masses, tenderness
- Carotids: pulsatile masses or obliterated pulse (Berry's sign)
- Lymph nodes

Percussion
- Retrosternal goitre

Auscultation
- Thyroid bruit (thyrotoxicosis)
- Carotid bruit (see Chapter 24, *Examination of the carotid artery*)
- Gurgling in pharyngeal pouch

To complete the examination...
- Perform Pemberton's test.
- Examine the oral cavity, ear, nose and throat.
- Visualise vocal cords directly.
- Examine thyroid status.

Thyroid status examination

Checklist

WIPER

Physiological parameters

General
- Weight status
- Mood: agitated, nervous, lethargic

- Hair: fine or coarse
- Clothing

Hands
- Pseudoclubbing of nails (thyroid acropachy)
- Onycholysis (Plummer's nails)
- Palmar erythema
- Palmar sweating
- Fine tremor
- Pulse: tachycardia, AF

Eyes
- Hair loss outer eyebrow
- Periorbital oedema
- Lid retraction (Dalrymple's sign)
- Exophthalmos/proptosis
- Chemosis/conjunctival injection
- Lid lag/ophthalmoplegia

Arms
- Proximal myopathy

Legs
- Pretibial myxoedema (Grave's disease)
- Slow relaxing ankle reflexes

Thyroid exam
- Full examination of neck and thyroid gland

To complete the examination...
Conclude on thyroid status: euthyroid/hyperthyroid/hypothyroid.

Examination notes

What questions need to be asked in the examination of a neck lump?

- Is it in the midline or lateral?
- Which triangle is it in?
- Is it solid or cystic?

What other questions may be useful?

- Is it pulsatile?
- Does it transilluminate?
- Is it exacerbated by coughing/blowing nose?

What groups of lymph nodes should be palpated?

- Submental, submandibular
- Pre- and postauricular
- Occipital and posterior triangle
- Jugular chain
- Supraclavicular

What are the specific examination points for the thyroid exam?

- Assess eye movements for evidence of thyroid eye disease:
    - lid lag
    - complex ophthalmoplegia
- Pretibial myxoedema.
- Proximal myopathy. Ask the patient to stand from the chair at the end of the examination. Assess use of hands to assist standing.
- Reflexes: assess for evidence of hyper-reflexia or hypo-reflexia.
- Assess voice for hoarseness – thyroid mass and hoarse voice is likely to be cancer.
- Assess swallowing.
- Assess for stridor.
- Pemberton's sign.

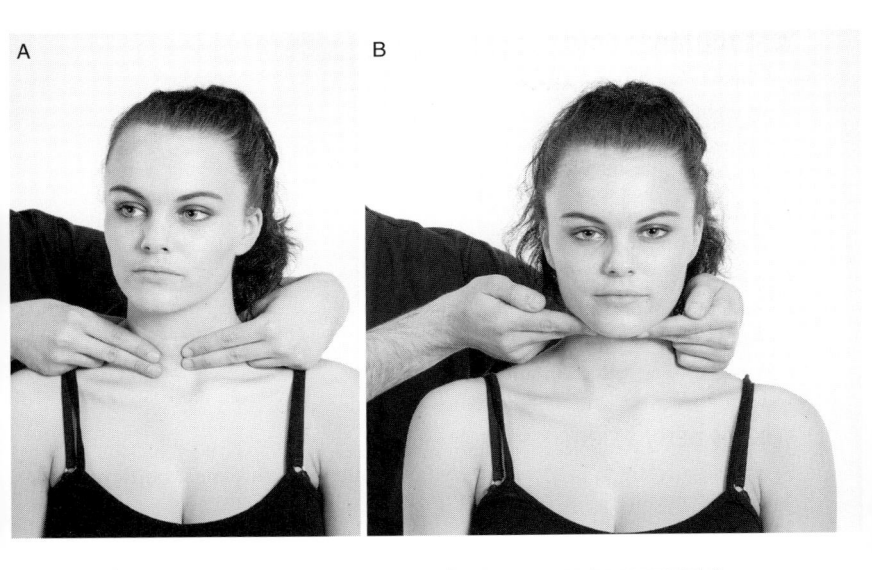

Chapter 36: Examination of the neck and thyroid | 311

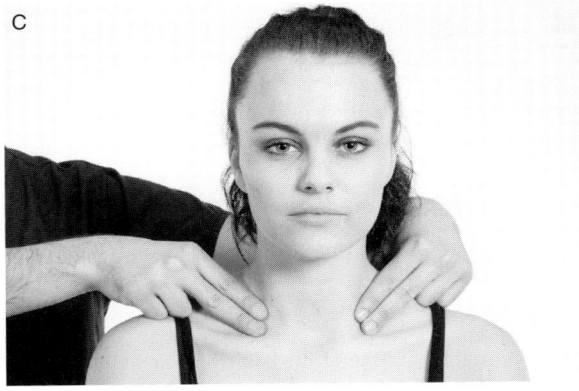

Palpation of the neck. Palpation of (A) the thyroid and (B, C) the lymph glands is performed with the patient sitting and the surgeon standing behind the patient.

What history points should be elicited for thyroid disease?
- Anxiety/mood
- Weight change
- Appetite
- Bowel habit
- Temperature preference
- Palpitations
- Visual disturbance
- Radiation exposure
- Family history
- Drug history – lithium/amiodarone

What is Berry's sign?
Berry's sign refers to obliteration of the carotid pulse in patients with malignant thyromegaly.

What is Pemberton's test/manoeuvre?
Rationale: To identify thoracic inlet obstruction/SVC compression. In the context of thyroid examination, this may be caused by a large retrosternal goitre compressing the thoracic inlet. Other causes include apical lung tumours and masses in the lower neck or upper mediastinum.

Technique: Patient is sitting on a chair. Elevate extended arms vertically above head.

Positive test: The patient develops facial redness/plethora (Pemberton's sign) and distended neck veins. It may be associated with shortness of breath or pre-syncope.

What is onycholysis?
Onycholysis is a distal separation of the nail from the nail bed.

What are the borders of the anterior triangle of the neck?
The anterior triangle is formed by the midline, the mandible and the anterior border of sternocleoidmastoid muscle.

What are the borders of the posterior triangle of the neck?
The posterior triangle is formed inferiorly by the clavicle, medially by the lateral border of sternocleoidmastoid and laterally by the medial border of the trapezius.

What structures are related to the parotid gland?
- Facial nerve: it travels through the gland but does not supply it; it may be damaged during parotid surgery.
- External carotid artery: the maxillary artery and superficial temporal artery arise within the parotid gland.

How can the different parotid gland tumours be differentiated?
- Pleomorphic adenoma:
    - commonest salivary gland tumour, slow-growing and painless
    - the tumour will classically deflect the earlobe laterally
- Adenocarcinoma of the parotid:
    - rare
    - facial nerve signs increase probability (due to direct invasion of the nerve)
- Warthin's tumour:
    - may be bilateral and is strongly associated with smoking
    - older patients

How would you investigate a thyroid mass?
A thyroid mass should be investigated using a triple assessment technique. This combines clinical examination, ultrasound scanning and targeted fine-needle aspiration (FNA) to achieve a diagnosis.

What are the complications of thyroidectomy?
- Hypocalcaemia due to damage/excision of parathyroid glands
- Damage to the recurrent laryngeal nerve leading to a hoarse voice
- Acute haemorrhage
- Airway obstruction

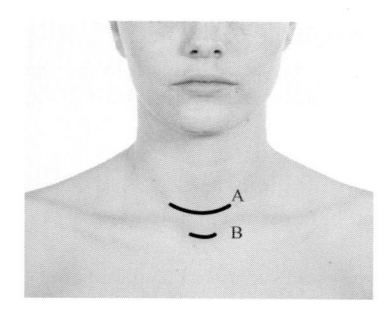

Neck scars. (A) Thyroidectomy or tracheostomy scar; tracheostomy scars heal by secondary intention and usually result in a broader scar compared to a thyroidectomy scar. (B) Mediastinoscopy scar.

What are the features of a branchial cyst?

- Embryological remnants of the second branchial pouch.
- Located on anterior border of sternocleoidmastoid at the level of the carotid bifurcation.
- Soft swelling that may fluctuate but may become infected and form an abscess.
- FNA – revealing the presence of cholesterol crystals is diagnostic.

What is a pharyngeal pouch?

- Diverticulum that arises through Killian's dehiscence (between inferior constrictor and cricopharyngeus).
- Presents with dysphagia, regurgitation of partially digested food.
- Clinical presentation is with a cervical lump. This may elicit gurgling when palpated.
- The diagnosis is confirmed by barium swallow.

What are the levels of the neck?

Levels of the neck describe specific regional lymph-node chains and are used in describing the extent of neck dissections:

Level 1 submental and submandibular triangles

Level 2 upper third of the jugular nodes

Level 3 middle third of the jugular nodes

Level 4 lower third of the jugular nodes

Level 5 posterior triangle nodes

Level 6 anterior compartment nodes (surrounding midline structures of the neck)

Level 7 superior mediastinum

Differential diagnoses

What are the causes of lymphadenopathy?

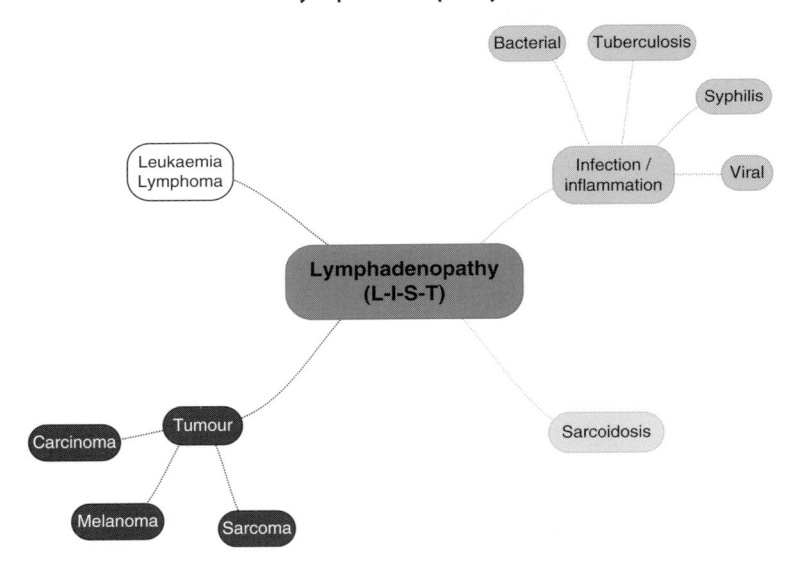

Lymphadenopathy (L-I-S-T)

- Leukaemia / Lymphoma
- Infection / inflammation
  - Bacterial
  - Tuberculosis
  - Syphilis
  - Viral
- Sarcoidosis
- Tumour
  - Carcinoma
  - Melanoma
  - Sarcoma

What are the causes of neck lumps?

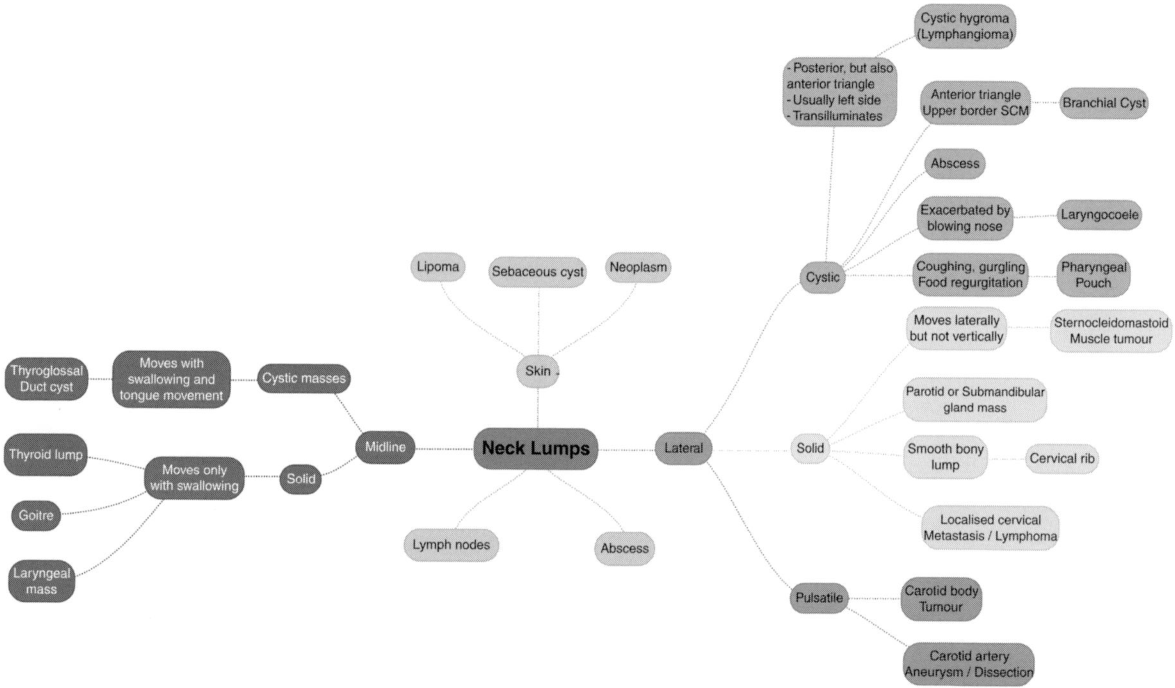

Neck Lumps

Skin
- Lipoma
- Sebaceous cyst
- Neoplasm
- Abscess
- Lymph nodes

Midline

Cystic masses
- Moves with swallowing and tongue movement
  - Thyroglossal Duct cyst

Solid
- Moves only with swallowing
  - Thyroid lump
  - Goitre
  - Laryngeal mass

Lateral

Cystic
- Posterior, but also anterior triangle
  - Usually left side
  - Transilluminates
  → Cystic hygroma (Lymphangioma)
- Anterior triangle, Upper border SCM → Branchial Cyst
- Abscess
- Exacerbated by blowing nose → Laryngocoele
- Coughing, gurgling, Food regurgitation → Pharyngeal Pouch

Solid
- Moves laterally but not vertically → Sternocleidomastoid Muscle tumour
- Parotid or Submandibular gland mass
- Smooth bony lump → Cervical rib
- Localised cervical → Metastasis / Lymphoma

Pulsatile
- Carotid body Tumour
- Carotid artery Aneurysm / Dissection

316

What are the causes of parotid masses?

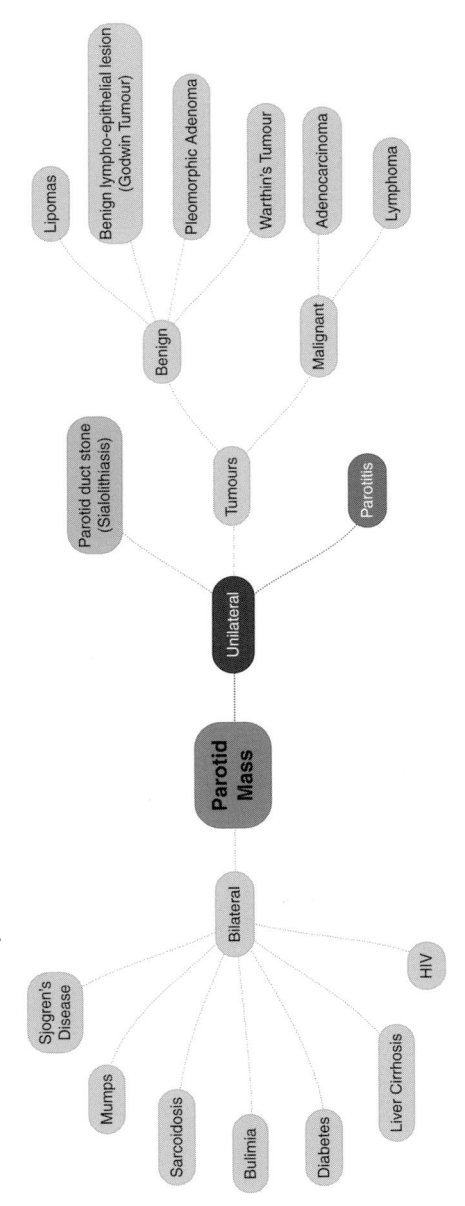

- **Parotid Mass**
  - **Unilateral**
    - Parotid duct stone (Sialolithiasis)
    - Tumours
      - Benign
        - Lipomas
        - Benign lympho-epithelial lesion (Godwin Tumour)
        - Pleomorphic Adenoma
        - Warthin's Tumour
      - Malignant
        - Adenocarcinoma
        - Lymphoma
    - Parotitis
  - **Bilateral**
    - Sjogren's Disease
    - Mumps
    - Sarcoidosis
    - Bulimia
    - Diabetes
    - Liver Cirrhosis
    - HIV

Section editor: Harry Bulstrode
Senior author: Diederik O. Bulters

Section 9 **Neurosurgery**

Chapter 37

Global neurological examination
Harry Bulstrode, Yezen Sheena and Diederik O. Bulters

Neurosurgical examination always seeks to localise pathology. Nevertheless, many common insults to the nervous system are diffuse in nature (e.g. meningitis and blunt head injury).

Obtunded and comatose patients in particular present a unique examination challenge. No single routine covers the assessment of these patients in contexts as diverse as the primary survey on the one hand, and confirmation of brainstem death on the other. You should look to the examiner for explicit or implicit pointers to guide your examination.

Examination of brain death

Testing is performed by two doctors who have held full registration with the GMC for more than 5 years. One must be a consultant, and neither should be part of the transplant team.
1. Correct:
    - Hypothermia
    - Hypoglycaemia
    - Neuromuscular blockade
    - Drug toxicity
2. Establish absence of:
    - Pupil reflex
    - Corneal reflex
    - Vestibulo-ocular reflex (see below)

Physical Examination for Surgeons, ed. Petrut Gogalniceanu, James Pegrum and William Lynn. Published by Cambridge University Press. © Cambridge University Press 2015.

- Oculocephalic reflex (see below)
- Gag reflex (on suction)
- Pain response (no peripheral response to cranial nerve stimulus or vice versa)
- Ventilatory effort – formal apnoea testing (see below)

3. Apply confirmatory tests if appropriate:
   - EEG
   - Angiography
   - Transcranial Doppler
   - Auditory brainstem evoked potentials

Assessment of brain death

Definition:
Irreversible loss of cerebral and brainstem function which can be confirmed by the absence of specific physiological responses and reflexes

Diagnosis not possible without prior correction of:
- Significant metabolic, electrolyte or endocrine disturbance
- Hypothermia <35C
- Hypotension
- Neuromuscular blockade, poisoning, drug intoxication

Mimics of brain death
- Locked in syndrome: Infarction of ventral pons — Vertical eye movements and blinking preserved
- Guillain Barre syndrome
- Severe hypothermia
- Anaesthetic/sedative effect

Criteria (UK – 1976 Conference of the Royal Medical Colleges)
- No pain response
- Pupils bilaterally fixed/unresponsive
- Corneal reflex absent bilaterally
- Oculo-cephalic reflex – absent (rotate the head sharply to exclude any 'doll's eye' maintenance of the point of gaze fixation)
- Vestibulo-ocular reflex – absent (ear canal irrigated with 20ml ice cold water, absence of eye deviation confirmed. Repeat with other ear after >5 mins)
- Apnoea test

Confirmatory tests (especially for children <1 year)
- Auditory brainstem evoked potentials
- EEG
- Cerebral angiography (no arterial filling at the skull base)
- Nuclear imaging
- Transcranial Doppler ultrasound

Examination notes

How is an apnoea test performed?

Preoxygenate with 100% O_2. Disconnect the ventilator (high-flow O_2 may be administered through a catheter).

Serial ABGs should be performed. A $pCO_2 > 6.7$ kPa without respiratory effort confirms apnoea. If hypoxia ($pO_2 < 8$ kPa) develops, the test must be stopped.

How is the vestibulo-ocular reflex elicited?

One ear canal is irrigated with ice-cold water. Eye deviation and nystagmus (slow phase towards the irrigated ear) should result if brainstem function is preserved. The test can be repeated on the other side after 5 minutes.

How is the oculocephalic reflex elicited?

The head is turned sharply to one side. The oculocephalic ('doll's eye') reflex entails eye movement as if to maintain the direction of gaze fixation despite movement of head.

Examining the level of consciousness

- Ensure the unconscious patient has had a primary survey and non-neurological causes of a low Glasgow Coma Scale (GCS) have been excluded.
- Assess GCS:
  - Speak to the patient and establish orientation in time, place and person:
    - What is the time?
    - What is the date?
    - Where are you?
    - What's my job?
  - A patient answering promptly and correctly has a GCS of 15.
- If GCS is < 15, proceed to:
  - Ask patient clearly and repeatedly to:
    - open the eyes
    - stick the tongue out

- If this fails to elicit a response, exert firm pressure over the supraorbital ridge:
  - Score M5 for localising only if the patient's hand reaches above the shoulder in response, otherwise M4 for withdrawal.
  - Score M3 for abnormal 'decorticate' flexion of elbows and wrists.
  - Score M2 for 'decerebrate' extensor posturing.

Glasgow Coma Scale: eyes, verbal, motor.

	1	2	3	4	5	6
Eyes n/4	Not opening	Open to painful stimulus	Open to voice	Open spontaneously		
Voice n/5	No response	Incomprehensible sounds	Inappropriate words	Confused speech	Lucid speech	
Motor n/6	No response	Abnormal extension	Abnormal flexion	Withdrawal	Localising	Obeying commands

> **Tip**
>
> Record and report any reduced GCS in full: e.g. 'E3 V4 M6' rather than '13'. This is much more informative for a clinician and avoids inconsistencies (e.g. an alert patient with an aphasia scoring 11).

> **Example**
>
> **Question:** What is the GCS of an unresponsive patient exhibiting abnormal flexion and making inarticulate sounds in response to pain, but not opening her eyes?
>
> **Answer:** The GCS is E1 V2 M3. It can help to remember that voice is scored out of 'V' or 5.

Examination notes

What indications are there for arranging CT following a head injury?

For adults who have sustained a head injury, the NICE criteria for performing a CT head scan **within 1 hour** are:[23]

- GCS less than 13 on initial assessment in the ED
- GCS less than 15 two hours post injury
- Suspected open or depressed skull fracture
- Any sign of basal skull fracture (haemotympanum, 'panda eyes', cerebrospinal fluid leakage from the ear or nose, Battle's sign)
- Post-traumatic seizure
- Focal neurological deficit
- More than one episode of vomiting

NICE criteria for performing a CT head scan **within 8 hours** are:

- Age 65 or older
- Any history of bleeding or clotting disorders
- Dangerous mechanism of injury (a pedestrian or cyclist struck by a motor vehicle, an occupant ejected from a motor vehicle or a fall from a height of greater than 1 metre or 5 stairs)

---

[23] National Institute for Health and Care Excellence. *Head injury: Triage, Assessment, Investigation and Early Management of Head Injury in Children, Young People and Adults.* NICE Guidelines CG 176, January 2014. http://www.nice.org.uk/guidance/CG176.

- More than 30 minutes retrograde amnesia of events immediately before the head injury

When is it reasonable to discharge patients on the day of a mild head injury?
- GCS 15 and no neurological deficits
- CT head (if indicated) is normal
- No drug or alcohol intoxication
- Accompanied by responsible adult
- Head injury advice provided

What is the lucid interval?
A patient who has sustained a blunt trauma to the head without significant primary brain injury may recover consciousness quickly and fully. If the injury results in damage to an intracranial blood vessel, the expanding blood clot can be accommodated initially. This is the lucid interval. According to the Monro–Kellie doctrine, as this compensation is exhausted, further enlargement of the mass leads to exponential increase in intracranial pressure akin to an intracranial compartment syndrome, resulting in 'coning': herniation of brain, loss of consciousness and death.

Classically the lucid interval precedes deterioration due to extradural haematoma, resulting from a temporal bone fracture with damage to the middle meningeal artery.

Assessment of meningism

History triad
- Headache
- Neck stiffness
- Photophobia

Examination
- Shine a light in the patient's eyes to confirm photophobia.
- Brudzinski's neck sign:
  - Flex the patient's neck gently.
  - Involuntary flexion of hips is observed.
- Kernig's sign:
  - Bend the hip and knee to 90°.
  - Attempted knee extension with the hip flexed is painful/resisted.

To confirm the diagnosis
- Consider CT head followed by lumbar puncture.

Examination notes

What are the principal causes of meningeal irritation?
- Infection
- Subarachnoid bleeding
- Chemical insult

> **Tip**
>
> The clinical signs associated with meningism have a low sensitivity.

Assessment of higher cognitive function

The most cursory assessment is to establish whether the patient is correctly orientated in time, place and person.

The 10-point Abbreviated Mental Test Score (AMTS) is a useful screen, whilst the 30-point Mini-Mental State Examination (MMSE) offers a more thorough evaluation.

Abbreviated Mental Test Score
- How old are you? (1 point)
- What time is it? (1 point)
- Ask patient to remember an address.
- What year are we in? (1 point)
- What is the name of this hospital? (1 point)
- Ask patient to recognise two persons (e.g. family member and nurse). (1 point)
- What is your date of birth? (1 point)
- Ask patient to recall a culturally acceptable notable date (e.g. end of World War II, coronation of the queen). (1 point)
- Ask patient to name a notable leader (e.g. queen, president, prime minister). (1 point)
- Count from 20 to 1. (1 point)
- Check the address that was given earlier. (1 point)

Examination notes

What patterns of aphasia are you aware of?

- Expressive aphasia:
    - Damage to Broca's area in the inferior frontal gyrus
    - An expressive deficit with failure to generate speech, but preserved comprehension
- Receptive aphasia:
    - Damage to Wernicke's area in the temporal lobe
    - A receptive deficit manifesting fluent, incomprehensible speech and impaired comprehension
- Conduction aphasia:
    - Due to damage to the arcuate fasciculus connecting Broca's and Wernicke's areas
    - Relatively preserved comprehension and speech generation, but impaired repetition

While the derivation of the terms *dysphasia* and *aphasia* implies respectively impaired and absent language function, the term aphasia is applied universally, and usually preferred, because of the potential for confusion between dysphasia and dysphagia.

How would you assess an aphasia at the bedside?

1. Establish comprehension (impaired in receptive aphasia):
    a. appropriate response to specific questioning
    b. obey multi-step directions
2. Establish ability to name objects (impaired in expressive aphasia). Be sure to distinguish dysarthria (difficulty articulating words) from expressive aphasia (difficulty finding words).
3. Establish ability to repeat phrases (impaired in conduction aphasia).

Comprehensive evaluation of aphasia depends on extensive standardised screening batteries administered by a neuropsychologist.

What are the cortical localising features?

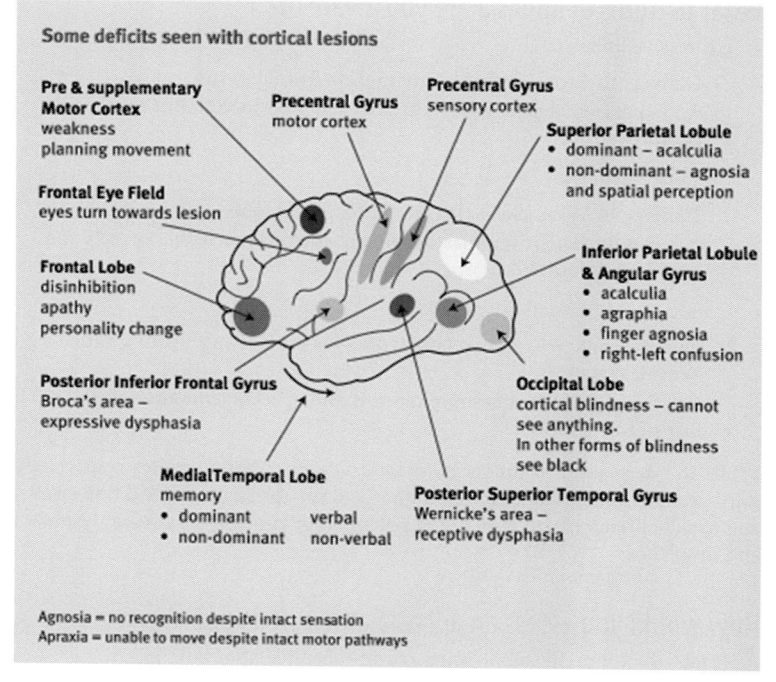

Some deficits seen with cortical lesions

Pre & supplementary Motor Cortex
weakness
planning movement

Precentral Gyrus
motor cortex

Precentral Gyrus
sensory cortex

Superior Parietal Lobule
- dominant – acalculia
- non-dominant – agnosia and spatial perception

Frontal Eye Field
eyes turn towards lesion

Frontal Lobe
disinhibition
apathy
personality change

Inferior Parietal Lobule & Angular Gyrus
- acalculia
- agraphia
- finger agnosia
- right-left confusion

Posterior Inferior Frontal Gyrus
Broca's area – expressive dysphasia

Occipital Lobe
cortical blindness – cannot see anything.
In other forms of blindness see black

Medial Temporal Lobe
memory
- dominant   verbal
- non-dominant non-verbal

Posterior Superior Temporal Gyrus
Wernicke's area – receptive dysphasia

Agnosia = no recognition despite intact sensation
Apraxia = unable to move despite intact motor pathways

Cortical localising features. Reproduced from Bulters D, Shenouda E. Assessment of neurological function. *Surgery (Oxford)* 2007; **25**: 501–4, with permission from Elsevier.

Differential diagnoses

What are the causes of seizures?

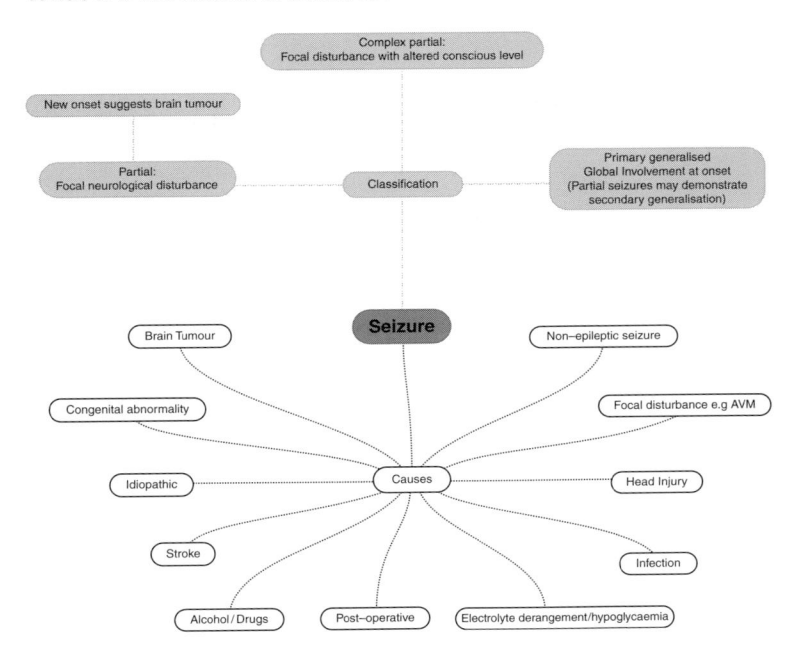

Classification:
- Partial: Focal neurological disturbance
  - New onset suggests brain tumour
- Complex partial: Focal disturbance with altered conscious level
- Primary generalised: Global involvement at onset (Partial seizures may demonstrate secondary generalisation)

Seizure — Causes:
- Brain Tumour
- Congenital abnormality
- Idiopathic
- Stroke
- Alcohol / Drugs
- Post-operative
- Electrolyte derangement / hypoglycaemia
- Infection
- Head Injury
- Focal disturbance e.g. AVM
- Non-epileptic seizure

What are the complications of head injuries?

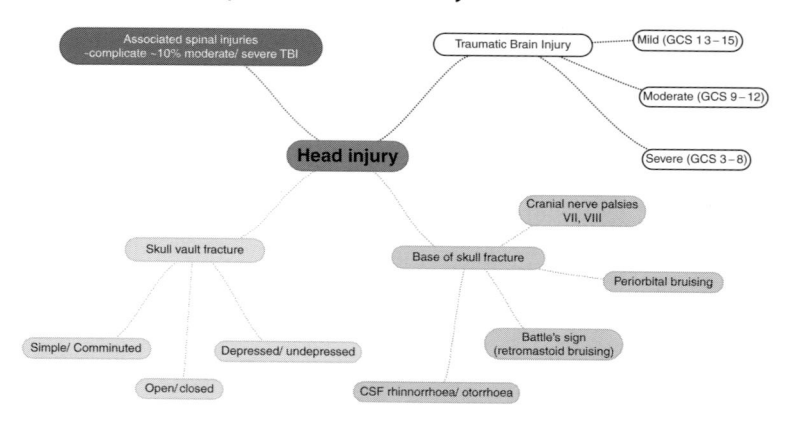

- **Head injury**
  - Associated spinal injuries - complicate ~10% moderate/ severe TBI
  - Traumatic Brain Injury
    - Mild (GCS 13–15)
    - Moderate (GCS 9–12)
    - Severe (GCS 3–8)
  - Skull vault fracture
    - Simple/ Comminuted
    - Depressed/ undepressed
    - Open/ closed
  - Base of skull fracture
    - Cranial nerve palsies VII, VIII
    - Periorbital bruising
    - Battle's sign (retromastoid bruising)
    - CSF rhinnorrhoea/ otorrhoea

What causes thunderclap headaches?

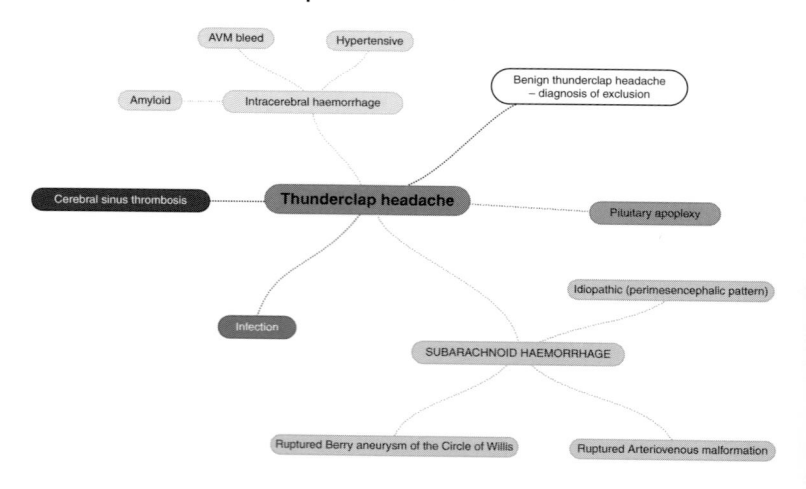

- **Thunderclap headache**
  - Intracerebral haemorrhage
    - AVM bleed
    - Hypertensive
    - Amyloid
  - Benign thunderclap headache – diagnosis of exclusion
  - Cerebral sinus thrombosis
  - Pituitary apoplexy
  - Infection
  - SUBARACHNOID HAEMORRHAGE
    - Idiopathic (perimesencephalic pattern)
    - Ruptured Berry aneurysm of the Circle of Willis
    - Ruptured Arteriovenous malformation

Chapter 37: Global neurological examination | 331

What is the differential for fever and headache?

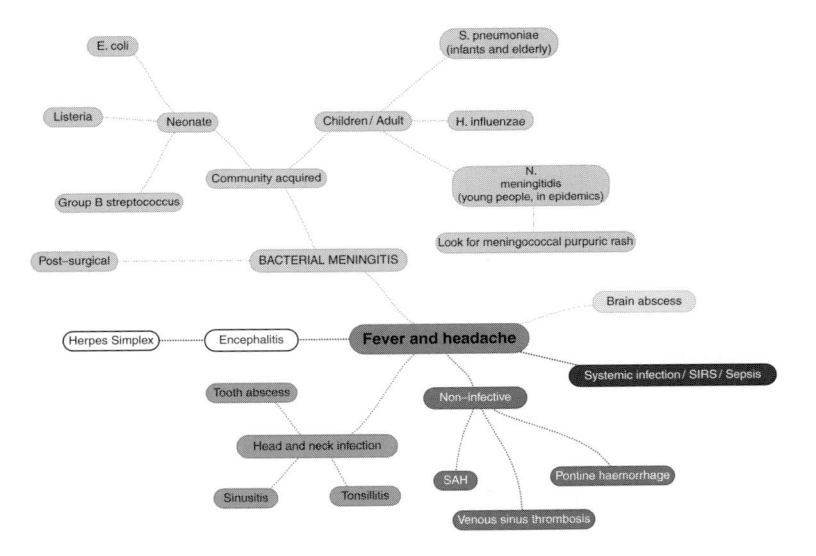

- **Fever and headache**
  - **BACTERIAL MENINGITIS**
    - Community acquired
      - Neonate
        - E. coli
        - Listeria
        - Group B streptococcus
      - Children / Adult
        - S. pneumoniae (infants and elderly)
        - H. influenzae
        - N. meningitidis (young people, in epidemics)
        - Look for meningococcal purpuric rash
    - Post-surgical
  - Encephalitis
    - Herpes Simplex
  - Brain abscess
  - Systemic infection / SIRS / Sepsis
  - Head and neck infection
    - Tooth abscess
    - Sinusitis
    - Tonsillitis
  - Non-infective
    - SAH
    - Venous sinus thrombosis
    - Pontine haemorrhage

/ Section 9 /

Chapter 38

Neurosurgery

Focal neurological examination

Harry Bulstrode, Yezen Sheena and Diederik O. Bulters

Neurological examination is traditionally divided into examination of the cranial nerves and examination of the peripheral nervous system. In fact the two routines are complementary, and serve a common primary goal: to localise pathology within the nervous system, central and peripheral. Together with an impression of the type of lesion, derived primarily from the history, this localising information is central to correct interpretation of subsequent cross-sectional imaging.

Examination of the cranial nerves

You may need to select appropriate components of the following examination routines according to the clinical scenarios and guidance provided by examiners. This is a test of frontal lobe function.

Checklist

CN I (olfactory nerve)
- Not routinely tested

CN II (optic nerve)
- Acuity: each eye individually
- Fields: four quadrants to confrontation
- Reflexes: accommodation; direct and consensual light reflex
- Ophthalmoscopy: visualise the disc, exclude papilloedema

CN III, CN IV, CN VI (oculomotor, trochlear, abducens nerves)
- Ask patient to report any double vision during testing.
- Instruct patient to keep the head still.

Physical Examination for Surgeons, ed. Petrut Gogalniceanu, James Pegrum and William Lynn. Published by Cambridge University Press. © Cambridge University Press 2015.

- Ask patient to follow finger with eyes and report any double vision.
- Move finger to all extremes of gaze in an H-shape, to confirm normal upgaze/downgaze in both eyes, in abduction and adduction.

CN V (trigeminal nerve)
- Assess fine touch sensation in the three divisions:
  - ophthalmic (Va) over temple
  - maxillary (Vb) over cheek
  - mandibular (Vc) over angle of mandible
- Confirm masseter/temporalis contraction on clenching teeth.
- Elicit corneal reflex and jaw jerk.

CN VII (facial nerve)
- Ask patient to:
  - raise eyebrows
  - close eyes tightly
  - puff out cheeks
  - show teeth

CN VIII (vestibulocochlear nerve)
- Test recognition of whispered speech in each ear individually.
- Weber's and Rinne's tests.

CN IX (glossopharyngeal nerve)
- Offer to test gag reflex.
- Prompt the patient to cough, looking for a strong cough.
- Prompt the patient to swallow, observing for symmetry.

CN X (vagus nerve)
- Observe palatal/uvula movements as patient says 'aah'.

CN XI (accessory nerve)
- Shrug shoulders against resistance.
- Turn head against resistance.

CN XII (hypoglossal nerve)
- Ask patient to stick tongue out and move it from side to side.

Examination notes: cranial nerves

What about the first cranial nerve?

Olfactory nerve function is not routinely tested. However, anosmia frequently complicates traumatic brain injury, and may be a feature of tumours (e.g. olfactory groove meningioma). Where appropriate, you could offer to test identification of coffee or vinegar, for example.

How would you assess visual fields to confrontation?

- Effective assessment requires the patient to maintain fixation centrally while identifying movement in four quadrants, upper and lower, left and right, and on both sides at once (to exclude neglect suggestive of parietal pathology). Testing each eye individually is key to fully appreciate any deficit.
- Key patterns to identify (see figure) are:
  - Bitemporal hemianopia (due to compression of the optic chiasm, classically by a pituitary tumour).
  - Superior quadrantanopia (temporal lobe pathology encroaching on Meyer's loop, part of the optic radiation).
  - Cortical lesions are characterised by macular sparing, since this part of the field is represented bilaterally.
- For completeness, further testing with a coloured pinhead can be offered to establish the extent of the blind spot and determine presence of scotomas.

What eye reflexes would you elicit?

- The pupillary light reflex should be assessed by shining a pen torch beam into each pupil in turn, observing prompt and equal constriction of the ipsilateral (direct reflex) and contralateral (consensual reflex) pupils.
- A *relative afferent pupillary defect (Marcus Gunn pupil)* indicative of unilateral retinal or optic nerve pathology is evidenced by alternating dilatation and constriction of both pupils as the beam is swung from the affected to the unaffected side and back again.
- The accommodation reflex comprises pupil dilatation on changing the patient's fixation from nearby ('concentrate on my finger tip') to a distant point ('and now the wall behind me'). Holmes–Adie pupil describes a tonically dilated pupil with an impaired light reflex but preserved accommodation response. It is a common finding, especially in young women.

Visual field deficits from lesions along the visual pathway

Locations on the left relate to deficits on the right. The lesions in the eye and optic nerve affect one eye only and may range from complete loss to a small deficit.

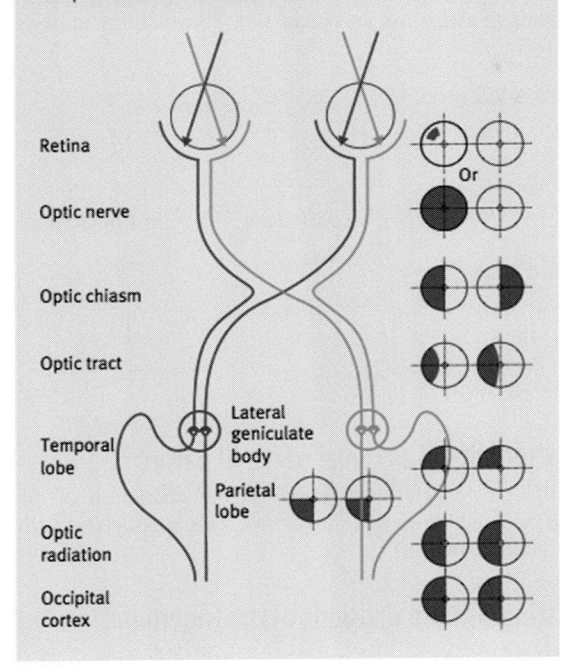

*Visual field deficits. Reproduced from Bulters D, Shenouda E. Assessment of neurological function. Surgery (Oxford) 2007; **25**: 501–4, with permission from Elsevier.*

What is the role of ophthalmoscopy in patients presenting with headache?

Ophthalmoscopy serves to identify:

- Papilloedema suggestive of sustained raised intracranial pressure (e.g. caused by a tumour or hydrocephalus). This may be absent in the context of acutely raised intracranial pressure, or there may be atrophic changes in longstanding chronic disease.
- Haemorrhage into the vitreous humour (Terson's syndrome) or other intraocular haemorrhage secondary to a subarachnoid haemorrhage.

How do you isolate the contributions of the individual muscles when testing eye movements?

On confrontation, ask the patient to fix his or her gaze on your finger while you draw a standard 'H' pattern in the air. If the patient is not able to keep the head still, use your free hand to stabilise the chin. The H-shape allows testing of vertical eye movements in abduction and adduction, to which the muscles contribute as follows:

Muscle	Nerve	Action	
Medial rectus	III	Adduction	
Lateral rectus	VI	Abduction	
		(In adduction)	**(In abduction)**
Superior rectus	III	(Intorsion)	Elevation
Inferior rectus	III	(Extorsion)	Depression
Superior oblique	IV	Depression	(Intorsion)
Inferior oblique	III	Elevation	(Extorsion)

What are the characteristics of a cranial nerve III palsy?

The patient suffers diplopia, which may be reduced on abduction of the affected eye. The eye is deviated 'down and out' at rest. This is associated with ptosis and mydriasis (pupil dilatation).

How would you distinguish the divisions of the trigeminal nerve on examination?

The divisions are tested using light touch stimulus:
- Va (ophthalmic): on the forehead
- Vb (maxillary): over cheekbone
- Vc (mandibular): on the mandible

Only Vc conveys a motor component, supplying the muscles of mastication.

How would you distinguish upper and lower motor neuron pathology in the facial nerve?

In upper motor neuron lesions the movement in the upper part of the face is spared because of bilateral supranuclear inputs to the nuclei controlling the frontalis and orbicularis oculi muscles.

Mild weakness may still manifest as an inability to 'bury' the eyelashes on forced eye closure.

What is Bell's phenomenon?

Bell's phenomenon is the upward rolling of the eye observed as the eyelid fails to close – this serves to protect the cornea when eye closure is impaired, typically due to lower motor neuron damage to the facial nerve.

How would you perform Weber's and Rinne's tests?

Weber's test (useful screening test): place a resonating tuning fork in the centre of the patient's forehead. The sound should be heard equally on each side.

- It will be heard more loudly in the unaffected ear in the context of sensorineural hearing loss.
- It will be heard more loudly in the affected ear in the context of conductive hearing loss.
- To differentiate between the two perform Rinne's test.

Rinne's test: place a resonating tuning fork on the mastoid process. Once sound can no longer be detected by the patient through the mastoid, place the tuning fork adjacent to the ear canal to determine whether residual vibrations are still heard. This compares bone and air conduction, respectively.

- To exclude a conductive hearing loss – air conduction should be louder than bone conduction.

For further details see Chapter 32, *Examination of the ear*.

How would you assess vestibular function?

Vestibular function can be assessed by:

- Gait examination: the patient will tend to veer towards the side of a unilateral vestibular lesion, especially when heel-to-toe walking.
- Romberg's test: ask the patient to stand with feet together and then to close the eyes. The examiner stands ready to catch them should they begin to fall. This usually occurs towards the side of the vestibular lesion.

How would you assess cranial nerves IX and X?

The gag reflex is subserved by the glossopharyngeal nerve (CN IX) as the afferent limb and the vagus nerve (CN X) as the efferent limb. However, it is unpleasant for the subject, so observing the patient's cough and swallow is the more appropriate routine screen in conscious patients.

What are you testing by asking the patient to turn the head to the right?

The left sternocleidomastoid muscle (CN XI) turns the head to the right, and the right SCM turns it to the left.

In which direction does the tongue deviate in the context of a CN XII lesion?

The tongue deviates to the side of the lesion on protrusion.

Differential diagnoses

What are the causes of eye movement abnormalities?

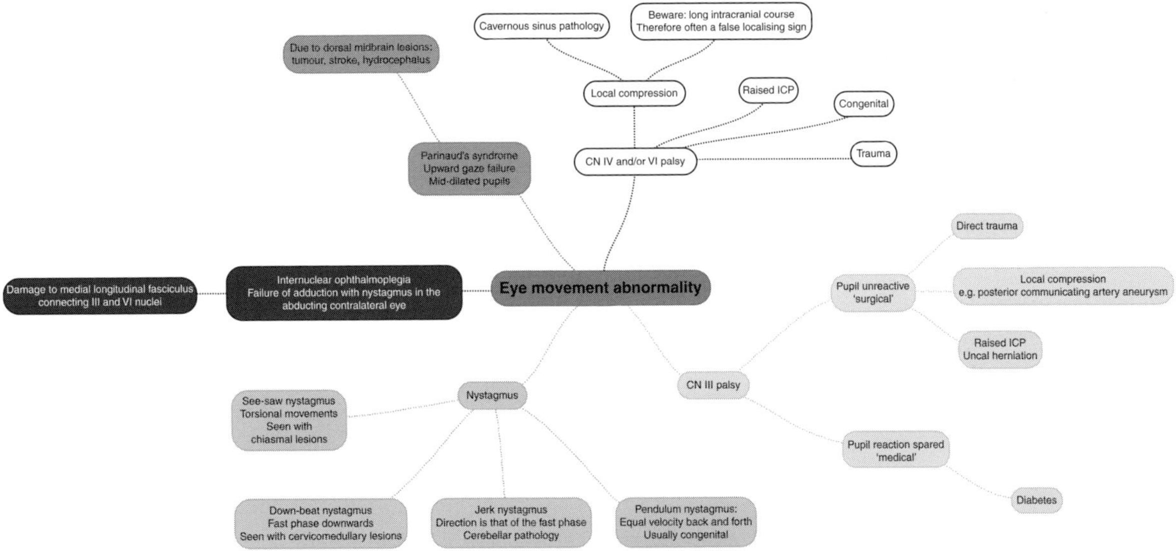

- **Eye movement abnormality**
  - **Internuclear ophthalmoplegia**
    Failure of adduction with nystagmus in the abducting contralateral eye
    - Damage to medial longitudinal fasciculus connecting III and VI nuclei
  - **Parinaud's syndrome**
    Upward gaze failure
    Mid-dilated pupils
    - Due to dorsal midbrain lesions: tumour, stroke, hydrocephalus
  - **CN IV and/or VI palsy**
    - Cavernous sinus pathology
    - Local compression
      - Beware: long intracranial course
      - Therefore often a false localising sign
    - Raised ICP
    - Congenital
    - Trauma
  - **CN III palsy**
    - Pupil unreactive 'surgical'
      - Direct trauma
      - Local compression e.g. posterior communicating artery aneurysm
      - Raised ICP
      - Uncal herniation
    - Pupil reaction spared 'medical'
      - Diabetes
  - **Nystagmus**
    - See-saw nystagmus
      Torsional movements
      Seen with chiasmal lesions
    - Down-beat nystagmus
      Fast phase downwards
      Seen with cervicomedullary lesions
    - Jerk nystagmus
      Direction is that of the fast phase
      Cerebellar pathology
    - Pendulum nystagmus:
      Equal velocity back and forth
      Usually congenital

What are the causes of a pupil abnormality?

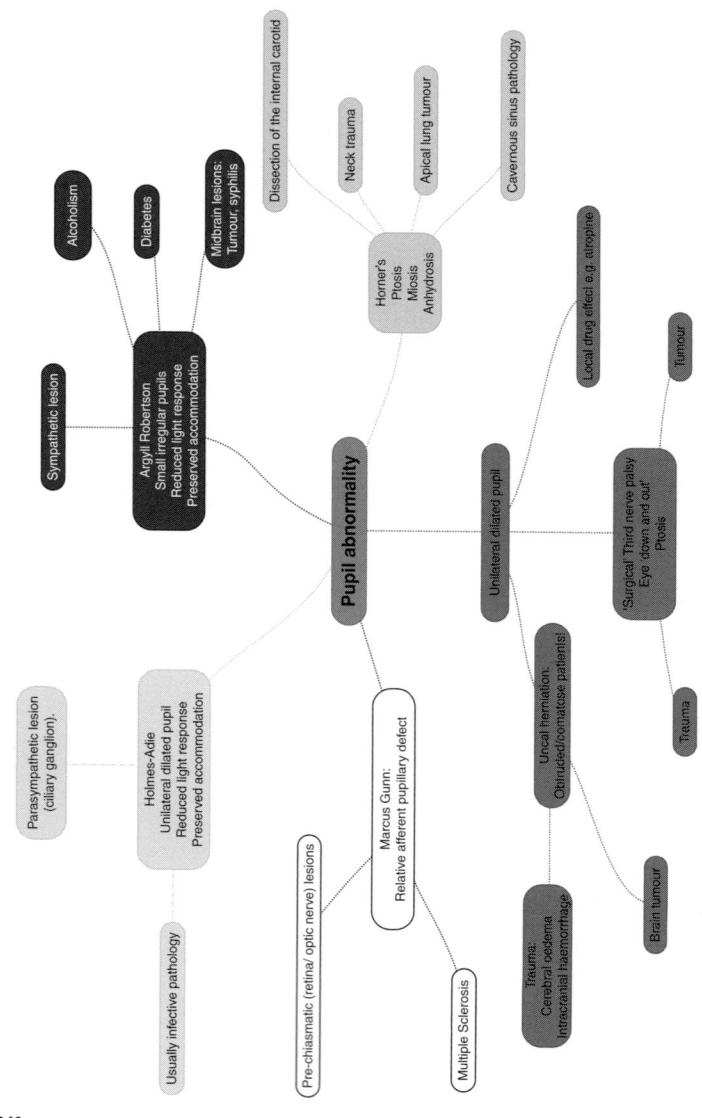

- **Pupil abnormality**
  - **Argyll Robertson**
    Small irregular pupils
    Reduced light response
    Preserved accommodation
    - Sympathetic lesion
    - Alcoholism
    - Diabetes
    - Midbrain lesions: Tumour, syphilis
  - **Horner's**
    Ptosis
    Miosis
    Anhydrosis
    - Dissection of the internal carotid
    - Neck trauma
    - Apical lung tumour
    - Cavernous sinus pathology
  - **Unilateral dilated pupil**
    - Local drug effect e.g. atropine
    - "Surgical" Third nerve palsy
      Eye 'down and out'
      Ptosis
      - Tumour
      - Trauma
    - Uncal herniation: Obtunded/comatose patients
      - Trauma: Cerebral oedema, Intracranial haemorrhage
      - Brain tumour
  - **Marcus Gunn:** Relative afferent pupillary defect
    - Pre-chiasmatic (retina/ optic nerve) lesions
    - Multiple Sclerosis
  - **Holmes-Adie**
    Unilateral dilated pupil
    Reduced light response
    Preserved accommodation
    - Parasympathetic lesion (ciliary ganglion)
    - Usually infective pathology

340

Examination of the peripheral nervous system: upper limbs

Checklist

WIPER and Physiological parameters
- Adequate exposure of neck and arms

Inspection
- Neck and arms:
  - wasting, fasciculation, contractures
  - scars over the cervical spine
  - skin stigmata (neurofibromas)
- Pronator drift

Tone
- Wrist, elbow and shoulder assessed in flexion and extension
- Normal/increased/decreased

Power
- Grade MRC 1–5 in all groups

Coordination
- Finger–nose

Reflexes
- Biceps, triceps, supinator
- Hoffmann's sign

Sensation
- Fine touch
- Joint position (proprioception)

Examination notes: upper limbs
What cervical spine scars should be identified?

- Posterior scars:
  - decompression, laminectomy
  - foramen magnum decompression (for Chiari malformation)
- Anterior scars:
  - decompression/discectomy

How is muscle power graded?

Medical Research Council (MRC) grading of muscle power.

5	Full and normal power against resistance
4	Overcomes gravity and moves against some resistance
3	Overcomes gravity but not resistance from the examiner
2	Active movement when gravity eliminated
1	Muscle contraction visible; no movement at the joint
0	No muscle contraction visible

How would you test the myotome/dermatome corresponding to this root level?

Upper limb neurology

Disc	Root	Myotomes	Dermatomes	Reflex
C4–5	C5	Shoulder abduction/deltoid	Lateral arm	Biceps
C5–6	C6	Elbow flexion/biceps	Lateral forearm, thumb and index finger	Brachioradialis
C6–7	C7	Elbow extension/triceps	Middle finger	Triceps
C7–T1	C8	Wrist flexion/long finger flexors	Medial forearm	—
T1–2	T1	Finger abduction/finger intrinsics	Medial arm	—

What is pronator drift?

Ask the patient to hold his or her arms out, palms up, and to close the eyes while maintaining this position. A 'drift' into pronation indicates pyramidal/upper motor neuron pattern weakness.

How do you elicit a Hoffmann's sign?

Technique: Hold the distal interphalangeal joint of the patient's middle finger between your thumb and middle finger and then depress the fingernail with your index finger. As your finger slips over the nail, the distal phalanx is released back into extension.

Positive test: Accompanying flexion of the other fingers of the hand.

Interpretation: Hyper-reflexia due to an upper motor neuron lesion affecting the limb.

Examination of the peripheral nervous system: lower limbs

Checklist

WIPER and physiological parameters
- Adequate exposure of back and lower limbs

Patient standing

Inspection (back and lower limbs)
- Wasting, fasciculation, fixed position/contracture
- Surgical scars: commonly lumbar decompression +/− fixation
- Gait and posture
- Romberg's test

Patient supine

Tone
- Roll legs
- Clonus

Power
- MRC grade 1–5
- Toes, ankles, knees, hips

Coordination
- Heel slide over shin

Reflexes
- Patella, ankle, plantar

Sensation
- Fine touch
- Joint position (proprioception): start with toes

Examination notes: lower limbs

How would you test the myotome/dermatome corresponding to this root level?

Lower limb neurology

Disc	Root	Myotomes	Dermatomes	Reflex
L1–2	L2	Hip flexion/iliopsoas (femoral nerve)	Medial thigh	—
L2–3	L3	Knee extension/quadriceps (femoral nerve)	Medial knee	—
L3–4	L4	Ankle dorsiflexion/tibialis anterior (deep peroneal nerve)	Medial ankle	Patella
L4–5	L5	Great toe extension/extensor hallucis longus (deep peroneal nerve)	Dorsum of foot	—
L5–S1	S1	Foot plantarflexion/Achilles tendon (tibial nerve)	Lateral ankle	Achilles tendon
Cauda equina	S2–4	—	Perianal sensation (saddle anaesthesia)	Anal wink, bulbocavernosus

What is clonus?

Clonus describes reflex repetitive muscle contraction in response to a stretch stimulus.

Sustained clonus at the ankle of more than five beats is considered pathological, indicating upper motor neuron pathology.

Describe the important gait abnormalities

- Antalgic gait – short weight-bearing time on the painful leg (any cause of limb pain)
- Spastic gait – 'scissoring' stiff movement, dragging feet; legs abnormally close together (upper motor neuron lesions, e.g. spinal cord compression, stroke)

- Ataxic gait – wide-based, unsteady (dorsal column/cerebellar pathology)
- Festinating gait – stooped, shuffling, short steps (Parkinson's)
- Myopathic gait – waddling (spinal muscle atrophy, muscular dystrophies)

How do you perform Romberg's test?

Rationale: To test proprioception and dorsal column function.

Technique:

- Ask the patient to stand still with feet together and eyes open.
- Unsteadiness in this situation may point to cerebellar ataxia, but is *not* a positive Romberg's.
- Prepare to catch the patient if they should lose balance, and ask them to close their eyes.

Positive test: Inability to maintain balance with the eyes closed points to exaggerated reliance on visual input because of a loss of proprioception. This may indicate damage to the dorsal columns.

Examination of suspected cauda equina syndrome (CES)

Your goals are to establish the nature and level of any deficit (remember that most disc protrusions will impinge on the nerve exiting at the root below), and to rule out upper motor neuron pathology (any indication of this will necessitate imaging above the lumbar region).

Checklist

1. Lower limb examination:
   - As detailed above.
2. Perineal examination:
   - Get a chaperone.
   - Explain what is intended and obtain verbal consent.
   - Position patient on the couch on his or her side.
   - **Sensation**: assess pinprick sensation over buttocks and perianal area bilaterally (saddle anaesthesia has 75% sensitivity for diagnosis of CES).
   - **Reflexes**: elicit reflex contraction of the anal sphincter by stroking the adjacent skin (anal wink) or applying pressure to the glans penis (bulbocavernosus reflex).
   - **Digital rectal examination**: assess passive tone and ability to squeeze. Is the rectum loaded with faeces? Urine retention commonly results from back pain and constipation without any cauda equine compression.
   - **Perform a straight leg raise** with the patient supine.
   - **Examine for a palpable bladder** (and perform a post-void bladder scan).

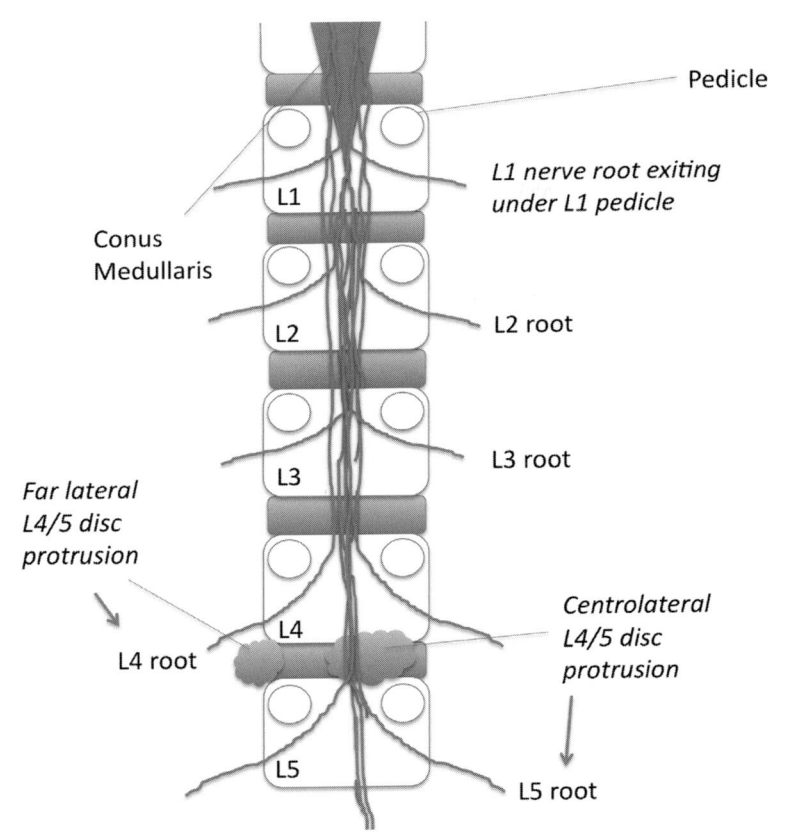

Chapter 38: Focal neurological examination | 347

Cauda equina anatomy: the lumbar spinal canal viewed from behind, with the posterior elements removed. The spinal cord terminates in the conus medullaris at L1. The nerve roots arising here comprise the cauda equina. Most disc prolapses compress only a single root, causing a lumbar radiculopathy. Commonly centrolateral disc prolapses (here at L4/5) will compress the transiting nerve root on its way to exit at the level below (here L5); occasionally a far lateral prolapse will compress the exiting nerve root at the higher level (here L4). A large central disc prolapse, especially in the context of a congenitally narrow spinal canal, can compress all the descending nerve roots to cause a cauda equina syndrome. Reproduced from Bulters D, Shenouda E. Assessment of neurological function. *Surgery (Oxford)* 2007; **25**: 501–4, with permission from Elsevier.

What are the immediate management priorities in a patient with spinal cord injury?

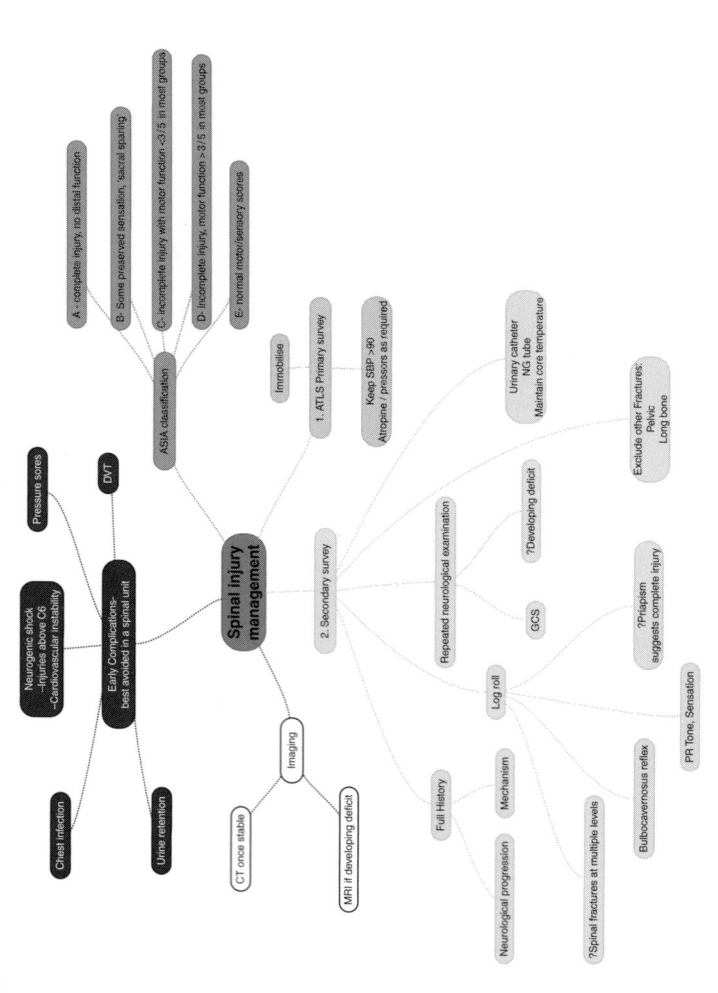

Spinal injury management

ASIA classification
- A - complete injury, no distal function
- B - Some preserved sensation, sacral sparing
- C - Incomplete injury with motor function <3/5 in most groups
- D - Incomplete injury, motor function >3/5 in most groups
- E - normal motor/sensory scores

1. ATLS Primary survey
- Immobilise
- Keep SBP >90
- Atropine / pressors as required

2. Secondary survey
- Urinary catheter
- NG tube
- Maintain core temperature
- Exclude other Fractures: Pelvic, Long bone
- Repeated neurological examination
- ?Developing deficit
- GCS
- ?Priapism suggests complete injury
- Log roll
  - Full History
  - Mechanism
  - Neurological progression
  - ?Spinal fractures at multiple levels
  - Bulbocavernosus reflex
  - PR Tone, Sensation

Imaging
- CT once stable
- MRI if developing deficit

Early Complications - best avoided in a spinal unit
- Pressure sores
- DVT
- Neurogenic shock
  - Injuries above C6
  - Cardiovascular instability
- Chest infection
- Urine retention

348

Localising the lesion

Motor system: type of weakness

UMN	Increased tone, increased reflexes, pyramidal pattern
LMN	Wasting, fasciculation, decreased tone, reduced reflexes
NMJ	Fatigued weakness, normal tone and reflexes
Muscle	Wasting, decreased tone, reduced reflexes

UMN: Upper Motor Neurone; LMN: Lower Motor Neurone; NMJ: Neuromuscular Junction.

Reproduced from Bulters D, Shenouda E. Assessment of neurological function. *Surgery (Oxford)* 2007; **25**: 501–4, with permission from Elsevier.

Motor lesions and their deficits

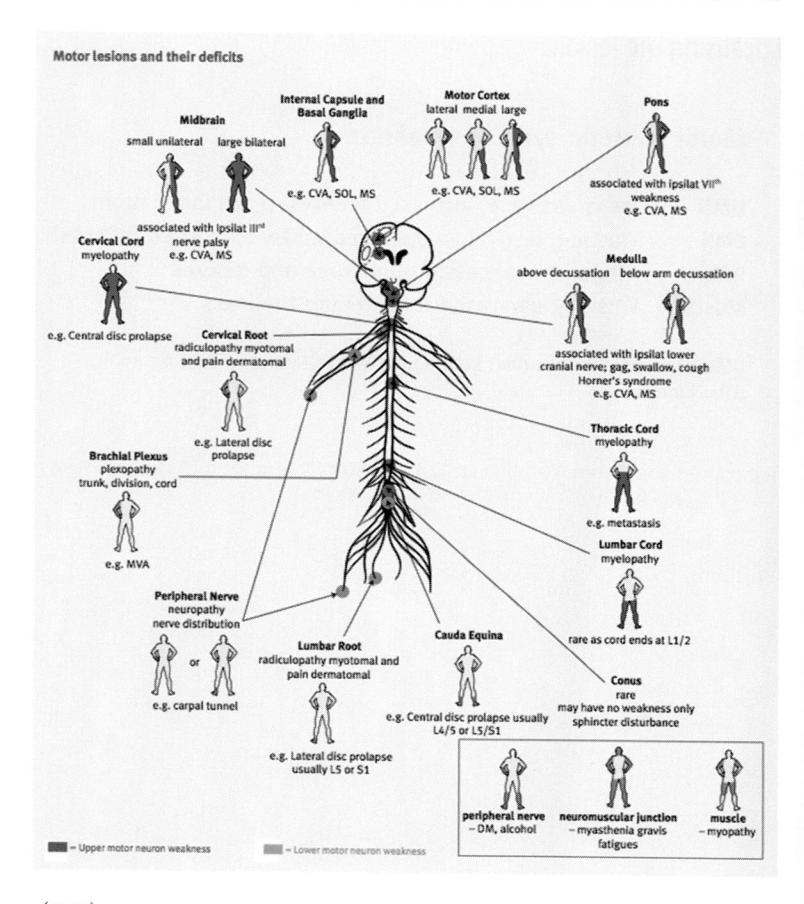

Midbrain
small unilateral — large bilateral
associated with ipsilat IIIrd nerve palsy
e.g. CVA, MS

Internal Capsule and Basal Ganglia
e.g. CVA, SOL, MS

Motor Cortex
lateral medial large
e.g. CVA, SOL, MS

Pons
associated with ipsilat VIIth weakness
e.g. CVA, MS

Cervical Cord
myelopathy
e.g. Central disc prolapse

Cervical Root
radiculopathy myotomal and pain dermatomal
e.g. Lateral disc prolapse

Medulla
above decussation — below arm decussation
associated with ipsilat lower cranial nerve; gag, swallow, cough
Horner's syndrome
e.g. CVA, MS

Brachial Plexus
plexopathy trunk, division, cord
e.g. MVA

Thoracic Cord
myelopathy
e.g. metastasis

Lumbar Cord
myelopathy
rare as cord ends at L1/2

Peripheral Nerve
neuropathy nerve distribution
e.g. carpal tunnel

Lumbar Root
radiculopathy myotomal and pain dermatomal
e.g. Lateral disc prolapse usually L5 or S1

Cauda Equina
e.g. Central disc prolapse usually L4/5 or L5/S1

Conus
rare
may have no weakness only sphincter disturbance

peripheral nerve – DM, alcohol

neuromuscular junction – myasthenia gravis fatigues

muscle – myopathy

■ = Upper motor neuron weakness   ■ = Lower motor neuron weakness

(*cont.*)

What are the causes of limb weakness?

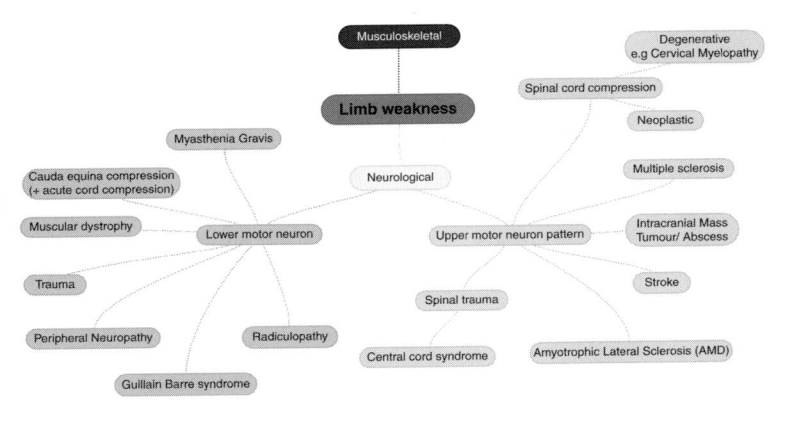

- **Limb weakness**
  - Musculoskeletal
  - Neurological
    - Myasthenia Gravis
    - Lower motor neuron
      - Cauda equina compression (+ acute cord compression)
      - Muscular dystrophy
      - Trauma
      - Peripheral Neuropathy
      - Radiculopathy
      - Guillain Barre syndrome
    - Upper motor neuron pattern
      - Spinal cord compression
        - Degenerative e.g Cervical Myelopathy
        - Neoplastic
      - Multiple sclerosis
      - Intracranial Mass Tumour/ Abscess
      - Stroke
      - Amyotrophic Lateral Sclerosis (AMD)
      - Spinal trauma
      - Central cord syndrome

What are the causes of spinal cord compression?

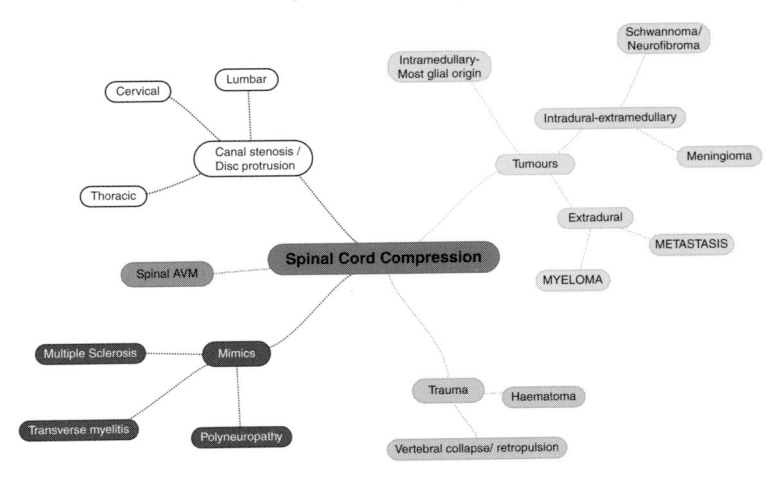

- **Spinal Cord Compression**
  - Canal stenosis / Disc protrusion
    - Cervical
    - Lumbar
    - Thoracic
  - Tumours
    - Intramedullary- Most glial origin
    - Intradural-extramedullary
      - Schwannoma/ Neurofibroma
      - Meningioma
    - Extradural
      - METASTASIS
      - MYELOMA
  - Trauma
    - Haematoma
    - Vertebral collapse/ retropulsion
  - Spinal AVM
  - Mimics
    - Multiple Sclerosis
    - Transverse myelitis
    - Polyneuropathy

What congenital abnormalities affect the hindbrain and spinal cord?

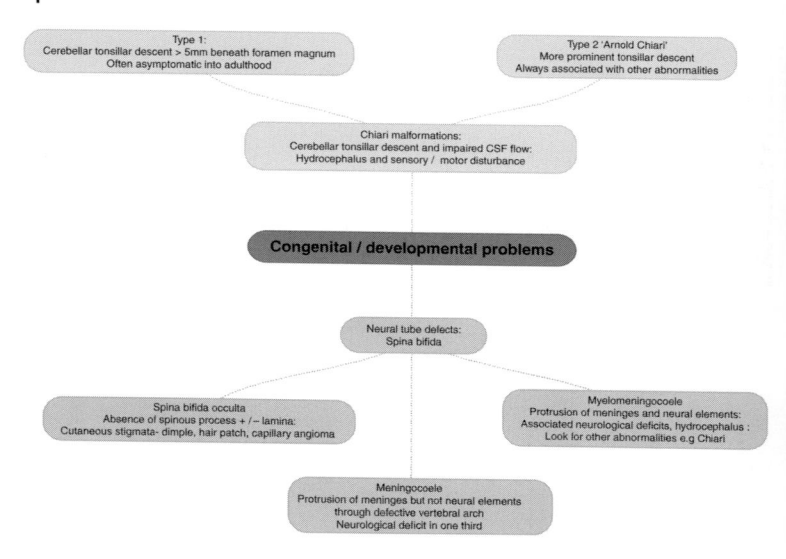

Congenital / developmental problems

- **Chiari malformations:**
  Cerebellar tonsillar descent and impaired CSF flow:
  Hydrocephalus and sensory / motor disturbance
  - **Type 1:**
    Cerebellar tonsillar descent > 5mm beneath foramen magnum
    Often asymptomatic into adulthood
  - **Type 2 'Arnold Chiari'**
    More prominent tonsillar descent
    Always associated with other abnormalities

- **Neural tube defects:**
  Spina bifida
  - **Spina bifida occulta**
    Absence of spinous process +/– lamina:
    Cutaneous stigmata- dimple, hair patch, capillary angioma
  - **Meningocoele**
    Protrusion of meninges but not neural elements through defective vertebral arch
    Neurological deficit in one third
  - **Myelomeningocoele**
    Protrusion of meninges and neural elements:
    Associated neurological deficits, hydrocephalus ;
    Look for other abnormalities e.g Chiari

Section editor: Yezen Sheena
Senior author: Henk Giele

Section 10 — Plastic surgery

Chapter 39

Examination of skin lesions and lumps

Edmund Fitzgerald O'Connor, Yezen Sheena, Petrut Gogalniceanu and Henk Giele

Checklist

WIPER
- Good light source. Lesion and loco-regional lymph nodes exposed.

Physiological parameters
- Ask: 'Where is the lesion?'
- Ask: 'Is the lesion painful?'

System
- **S-E-I-S** (Site, External, Internal, Surroundings)

Skin type
- Fitzpatrick classification of skin type

Site
- Location of lesion
- Number of lesions

External features
- Size (in cm)

Physical Examination for Surgeons, ed. Petrut Gogalniceanu, James Pegrum and William Lynn. Published by Cambridge University Press. © Cambridge University Press 2015.

- Shape:
    - smooth or irregular edge
    - flat or raised profile
- Surface:
    - skin: intact or ulcerated skin, skin adnexae
    - colour/pigmentation and telangiectasia
    - colour distribution: regular vs. irregular
    - discharge: blood, pus, lymph
- Scars from previous surgery (skin lesions or lymphadenectomy)

Internal
- Consistency: soft, hard
- Content: gas (crepitus), fluid (fluctuant and transilluminable), solid (non-transilluminable)
- Dynamic interaction: pulsatile, reducible, indentable, compressible
- Mobility and attachment to surrounding structures (above, below and laterally)
- Percussion: dull or resonant (gas, fluid, solid)
- Auscultation: bruits, bowel sounds

Surroundings
- Assess surrounding skin: normal or satellite lesions.
- Palpate for local, regional, general lymphadenopathy.
- Assess nerves: local and distal sensory and motor functions.
- Assess vascular supply of lesion: capillary refill time and pulses.
- Palpate liver for an irregular edge or enlargement and vertebral spine for tenderness if concerned about metastatic deposits.

Examination notes

Tip

The examination of a lump is very poorly done in general, due to a lack of a systematic or anatomical way of approaching the lesion. Palpation in particular needs to be structured as described above in order to avoid redundant gestures.

What is the system for examining a skin lump?

S-E-I-S:

Skin (type) and **S**ite (inspection)

External features (inspection)

Internal features (inspection and palpation)

Surroundings: skin, local, regional or distal lymph nodes (inspection, palpation and movement)

> **Tip**
>
> Beware the melanoma patient with a prosthetic eye or ear.

What are the principal questions in assessing a skin lesion?

- Where is the lesion located on the body?
- What does the lesion look like externally?
- What is inside the lesion?
- What is the anatomical plane of the lesion?
- Does it arise from:
    - skin?
    - subcutaneous tissues?
    - underlying tissues (blood vessels, nerves, tendons muscles and bones)?
- Is the lesion likely to be benign or malignant?

How should the site be described?

The position of the lesion should be given by distance from two fixed reference points (e.g. 'The lesion is found 3 cm from the lateral canthus of the left eye and 2 cm superior to the left zygomatic arch').

What is the purpose of auscultation?

- Identify bruits from vascular malformations or arteriovenous fistulas.
- Identify presence of bowel sounds.

What are the common malignant skin lesions?

1. Basal cell carcinoma (BCC).
2. Squamous cell carcinoma (SCC).
3. Malignant melanoma (MM).

What are the rarer malignant skin lesions?

1. Merkel cell tumour
2. Dermatofibrosarcoma protuberans (DFSP): high rate of local recurrence
3. Eccrine porocarcinoma
4. Leiomyosarcoma

What are the common benign skin lesions?

1. Naevi
2. Seborrhoeic keratosis
3. Actinic keratosis (precancerous lesion: 2–5% will go on to become SCC)
4. Dermatofibromas

> **Tip**
>
> Pigmented benign lesions should be assessed with a view to excluding malignant melanoma.

How should lesions be described?

- Use dermatologically accurate terms. Ask: Is it raised or flat? Is it over or under 1 cm?
- Flat circumscribed area of altered skin colour:
  - macule < 1 cm
  - patch > 1 cm
- A solid raised circumscribed skin lesion:
  - papule < 1 cm
  - nodule > 1 cm
- When estimating size use a ruler or TBSA for larger lesions.

What are the 'red flag' features of MM?

Suspicion should be raised about pigmented lesions with the following features:

Asymmetry
Border (irregular)
Colour (very dark or heterogeneous/variegated)

Diameter (> 6 mm)

Evolution (any relatively recent changing moles or additional features like itchiness/bleeding is suspicious)

Any of the above merits low threshold for diagnostic excision biopsy (2 mm margin).

How do you differentiate between SCC and BCC?

- Basal cell carcinomas or 'rodent ulcers' commonly appear raised with a pearly 'transluescent' edge and telangiectasia.
- Squamous cell carcinomas are classically crusted patches with ulceration (but may have raised 'everted' edges).
- Telangiectasias are potentially very subtle and require close inspection. Gently stretch the skin around the lesion and look for blanching vessels within or crossing the lesion.

> **Tip**
>
> SCCs can arise from chronic skin irritation (Marjolin's ulcer), so have a low threshold for incision biopsy of 'non-healing' ulcers near chronic wounds or fistulas.

What is the Fitzpatrick classification?

The Fitzpatrick scale classifies skin colour and its susceptibility to UV damage:

Type I	Light; pale (red hair). Always burns, never tans.
Type II	White; fair (blonde hair). Usually burns, tans with difficulty.
Type III	Medium; beige skin. Sometimes burns, gradually tans light brown.
Type IV	Olive-brown (dark hair). Rarely burns, easily tans moderate brown.
Type V	Dark brown. Very rarely burns, tans very easily.
Type VI	Black. Never burns, tans very easily, deeply pigmented.

Use this classification to accurately describe the patient's skin type, as it correlates to the risk of developing sun damage and malignancies.

What is the role of the dermatoscope?

Hand-held dermatoscopes usually magnify ×10 and use polarised light (minimising skin reflection). When used by trained clinicians they can improve

diagnostic accuracy of superficial skin lesions by identifying pathognomonic signs of different skin cancers:
- BCC: asymmetrical 'arborising' vessels
- SCC: glomerular/pinpoint vessels
- MM: blue-grey veil, pseudopodia, irregular dots and globs

Why should sensory and motor function be tested?

Sensory and motor assessment is important to identify potential invasive lesions and tissue viability.

# Section 10: Plastic surgery

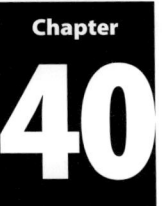

Chapter 40: Examination of scars

Edmund Fitzgerald O'Connor, Yezen Sheena and Henk Giele

Checklist

WIPER

Physiological parameters

Look
- Anatomy: **S**ite, **O**rientation, **L**ength, **C**olour, **C**ontracture
- Healing status: fresh, healing, healed, mature
- Healing method: primary or secondary intention
- Pathological scarring: hypertrophic or keloid changes, scar widening or stretching
- Infection: sinuses, fistulas, granulation or discharge
- Signs of surgical correction (e.g. z-plasty)

Feel
- Tenderness
- Thickness, pliability
- Adherence
- Evidence of malignant occurrence or recurrence

Move
- Mobility of scar
- Mobility and laxity of surrounding skin
- Associated functional impairment (test related muscles, joints and nerves)

Physical Examination for Surgeons, ed. Petrut Gogalniceanu, James Pegrum and William Lynn. Published by Cambridge University Press. © Cambridge University Press 2015.

> *To complete the examination...*
> - Assess regional lymph nodes.
> - Obtain formal function assessment by occupational therapist/physiotherapist as required.

Examination notes

How do wounds heal?

Skin scarring is the normal and inevitable outcome of cutaneous wound healing. Wound healing follows a sequence of overlapping phases: haemostasis, inflammation, proliferation and remodelling.

What factor must be considered on inspection?

- **Cause**: Consider underlying medical comorbidities that led to the scar, but never assume the surgical procedure if this information has not been given.
- **Colour**: An assessment of the colour of the scar may indicate its age. Wound healing has defined sequential yet overlapping stages within which the scar will change in colour. As a scar passes from the proliferative phase through to remodelling and finally into a mature scar so its colour will decrease in red pigmentation. A variegated pink scar is younger than a homogeneous white scar.
- **Location**: The position of the scar indicates potential functional complications. If the scar is over a joint there is a risk of contractures causing decreased range of movement. Assess for underlying neurovascular function and deficits following surgery or injury: for example, periorbital scars may be associated with ectropion directly from cicatricial healing, or weakness due to damage to the temporal branch of the facial nerve (CN VII), or a sensory loss due to trigeminal nerve (CN V1) injuries.
- **Closure**: The presence of suture marks may give an indication as to the type of incision or the wound treated. Planned elective surgery is less likely to use interrupted non-absorbable sutures, whilst trauma surgery or infected wound treatment would. A wide, irregular scar may have healed by secondary intention. These are not definitive rules.

What are the differences between hypertrophic and keloid scarring?

- Hypertrophic scarring is defined as an abnormally **raised**, pink, persistent scar tissue **within the boundaries of the original wound**.
- Keloid scars are significantly abnormally **raised**, persistent scars that extends **beyond the wound's boundaries**.

What is the relevance of scar tenderness?

A tender scar might indicate recent injury/surgery, tethering to underlying structures, neuropathy or underlying infection.

How can scars be classified and assessed?

The Vancouver Scar Scale (VSS) is used widely to provide an objective clinical assessment of scars, based on vascularity, pigmentation, pliability and height.[24]

> **Tip**
>
> Connective tissue disorders such as Ehlers–Danlos syndrome can cause abnormal wound healing and stretched or hypertrophic scarring.

---

[24] Sullivan T, Smith J, Kermode J, McIver E, Courtemanche DJ. Rating the burn scar. *J Burn Care Rehabil* 1990; **11**: 256–60.

Section 10 **Plastic surgery**

Chapter 41

Examination of flaps and grafts

Edmund Fitzgerald O'Connor, Yezen Sheena and Henk Giele

Checklist

WIPER

Physiological parameters

General
- Note any scars, deformities or skin lesions. Offer to inspect the whole body.

Inspection
- Identify any flaps and grafts, and describe any scars present (see Chapter 40, *Examination of scars*).
- Comment on the location.
- Flap:
  - site and size
  - type of flap: local, regional or distant
  - phase of healing: well-healed, immaturity of scar, adequacy of outcome
  - check donor sites or exposure scars
- Graft:
  - site, size and colour match of graft
  - type of graft:
    - pattern of scarring: split-thickness skin graft (STSG) or full-thickness skin graft (FTSG)
    - cobblestone or crocodile skin appearance (derived from a meshed graft)

Physical Examination for Surgeons, ed. Petrut Gogalniceanu, James Pegrum and William Lynn. Published by Cambridge University Press. © Cambridge University Press 2015.

- healing: graft take as a percentage
- bed of flap: muscle flap/native muscle/fat
- Check common graft donor sites:
  - upper thighs for STSG
  - inner upper arms, supraclavicular fossa, retroauricular, groins for FTSG

Palpation
- Consistency: thickness, pliability, contour
- Vascular supply: colour, capillary refill
- Neurology: sensation
- Base:
  - firm (recurrent disease or scarring)
  - fluctuant (seroma or haematoma)

To complete the examination...
- Inspect for donor sites and any other scars/skin lesions.
- Offer to palpate regional lymphatic drainage sites if previous cancer excisions.

Examination notes

What is the system for inspecting flaps and grafts?
S-T-H-D:
- **S**ite
- **T**ype
- **H**ealing
- **D**onor site

What is the difference between a flap and graft?
- A skin graft consists of skin tissue taken from one area of the body and transferred to another, being dependent on the recipient site for blood and nutrients.
- A flap consists of tissue taken from one area of the body and transferred to another, bringing with it its own source of blood and nutrients.

What are the different types of grafts?
Split-thickness skin graft (STSG)
- Split-thickness skin grafts consist of epidermis and a variable amount of dermis.
- STSGs are able to resurface larger areas than full-thickness grafts.

- A meshed STSG can give a characteristic cross-hatched or pebbled appearance. It has a higher chance of developing hypertrophic scarring. Meshing allows for a larger defect area to be covered.

Full-thickness skin graft (FTSG)
- Full-thickness skin grafts contain the entire epidermis and dermis.
- FTSGs are thicker, and more robust, pliable and normal than STSGs.
- They are usually taken from donor areas with sufficient laxity, allowing direct closure.
- The general principle with FTSGs is to replace like with like. In a facial FTSG inspect for common facial donor sites in the preauricular, postauricular or supraclavicular areas.

How are flaps assessed and described?

Flaps can be classified by the 5 Cs:
- **Circulation**: random-pattern blood supply, axial blood supply (flap dependent on a named vessel or perforator)
- **Composition**: cutaneous, fasciocutaneous, fascial, musculocutaneous, muscle, osseocutaneous, osseous
- **Contiguity**: local, regional and distant (pedicled and free)
- **Contour**: the method in which they are transferred into the defect – transposition, advancement rotation
- **Conditioning**: delay principle

A **local flap** is defined as tissue moved with its own source of blood and nutrients which shares a common edge with or is directly adjacent to the defect being reconstructed.

What are the different types of local skin flaps?

- **Advancement**: tissue is advanced forward to close a defect, utilising laxity within the skin.
- **Transposition**: the movement of adjacent tissue for reconstruction, leaving a defect requiring closure with a different method.
- **Rotation**: tissue rotated around a pivot point for defect closure, with the ability to close the donor site.
- **Pedicled**: tissue moved from a distant site to which they remain attached via nutrient vessels.
- **Free**: tissue taken from one area of the body and moved to another with its own blood vessels detached and anastomosed at the recipient site.

How are free flaps identified?
- Free flaps may be identified as discrete areas that slightly differ from the surrounding tissues, usually with a contour or skin character change.
- Free flaps may have a corresponding donor site scar.
- Donor site scars can be linear (if direct closure was possible) or contain a skin graft.

What are the common reasons for free flap reconstruction?
- Head and neck: skin cancer excision, aerodigestive cancers
- Chest: breast cancer reconstruction
- Lower limb trauma: open tibial fractures

What are the common cutaneous (fascio- or myocutaneous) free flap donor sites?
- Lateral thigh: anterolateral thigh (ALT) flap
- Lower abdomen: deep inferior epigastric perforator (DIEP) flap or rectus abdominus flap
- Back: latissimus dorsi (LD) flap or scapula flap
- Forearms: radial forearm flap (RFF)
- Groins: groin flap

What are the common muscle free flap donor sites?
- Back: latissimus dorsi
- Inner thigh: gracilis
- Abdomen: rectus

What do you understand by the term the 'reconstructive toolbox'?

Flaps and grafts are two tools in the reconstructive surgeon's so-called 'toolbox' of wound management. Many factors must be considered in choosing the best solution, tailored to each patient's tissue defect.

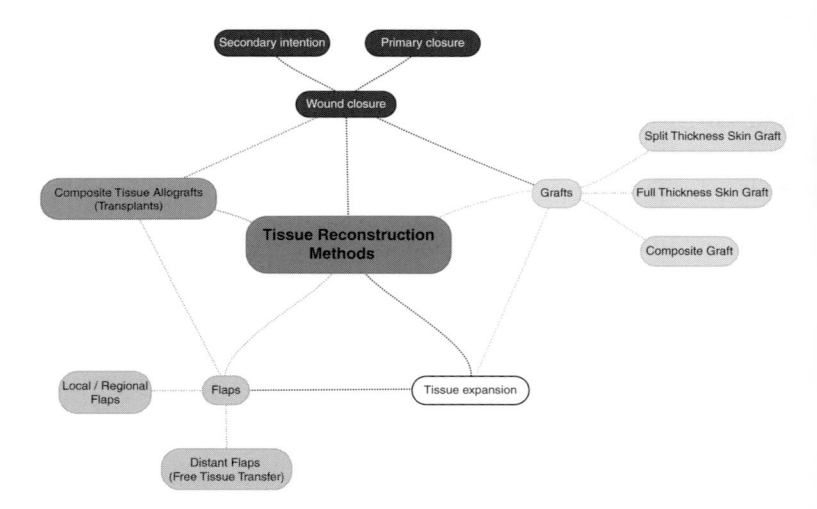

- **Tissue Reconstruction Methods**
  - Wound closure
    - Secondary intention
    - Primary closure
  - Grafts
    - Split Thickness Skin Graft
    - Full Thickness Skin Graft
    - Composite Graft
  - Composite Tissue Allografts (Transplants)
  - Flaps
    - Local / Regional Flaps
    - Distant Flaps (Free Tissue Transfer)
  - Tissue expansion

Section 10 **Plastic surgery**

Chapter 42

Examination of burns

Yezen Sheena, Edmund Fitzgerald O'Connor, Petrut Gogalniceanu and Henk Giele

Acute burns

Checklist

WIPER

Physiological parameters

General
- Resuscitate patient.
- ITU support: airway, hydration, analgesia and antibiotics.
- Comment on dressings already applied.

Look
- Site of the burn
- Airway compromise risk factors: singed nasal hairs, perioral burns, blistered palate, swelling of tongue or naso-oral mucosa, hoarse voice due to laryngo-oedema, swollen uvula
- Percentage of total body surface area (TBSA) burnt
- Circumferential burns to chest or limbs
- Depth of burn:
  - superficial (epidermal)
  - superficial partial-thickness (superficial dermal)
  - deep partial-thickness (deep dermal)
  - full-thickness
- Assess any structure(s) involved at the base of the burn.

Physical Examination for Surgeons, ed. Petrut Gogalniceanu, James Pegrum and William Lynn. Published by Cambridge University Press. © Cambridge University Press 2015.

Feel
- Sensation/tenderness
- Capillary refill time in burn, peripheral and centrally
- Moist or dry burn
- Assess peripheral pulses
- Assess chest movements if any circumferential burns
- Identify compartment syndrome in circumferential limb burns

Move
- Movement of underlying joints

Old burns

Checklist

WIPER

Physiological parameters

General
- Tracheostomy scar
- Fitted pressure garments/splints

Look
- Site affected by the burn
- Extent of burn
- Burn and donor sites: graft/flap healing status, colour, contour, contracture, cosmetic result

Feel
- Burn and donor sites for healing result: thickness scars, texture, sensation, tenderness, pliability

Move
- Assess contraction of scars around joints, testing ROM.
- Assess functional impairment of local structures.

To complete the examination...
- Assess neurovascular status of loco-regional tissue involved.

Examination notes
What is a burn?
A burn is the coagulative necrosis of tissue due to a thermal, chemical, electrical, friction or radiation insult.

What are the guidelines for the management of burns?
1. Advanced Trauma Life Support (ATLS)[25]
2. Emergency Management of Severe Burns (EMSB) principles[26]

One must accurately assess the burn size and depth, as this will determine further specialist management.

> **Tip**
>
> The size and depth of a burn is dynamic/progressive according to Jackson's three-zone model:
>
> 1. Coagulation: necrosis
> 2. Stasis: surrounding 'penumbra' potentially salvageable with correct resuscitation
> 3. Hyperaemia: increased perfusion peripheral areas usually recover

How is burn depth estimated?
- Superficial burns (epidermal injury only): erythema with no blistering.
- Partial-thickness burns (dermal injuries):
  - blisters:
    - de-roofed blisters: wet, sensate bed and blanch on direct pressure
    - deep dermal (reticular dermis): fixed staining of thrombosed capillaries; reduced sensation
- Full-thickness burns (entire dermis and adnexal structure destroyed): charred leathery appearance, insensate and soft tissue is devitalised; may extend deeper (bone).

---

[25] Committee on Trauma, American College of Surgeons. *ATLS: Advanced Trauma Life Support Program for Doctors*, 8th edn. Chicago: American College of Surgeons, 2008.

[26] Hettiaratchy S, Papini R. Initial management of a major burn: I. overview. BMJ 2004; **328**: 1555–7. Herndon DN, ed. *Total Burn Care*, 4th edn. London: Saunders, 2012.

How can a burn size be estimated?

There are different methods of assessing the total body surface area (TBSA), but excluding erythema.

- Very small burns are best described in terms of their measured dimensions (like any other lump or skin lesion).
- Slightly larger burns may be estimated using the *palm rule* (the patient's hand including fingers is 0.8–1% TBSA).
- Large burns can be estimated using the *rule of nines*. This allocates 9% TBSA for the head and neck, and for each upper limb; 18% for the front, the back of torso and each lower limb; 1% for genitalia. Beware that this rule needs to be modified for children and obese adults.
- An alternative method uses a Lund and Browder chart.

What life-threatening emergencies must be identified on clinical examination of the burns victim?

- Airway compromise and inhalation injuries
- Compartment syndrome
- Hypovolaemia/hypothermia/hypoglycaemia
- Sepsis
- Carbon monoxide/cyanide poisoning

What are the criteria for burn centre transfer?

- Any full-thickness, circumferential or inhalation burns
- Partial-thickness burns > 5% in child or 10% in an adult
- Special areas (hands, feet, genitalia, perineum, flexures, neck, face)
- Chemical, electrical (including lightning strikes), high-pressure injection/steam
- Concomitant trauma, pre-existing medical comorbidity or pregnancy
- Vulnerable adults and patients with mental health problems
- Extremes of age, suspected NAI (non-accidental injury) or any other concerns

Section 10

Plastic surgery

Chapter 43

Examination of the hands

Yezen Sheena, Edmund Fitzgerald O'Connor, Petrut Gogalniceanu and Henk Giele

Checklist

WIPER
- Hands on a pillow on the patient's lap

Physiological parameters
- Ask if there is any pain

Systemic observations
- Aids/splints
- Ears: gouty tophi
- Face: scleroderma, acromegaly, hypothyroidism
- Elbow extensor surfaces: rheumatoid nodules, psoriasis plaques

Look
- **Skin**: scars, palmar erythema, finger pulp infarcts, cyanosis, nail changes
- **Soft tissues**: muscle wasting, swelling around tendons
- **Bone**: Heberden's and Bouchard's nodes (OA), square wrists and finger deformities in RA (z-thumb, swan neck and ulnar drift deformities), joint subluxations

Feel
- **Skin**: temperature, tenderness

Physical Examination for Surgeons, ed. Petrut Gogalniceanu, James Pegrum and William Lynn. Published by Cambridge University Press. © Cambridge University Press 2015.

- **Soft tissues**:
  - nodules, cords and fascial contractures (Dupuytren's)
  - joints: tenderness, swelling, mucous cysts, ganglions
  - tendons: boggy swelling (tenosynovitis), ruptures
- **Bone**: bone tenderness, crepitus, instability

Vascular
- Radial and ulnar pulses
- Capillary refill time
- Allen's test (see Chapter 26, *Arterial examination of the upper limbs*)

Sensory nerves
- **Median**: palmar thenar eminence and radial 3.5 fingers
- **Ulnar**: palmar hypothenar eminence and ulnar 1.5 digits
- **Radial**: dorsum of hand first web space

Motor nerves
- **Median**:
  - thumb abduction ('palm up, thumb vertical')
  - thumb and index finger: 'OK sign'

- **Ulnar**:
  - interossei PAD/DAB:[27] cross fingers test
  - adductor pollicis: Froment's (thumb-paper test)
  - abductor digiti minimi: little fingers pressed against each other

- **Radial**:
  - extensor pollicis longus: 'flat palm down on table, lift thumb'
  - extensor digitorum communis: extension of four digits

Move
- Test active then passive ROM with a view to identifying neurological, tendon or joint stiffness, crepitus, triggering, instability.
- Assess MRC power grading for each muscle or composite movement as required (see Chapter 38, *Focal neurological examination*).
  Ask patient to make a fist, then to extend all the fingers.

---

[27] PAD, palmar interossei adduct; DAB, dorsal interossei abduct.

- **Wrists**:
  - extension and flexion
  - radial and ulnar deviation
  - supination and pronation
- **Thumbs**:
  - opposition, abduction and adduction, flexion and extension
- **Fingers**:
  - assess alignment/posture/triggering of fingers with movement
  - FDS: fix other fingers in extension → assess PIP joint flexion[28]
  - FDP: fix each PIP joint → test DIP joint flexion[29]
  - interossei: palmar adduct and dorsal abduct fingers (PAD/DAB)
  - extensors: assess lag (dropped finger sign)

Special tests

- Assessment for nerve entrapments (compression neuropathies) – Phalen's sign
- Thumb MCP joint ulnar collateral ligament stability assessment
- Finkelstein's test for De Quervain's tenosynovitis

To complete the examination...

- Examine elbow, shoulder and neck.
- Formally measure any ROM deficit using a goniometer.
- Assess hand function: key grip, writing, button shirt.
- Obtain orthogonal views of hand x-rays (should include adjacent joints).
- Consider further imaging, neurophysiology, or other investigations.
- Full neurological assessment (see Chapter 38).

---

[28] FDS, flexor digitorum superficialis; PIP, proximal interphalangeal.
[29] FDP, flexor digitorum profundus; DIP, distal interphalangeal.

Examination notes
What are the common scars of the hand?

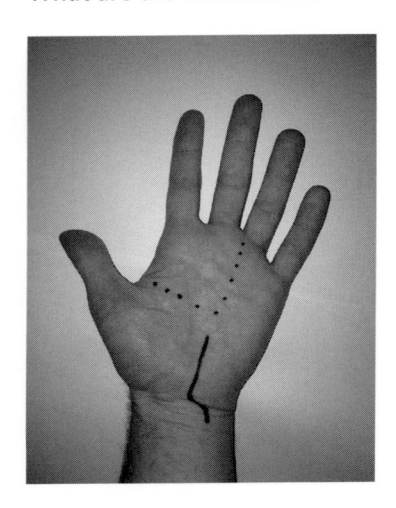

Carpal tunnel decompression scar. Radial border of the ring finger and Kaplan's cardinal line are the key landmarks shown (dotted lines). **If the incision needs to be extended proximally past the distal wrist crease,** the proximal end should **not** go radially, but should be extended towards the ulnar side. This is needed to avoid the cutaneous branch of the median nerve, which is found just radial to palmaris longus.

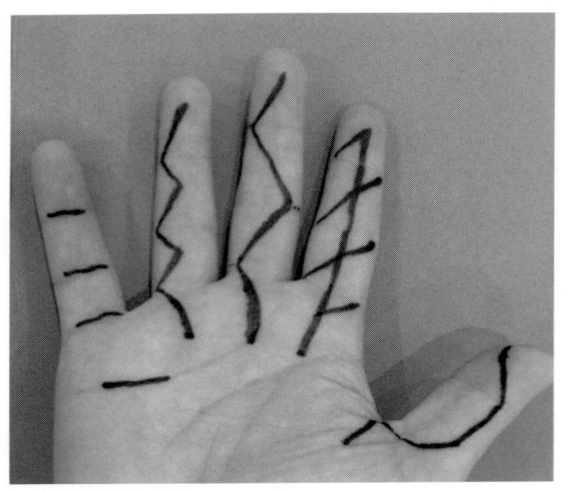

Palmar incisions: thumb, mid-lateral mixed with Bruner; index, Skoog incorporating Z-plasties; middle, Bruner; ring, Littler; little, McCash.

What is the sequence of joints in the hand, from proximal to distal?
- Radiocarpal joint
- Mid-carpal joint
- CMC (carpometacarpal) joint
- MCP (metacarpophalangeal) joint
- PIP (proximal interphalangeal) joint
- DIP (distal interphalangeal) joint

What are the common hand deformities?
- Dupuytren's contractures
- Rheumatoid hands
- Arthritic: OA, psoriatic or seronegative (SLE) arthritides
- Dropped 'mallet' finger (extensor tendon rupture)

What are the common finger deformities?
- Swan neck: hyperextended PIP joint, flexed DIP joint (common in RA)
- Boutonniere: flexed PIP joint, hyperextended DIP joint (common in RA)
- Mallet: flexed (unable to actively extend) DIP joint (distal extensor insertion rupture)
- Bouchard's nodes: PIP joint osteophytes in OA
- Heberden's nodes: DIP joint osteophytes in OA
- Finger (MCP joint) ulnar deviation in RA
- Trigger finger: finger gets stuck in flexion due to tendon nodule stuck under A1 pulley

What are the examination findings in Dupuytren's disease?
- Palmar pits, palmar Dupuytren's nodules and cords and dorsal knuckle (Garrod's) pads.
- Contraction of the palmar or digital fascia with resulting flexion deformity of MCP and PIP joints, commonly of little and ring fingers.
- Pathological cords are: pre-tendinous (palmar), central (digital), lateral (lateral digital), spiral around digital nerve (combination of aforementioned), natatory (web-space).
- Associated with penile fibrous plaques (Peyronie's disease), plantar fibromatosis (Ledderhose's disease) and frozen shoulder.

> **Tip**
>
> Hueston's tabletop test is positive if the patient is unable to place all fingers flat on a table, signifying flexion contractures that merit surgical correction.

What scars can be seen in patients who have had surgery for Dupuytren's disease?

- Longitudinal or transverse (to access > 1 ray) palmar and digital skin incisions. Fasciectomy involves excision of diseased fascia to the affected digit (limited) or all palmar fascia (radical). Skin closure by z-plasty or skin graft.
- Skin and fascia excision (dermofasciectomy with FTSG) may reduce recurrence.

What are the examination findings in rheumatoid arthritis?

A symmetrical polyarthropathy (90% hand involvement) with extra-articular manifestations.

- Rheumatoid nodules on extensor aspect elbows (prognostic of severe disease).
- Joint and tendon synovitis (warm, boggy swelling when active disease).
- Wrists: limited extension/supination from caput ulnae syndrome with dorsally prominent ulna head, and palmar subluxed wrist.
- Tendons: extensor tendon attrition ruptures over ulnar styloid (Vaughan–Jackson lesion).
- Fingers: z-thumb, Boutonnière, swan neck and ulnar drift deformities.

What are the features of osteoarthritis?

- Heberden's and Bouchard's nodes
- 'Squaring' deformity of the wrists
- Crepitus on joint movement
- Stiffness, tenderness and reduced ROM

> **Tip**
>
> **The patient is always seen in the anatomical position: hands opened and supinated, fingers pointing to the floor, palms facing forwards.**
>
> Remember that thumb abduction occurs anteriorly, away from the palmar plane. Adduction is the opposite movement, towards the palm.
>
> Extension occurs laterally/radially away from the palm. Flexion is the opposite movement towards the palm.
>
> Opposition is a complex composite movement involving abduction, flexion and circumduction to bring thumb to finger pulps.

> **Mnemonic for thumb movements**
>
> **FAB REX:**
> Forward abduction
> Radial extension

How can individual peripheral nerves of the hand be examined?

Nerve	Median	Ulnar	Radial
Look	• Wasting of thenar eminence • Extended index and thumb in high median or anterior interosseous (AIN) palsy	• Wasting small muscles of hand especially 1st dorsal interosseous • Posture of hand with extended MCP joints, ulnar claw	• Failure of extensor mechanism: fingers flexed, wrist drop (depending on level)
Feel	• Altered sensibility palmar radial 3½ fingers (thenar mass normal if CTS)	• Altered sensibility palmar and dorsal aspect of 5th finger and half ring finger	• Altered sensibility dorsal 1st web space and dorsum thumb
Move	• Weak thumb abduction/opposition. Weak FPL and FDP (OK sign)	• Weak PAD/DAB • Unable to cross fingers. Froment's sign positive • Unable to flex MCP joints whilst extending IP joints • If high ulnar palsy weak FDP to little and ring	• Weak extensors of the MCP and wrist
Lesion type and level	• Compressive: carpal tunnel/AIN/pronator syndromes • Trauma	• Compressive: Guyon's canal/cubital tunnel syndrome • Trauma	• Compressive: 'Saturday night palsy' • Trauma: shoulder dislocation, humeral fractures

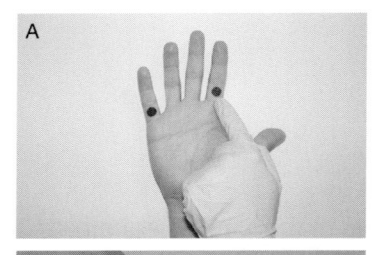

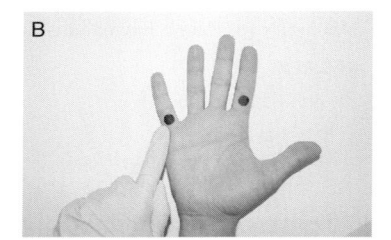

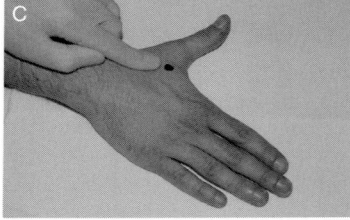

Testing sensory function of (A) median, (B) ulnar and (C) radial nerves in the hands.

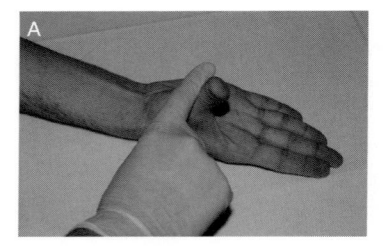

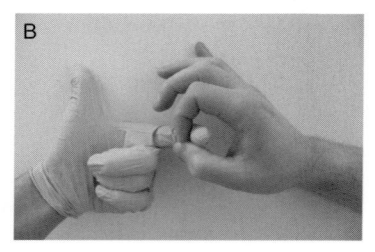

Testing motor function of the median nerve in the hand: (A) resisted thumb abduction and (B) OK sign (FPL in thumb and FDP in index finger).

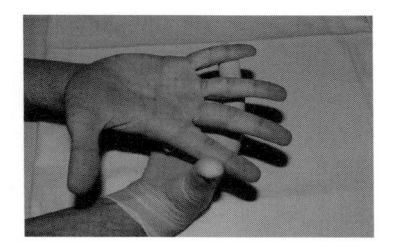

Testing motor function of the ulnar nerve in the hand: finger abduction.

What is Froment's sign?

It tests the ulnar nerve innervation of the adductor pollicis and first dorsal interosseous muscles. Ask the patient to hold a piece of paper between thumb and index finger whilst you attempt to pull it away with gradually increasing strength. The test is positive if the patient has to compensate for weakness in the ulnar nerve muscles by utilising the median-nerve-innervated FPL (flexing thumb IP joint).

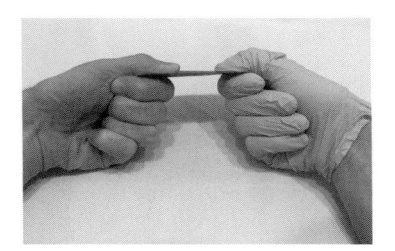

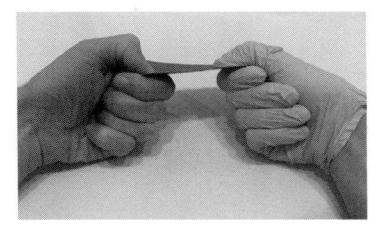

Froment's sign: (A) normal: ulnar nerve intact; (B) abnormal: ulnar nerve lesion with compensation by FPL.

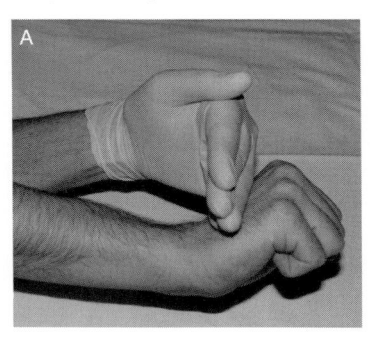

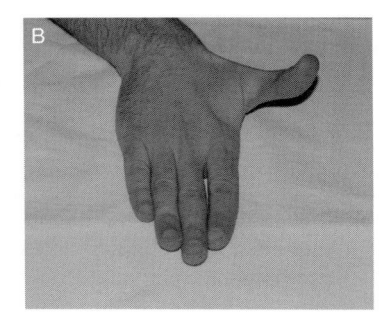

Testing motor function of the radial nerve in the hand: (A) wrist extension, and (B) abduction and extension of the thumb.

> **Tip**
>
> **How can the motor nerves of the hand be quickly screened?**
> Median: 'OK' sign (thumb and index opposition)
> Ulnar: cross index and middle fingers (finger adduction)
> Radial: 'thumbs up' sign ('going up' sign)

What are the common nerve entrapment neuropathies?
- Carpal tunnel: median nerve at the wrist under the transverse carpal ligament
- Cubital tunnel: ulnar nerve at the elbow under Osborne's ligament

How do you examine for carpal tunnel compression?
- Median nerve compression at wrist (carpal tunnel) causing pain, paraesthesia and weakness
- Look: thenar wasting
- Feel: loss of thenar muscle bulk on contraction and resisted thumb abduction, altered sensation in radial 3½ fingers
- Move: weak thumb abduction
- Special tests: Tinel's/Phalen's/Durkan's tests

What is Tinel's sign?
Light tapping (percussion) over irritated nerves anywhere in the body elicits pain or paraesthesia sensation in that nerve's distribution. It can be used to detect nerve regrowth after injury, or as a sign of a compression site. Some correlate speed of positivity with severity of irritation, but the test should be performed for 20 seconds.

What is Phalen's manoeuvre?
- The wrists are placed in maximal flexion (dorsum of hands pressed against each other) for 30 seconds which increases pressure in the carpal tunnel. Alternatively hold the wrist with pressure over the transverse carpal ligament (Durkan's test) and keep the wrist flexed and elevated. This posture increases the pressure within the carpal tunnel and increases the sensitivity of Phalen's sign.
- Positive test: pain or paraesthesia sensation in median nerve distribution is suggestive of carpal tunnel syndrome.
- The reverse Phalen's places hands in maximal wrist extension (Prayer sign). This also raises pressure in the carpal tunnel, provoking symptoms.

How do you examine for cubital tunnel syndrome?
- Cubital tunnel syndrome consists of ulnar nerve compression around the elbow (medial epicondyle) causing sensory and motor changes in the ulnar nerve distribution.
- Look: ulnar guttering, claw-hand deformity.
- Feel: wasting 1st dorsal interosseous and hypothenar muscles, altered sensation in ulnar 1.5 digits (including dorsally, which is normally spared in distal lesions like Guyon's canal).
- Move: PAD/DAB and test power of abductor digiti minimi and adductor pollicis.
- Special tests: Tinel's positive at elbow, Froment's positive and exacerbation of symptoms during elbow flexion whilst applying pressure over the nerve as it travels through the medial epicondylar groove.

What causes clawing of the hand?
- An ulnar nerve injury can result in clawing, characterised by hyperextension of the MCP joints and flexion of the IP joints of the ulnar two digits due to denervation of the ulnar intrinsic muscles including the lumbricals (which normally flex the MCP joints while extending DIP joints). The index and middle fingers do not claw despite loss of their interossei due to the action of their median-innervated lumbricals.
- Clawing is most severe with lower ulnar nerve injuries, as more proximal lesions would also denervate the ulnar two FDPs and therefore lead to a paradoxically milder clawing, as less flexion is possible. This is called the 'ulnar paradox'.

How and where are the nerves of hand commonly injured?
- Median nerve: C5, C6, C7 (lateral cord) and C8, T1 (medial cord)
    - Wrist lacerations cause thenar muscle wasting and loss of sensation over the radial 3½ fingers only.
    - Distal humeral fractures in children cause median, including anterior intraosseous, nerve injury,
- Ulnar nerve: C8, T1 (medial cord)
    - Wrist lacerations cause significant 'claw hand' and loss of sensation over medial 1½ fingers.
    - Elbow lacerations, dislocations or fractures of the medial humeral epicondyle cause radial deviation of wrist on flexion and milder hand clawing.

- Radial nerve: C5–C8, T1 (posterior cord)
  - Fracture of midshaft of humerus causes wrist drop and paraesthesia on the dorsum of the hand over the thumb and first web space.
  - Distal forearm (superficial radial nerve) trauma causes sensory loss only.

> **Tip**
>
> Understand that nerve root compression (radiculopathies) must be differentiated from peripheral compression neuropathies (e.g. a C6/7 with carpal tunnel syndrome, C8 with ulnar nerve entrapment). The 'double crush' and 'reverse double crush' phenomena have been described, referring to increased neuropathy susceptibility from a second compression site, either more proximal or more distal, respectively.

Section editor: Hardi Madani
Senior authors: John Curtis, Helen Marmery

Section 11: Surgical radiology

Chapter 44: Principles of plain film

Hardi Madani, Petrut Gogalniceanu, James Pegrum, John Curtis and Helen Marmery

Plain film consists of a single-shot image using x-rays.

What are the different densities in x-rays?

- Black – gas
- White – calcified structures
- Grey – soft tissues
- Darker grey – fat
- Intense white – metallic objects

What are the basics that must not be missed?

Always check:

- Name of patient, date of birth and date – this may give information about patient's age and gender, which could elucidate the underlying pathology.
- Adequacy of imaging: does the x-ray cover the entire area of interest?
- Orientation of film: right vs. left – 'R' label on corner of film.
- Position of patient. For example, a pneumothorax will look different on supine chest x-ray vs. erect film; air under the diaphragm will not be seen in a chest x-ray of a patient lying flat.
- Cervical spine: multiple standardised views (see Chapter 49, *Cervical spine x-ray*).
- Distal limbs: minimum of two views. If only one view is shown, ask for a second view.

Physical Examination for Surgeons, ed. Petrut Gogalniceanu, James Pegrum and William Lynn. Published by Cambridge University Press. © Cambridge University Press 2015.

What are the rules of 2?
- 2 sides: in paired structures (e.g. limbs) always compare the affected structure with the contralateral one, which may be normal.
- 2 views: obtain two views of the same structure, e.g. anteroposterior and lateral.
- 2 times: view images of the same structure at two different points in time: compare current images with previous ones.
- 2 joints (in orthopaedics): view the joint above and the joint below the one of interest.
- 2 readers: get a second opinion.

What is fluoroscopy?
- An imaging modality that uses continuous x-ray exposure to get dynamic imaging
- Has the capacity to save representative images
- Contrast material used to help differentiate pathology. Examples:
    - barium studies in swallow or enemas
    - intravenous iodinated contrast in vessels for arterial delineation
- Describe image as a single shot or series
- Always compare to previous imaging

What are the rules for describing orthopaedic radiographs?
As a general rule we advise surgeons to comment on three aspects:
- Views: comment on technical adequacy of radiograph as well as whether it is the appropriate method of visualising the pathology that is clinically suspected.
- Anatomy: describe key bones and bony eminences that should be examined – 'relevant negatives'.
- Pathology: look for specific injuries:
    - fractures and osteoporosis
    - osteomyelitis
    - lytic lesions
    - joint deformities, osteoarthritis or rheumatoid arthritis
    - foreign objects
    - surgical implants: nails, screws or plates

What are the radiological features of osteoarthritis?
LOSS:
 Loss of joint space
 Osteophyte formation
 Subchondral sclerosis
 Subchondral (s)cysts

Section 11 Surgical radiology

Chapter 45 Chest x-ray

Hardi Madani, Petrut Gogalniceanu, John Curtis and Helen Marmery

Introduction

'This is a chest radiograph in AP/PA erect/supine view with no/some rotation. It is (is not) adequate.'

Summary

Examination sequence **ABCDEF**:

- **A** Address
- **A** Adequacy of film
- **A** Airway
- **B** Breathing
- **B** Bones
- **B** Breasts
- **C** Circulation
- **D** Diaphragm
- **D** Danger areas
- **E** Everything else
- **F** Foreign objects

Physical Examination for Surgeons, ed. Petrut Gogalniceanu, James Pegrum and William Lynn. Published by Cambridge University Press. © Cambridge University Press 2015.

Checklist

Address
- Name and date of birth of patient

Adequacy
RIPO:

- **R**otation – symmetrical distances between spinous processes and clavicular heads
- **I**nspiration – 5–6 anterior ribs cross the mid-clavicular line and diaphragm
- **P**enetration – vertebral bodies seen behind heart
- **O**rientation – PA usual, AP if patient is unwell

Airway
- Trachea:
  - central or deviated
  - carina: position and angle (widened by malignant carinal lymphadenopathy)
  - endotracheal tube: tip should be 2 cm above carina
- Branches:
  - inhaled foreign body: commonly right lower lobe, although may affect any lobe

Breathing (lung fields)
- Mediastinal shift: tension pneumothorax
- Lung parenchyma:
  - increased lucency (black): pneumothorax (absent lung markings), bullae, COPD
  - increased opacity (white): consolidation, pulmonary oedema, collapse, effusion, haemothorax, empyema
- Lobar involvement: ill-defined edges:
  - right middle lobe: poor definition of right heart border
  - right lower lobe: poor definition of right hemi-diaphragm
  - left upper lobe/lingual lobe: poor definition of left heart border
  - left lower lobe: poor definition of left hemi-diaphragm
- Hila: position (usually left higher than right), size, masses

Bones
- Fractures: ribs, sternum, clavicles, humerus, scapulae, vertebrae
- Dislocations: humerus, clavicles

Breast (in women)
- Present/absent (only relevant if at least one breast is seen)
- Breast implants

Circulation
- Mediastinum: pericardial effusion, pneumopericardium, left lower lobe collapse, hiatal hernia
- Heart size > 50% of thoracic diameter on PA radiograph = cardiomegaly
- Aorta: widened (aneurysm, dissection, unfolded)

Diaphragm
- Above diaphragm: loss of costophrenic angle (effusion, consolidation, lower lobe collapse)
- Below diaphragm:
  - air below diaphragm: hollow viscus perforation, Chilaiditi's sign[30]
  - air below the diaphragm is physiological if on the left side and part of gastric bubble (air in fundus of stomach). However, free air may be seen under the left diaphragm alone and must not be ignored
- Diaphragm itself:
  - right higher than left because of liver
  - hemi-diaphragm elevation: phrenic nerve palsy, perihepatic/perisplenic abscess, consolidation or tumour causing superior traction
  - diaphragm may be flat in hyperexpansion of the chest (COPD)

Danger areas
LUSH:

- **L**ines behind mediastinum (hiatal hernias, left lower lobe collapse)
- **U**pper lobe/apical lung lesions (apical TB, cancer or bullae)
- **S**ubtle pneumothorax: check again!
- **H**umeral fractures or dislocations

---

[30] Chilaiditi's sign is a form of pseudo-pneumoperitoneum. The presence of colonic gas in a loop of large bowel interpositioned between the liver and diaphragm may give the impression of visceral perforation (pneumoperitoneum).

Chapter 45: Chest x-ray | 389

Everything else/emphysema
- Surgical emphysema

Foreign objects

A: Endotracheal tube, tracheostomy cannula
B: Chest drains
C: CVP line, Hickman lines, pacemakers, implantable defibrillators, sternotomy wires
Other: Bullets, knives, swallowed coins, breast implant side ports

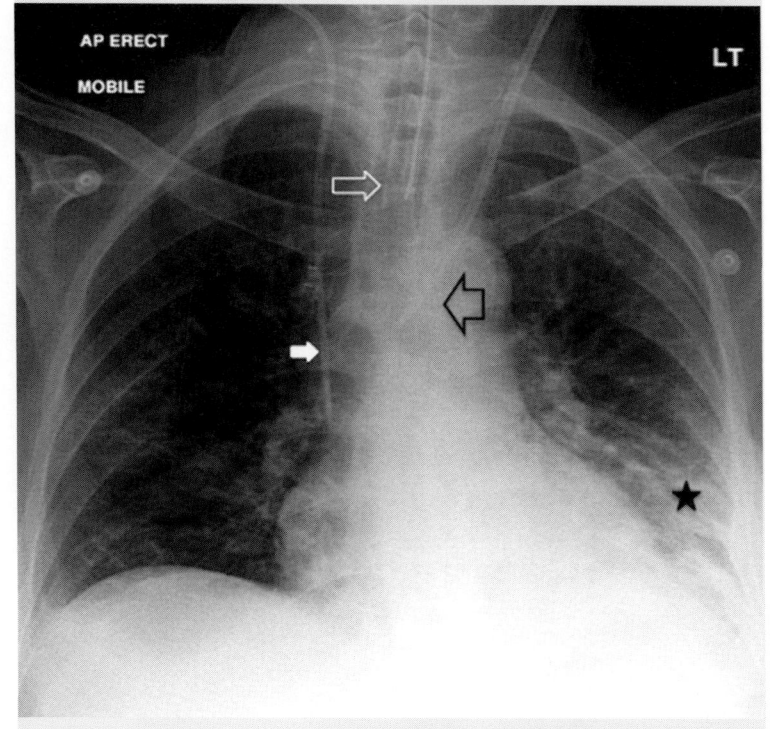

Chest radiograph showing right central venous line (solid white arrow) and ET tube (hollow white arrow) in correct positions. A left central line, which only reaches the brachiocephalic vein, requires repositioning (hollow black arrow). Note the left mid and lower zone consolidation (star).

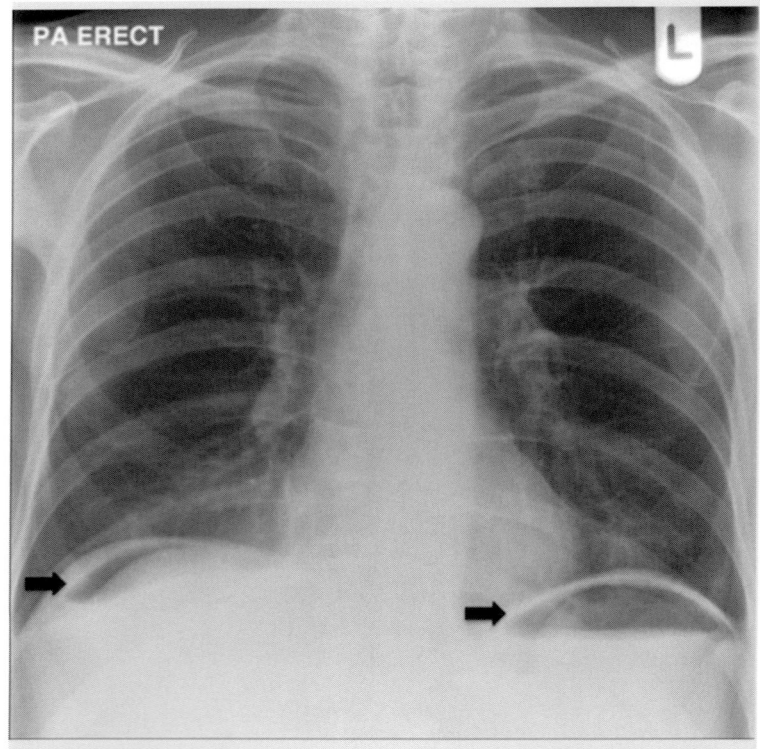

Chest radiograph showing free air below both hemi-diaphragms (arrows) from perforated abdominal viscus.

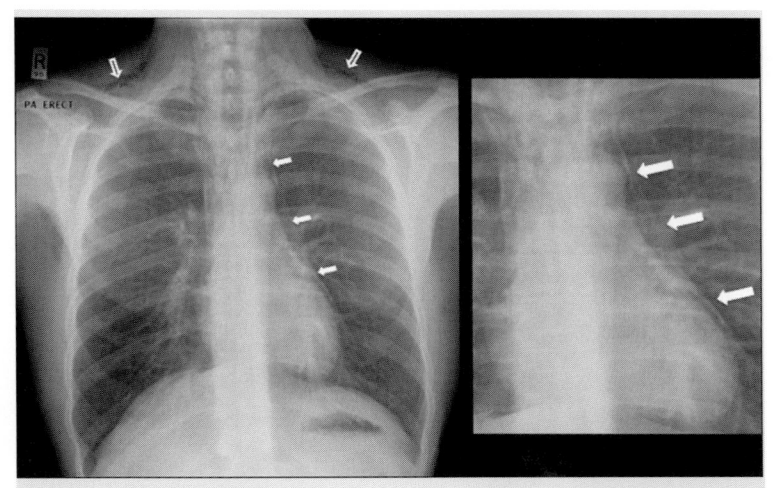

Chest radiograph shows surgical emphysema (hollow arrows) and air outlining the heart border and mediastinum (solid arrows), consistent with pneumomediastinum. This was caused by excessive vomiting (Boerhaave's syndrome).

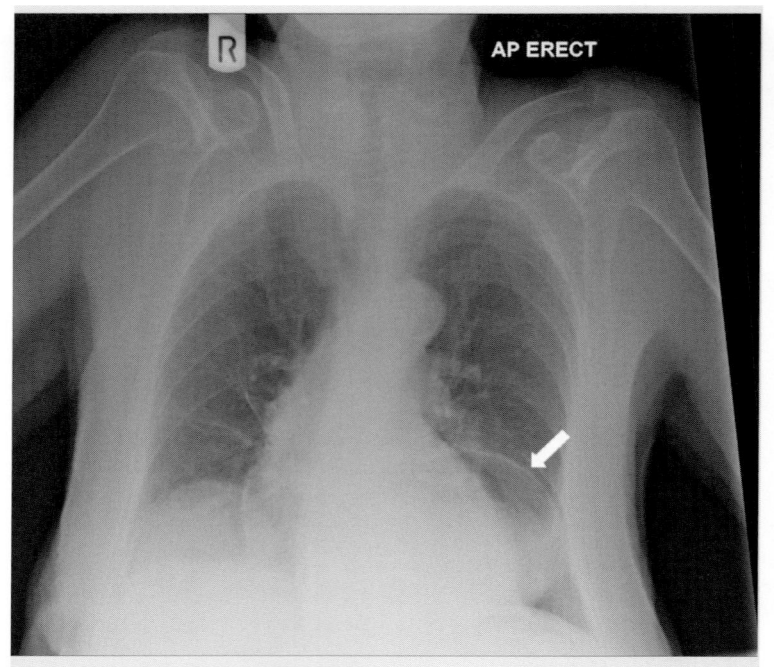

Chest radiograph demonstrating hiatus hernia: stomach present in the thorax.

Chapter 45: Chest x-ray | 393

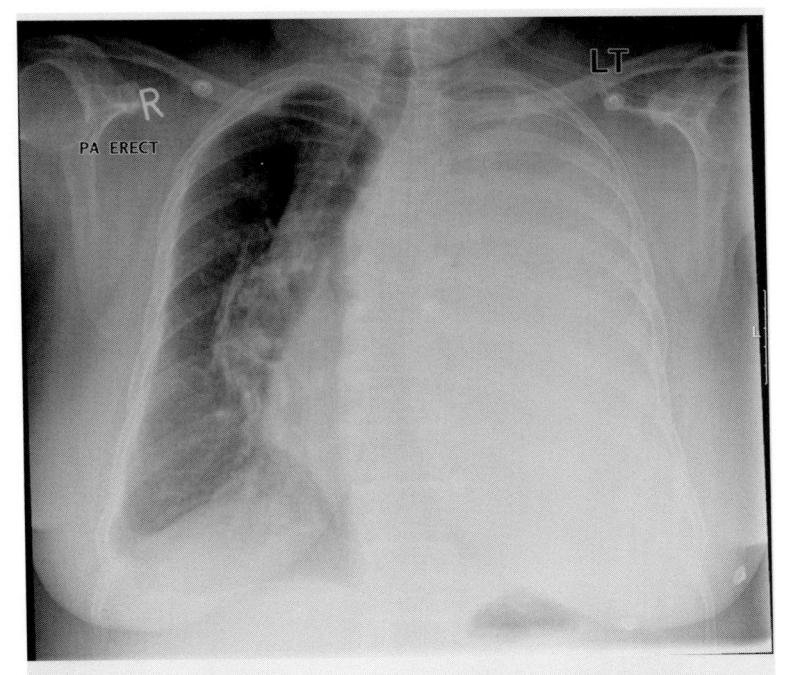

Chest radiograph demonstrating a very large left-sided pleural effusion causing midline shift of the mediastinum to the right. Note also tracheal deviation to the right

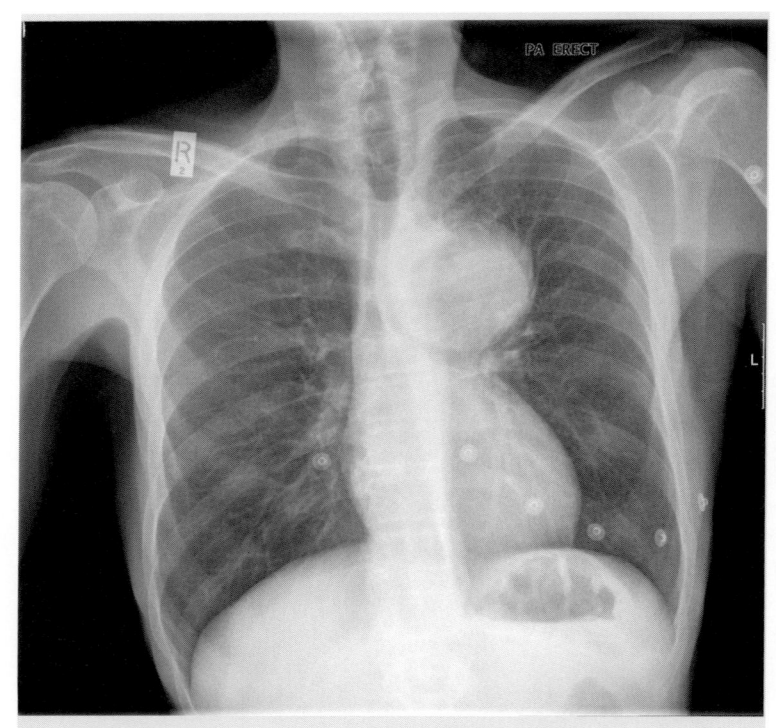

Mass in the hilum of the lung (lymphoma) causing compression of the trachea. This may represent impending airway compromise.

Examination notes

What are the correct positions of the following lines?

- ET tube – 2 cm above carina
- NG tube – below diaphragm overlying stomach bubble
- Central line – superior vena cava (SVC) above the level of the right atrium; beyond SVC/right atrial border signifies incorrect placement
- Pacemaker – leads overlying left or right cardiac shadow

Tip

If no obvious abnormality is seen, try the system described. If the system reveals nothing, consider the following six easily missed 'review areas' (**start low and aim high**):

1. Under diaphragm – free air or fluid – loss of normal diaphragm curve
2. Behind heart – left lower lobe collapse
3. Hila – enlarged nodes, mass, dissection
4. Apices – mass, TB
5. Humerus and scapula – fracture or bone metastases
6. Clavicles – easy to miss lung tumour projected over the clavicle, eroding clavicle or fractures

Section 11 Surgical radiology

Chapter 46

Abdominal x-ray

Hardi Madani, Petrut Gogalniceanu, John Curtis and Helen Marmery

Introduction

'This is an abdominal x-ray with the entire abdomen and pelvis imaged.' Although unlikely, mention if there are any intra-abdominal areas not imaged.

Summary

ABCS:

- **A** Address
- **A** Adequacy
- **A** Artefacts
- **A** Air
- **B** Bowel
- **B** Bone
- **C** Calcification
- **S** Soft tissues and viscera

Checklist

Address
- Name and date of birth

Adequacy
- Lung bases to pubic bone
- Lateral edges of abdominal wall

Physical Examination for Surgeons, ed. Petrut Gogalniceanu, James Pegrum and William Lynn. Published by Cambridge University Press. © Cambridge University Press 2015.

Artefacts

- Intrauterine devices
- Surgical instruments
- Intrabdominal drainage tubes
- Stents (biliary tree/ureteric/aortic/colonic)
- Foreign objects: buttons, coins, body piercings

Air (extraluminal gas)

- Pneumoperitoneum: free air under the diaphragm; evidence of hollow viscus perforation[31]
- Rigler's sign[32]
- Biliary tree (pneumobilia):
  - normal after biliary surgery
  - fistula between bowel and biliary tree
  - biliary sepsis, e.g. cholangitis
- Bowel wall:
  - bowel ischaemia or necrotising enterocolitis (pneumatosis coli/intestinalis)
  - toxic megacolon
- Portal vein: the presence of gas in the portal vein indicates bowel ischaemia or mesenteric sepsis. Portal venous gas is unlike biliary tract gas in that it is more difficult to see on AXR and will branch out to the periphery of the liver. Biliary tract gas tends to be more central in position.
- Pseudopneumoperitoneum: intraluminal (usually colonic) gas in a loop of intestine interpositioned between liver and right hemi-diaphragm (Chiliaditi's sign).

Bowel (bowel gas pattern)

- Obstruction:
  - distended bowel loops
  - volvulus/closed loop obstruction

---

[31] Air under diaphragm cannot be ruled out unless an erect chest x-ray is obtained.

[32] Rigler's sign is seen in the presence of free intraperitoneal air. This is characterised by visualisation of both the luminal and serosal surfaces of the intestinal wall ('both sides of the bowel wall' sign). Normally, only the luminal wall should be seen, as it is the only surface in contact with air.

- Faeces and constipation:
  - mottled appearance within lumen of the bowel
- Toxic megacolon

Bone
- Vertebrae: crush fractures, bamboo spine, Paget's disease, malignancy
- Hips: fractures, osteoarthritis
- Pelvis: fractures of pelvis, femoral heads and necks, metastases or primary malignancy, Paget's disease

Calcifications
- Kidneys and ureters: staghorn calculus, renal, ureteric and vesical stones
- Gallstones
- Appendicolith
- Aorta, iliacs and splanchnic vessels: atherosclerosis
- Pancreas: chronic calcific pancreatitis
- Fibroids
- Prostate

Soft tissues
- Liver contour
- Spleen contour
- Kidney contour (between T12 and L2)
- Psoas muscle shadows: if one is obliterated, it suggests retroperitoneal pathology (abscess, haemorrhage)
- Bladder: calcified or containing air (schistosomiasis, TB)
- Soft tissue: loss of peritoneal lines, surgical emphysema, bacterial infection with gas-forming organisms

Examination notes

What are the principles of fluoroscopy?

Barium or ionic water-soluble (gastrografin) contrast agents are given rectally in order to define large bowel pathology. Non-ionic water-soluble contrast agents are given orally. Non-ionic agents are less likely than ionic agents to induce pulmonary oedema if aspirated.

Common examples:

- Swallow → oesophagus: for malignancy, strictures, perforations (water-soluble contrast media).
- Meal → stomach and duodenum: for congenital malrotation or stenosis.
- Small bowel meal → useful for inflammatory bowel disease or proximal obstruction. The small bowel meal is less useful for distal obstruction, as the barium is diluted by the intestinal fluid.
- Enema → large bowel: for malignancy, strictures or polyps – largely superseded by CT virtual colonoscopy. Gastrografin enemas can be used to assess anastomotic leaks or to define pathology such as sigmoid volvulus if there is doubt about the diagnosis.

What are the features of small bowel obstruction?

- 'String of beads' sign.
- Bowel diameter > 3 cm.
- Central 'sausages' appearance.
- Valvulae conniventes (horizontal lines across entire diameter of bowel).

What are the features of large bowel obstruction?

- Peripheral/'picture frame' appearance.
- Diameter of bowel > 5 cm.
- Haustra (horizontal lines that do not cross entire diameter of bowel, interrupted by taeniae coli).
- If there is evidence of large bowel obstruction but no gas in the small bowel, the ileocaecal valve is likely to be patent. This means the large bowel cannot decompress itself into the small bowel and the risk of large bowel perforation is higher.
- Inflamed thumbprinting of the bowel wall (mucosal oedema).
- Pipe-like in 'burned out' UC.
- Dilated in toxic megacolon.

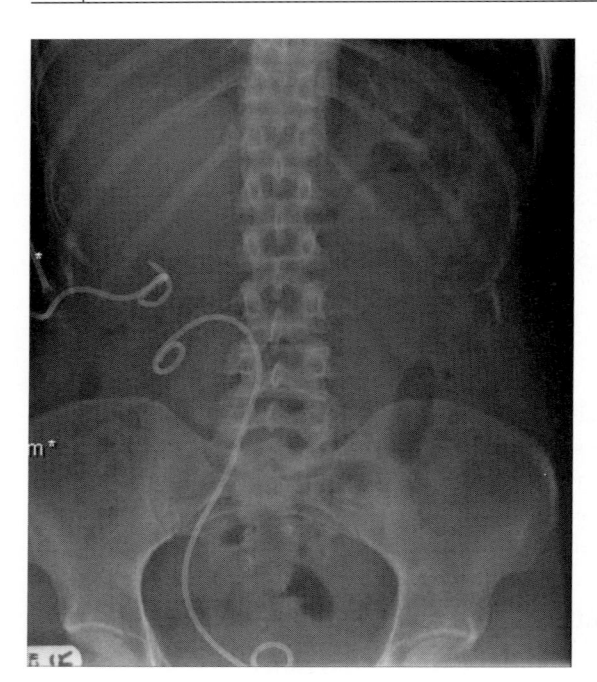

Abdominal radiograph with right JJ stent and nephrostomy tube in situ.

Chapter 46: Abdominal x-ray | 401

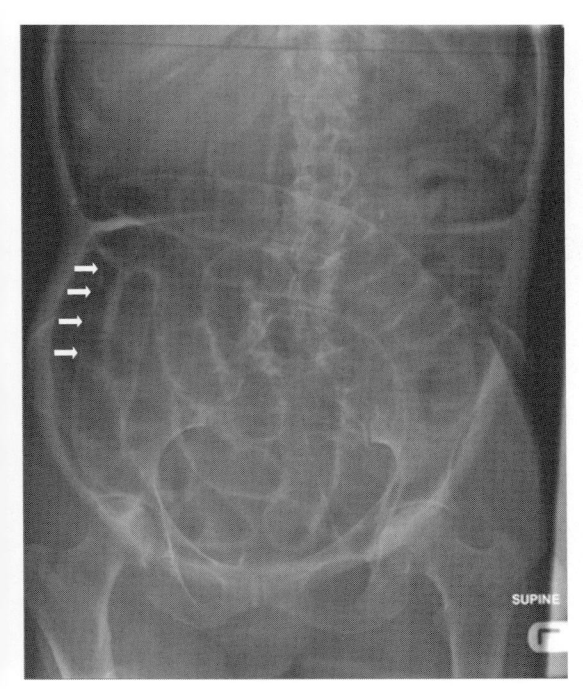

Abdominal radiograph shows dilated small bowel loops with air on both sides of well-defined bowel wall (arrowheads), consistent with pneumoperitoneum (Rigler's sign).

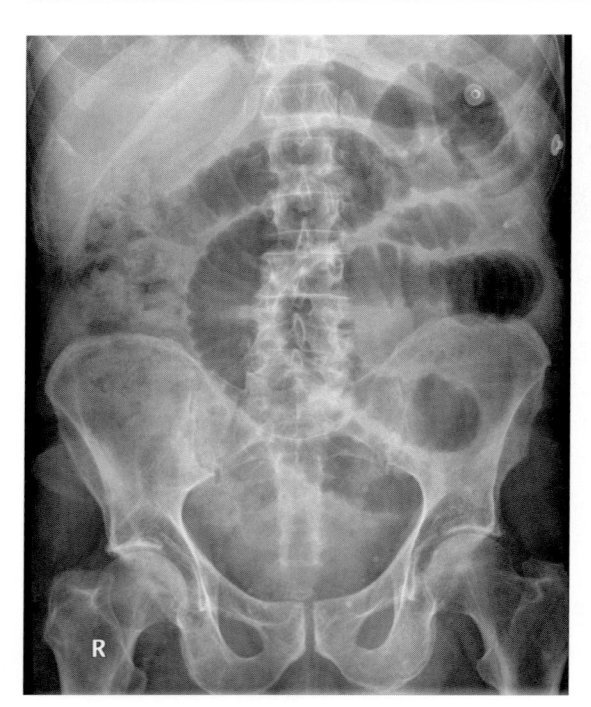

Abdominal radiograph shows multiple dilated loops of small bowel, due to a left inguinal hernia (not shown) causing bowel obstruction.

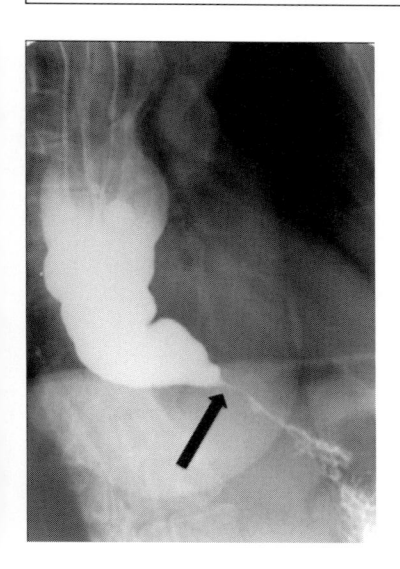

Selected single static image of barium swallow showing a dilated distal oesophagus with smooth, tapered narrowed or 'bird beak' appearance (arrow), consistent with achalasia.

Section 11: Surgical radiology

Chapter 47

Mammogram

Hardi Madani, Helen Marmery and Trupti Kulkarni

Introduction

'This is a mammogram in CC/MLO projection showing the right/left breast.'

Views

Standard projections include:

- Craniocaudal view (CC): does not capture much of the axillary or upper chest breast tissue
- Mediolateral-oblique view (MLO): images axillary and upper chest breast tissue

Summary

ABCDE:

- A Areola and skin
- B Breast tissue
- C Calcification
- D Distortion
- D Ducts
- E Edges and nodes

Physical Examination for Surgeons, ed. Petrut Gogalniceanu, James Pegrum and William Lynn. Published by Cambridge University Press. © Cambridge University Press 2015.

Checklist

Areola and skin

- Nipple inversion, retraction, distortion
- Skin thickening:
  - unilateral causes: inflammation, cancer, post radiotherapy
  - bilateral causes: CCF or other causes of peripheral oedema
- Skin retraction.

Breast tissue

- Size and shape disparity (R vs. L)
- Breast implants
- Density:
  - fibroglandular: young women, dense or 'white'
  - fatty: older women, less dense or 'grey'
- Focal masses
  - density
  - margins: circumscribed vs. microlobulated
  - shape

Calcification

- Microcalcification
- Popcorn-like: fibroadenoma
- Rim or eggshell: cyst or fat necrosis
- Suture calcification: post-surgical changes

Distortion

- Tumour, radial scar, benign sclerosing adenosis
- Post surgical, biopsy or radiotherapy changes

Ducts

- Ductal ectasia: prominent ducts in a retroareolar location
- Plasma cell mastitis: rod-like calcification
- Intraductal papilloma: retro/periareolar usually well-defined lesion as seen on mammogram

Edges

- Axillary nodes: metastatic or inflammatory
- Pectoralis muscle irregularity: postoperative scarring

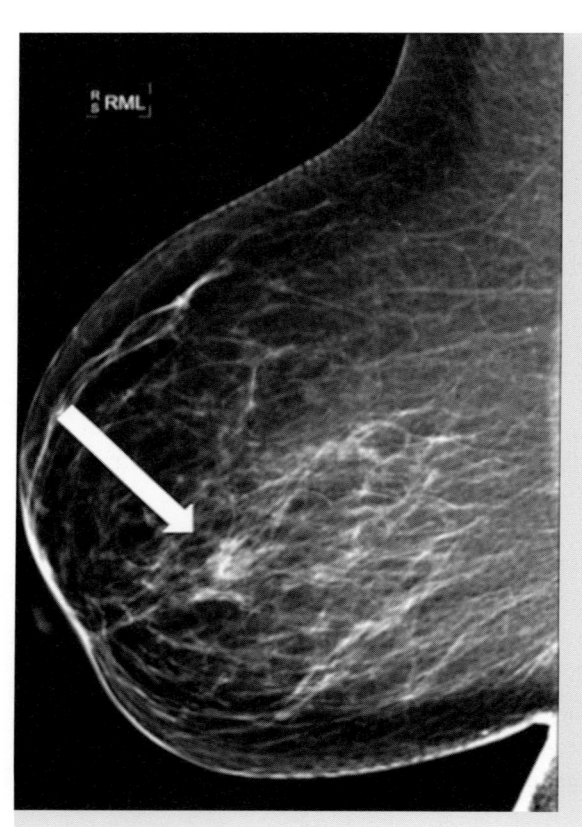

Mammogram of the right breast in right mediolateral (RML) view, showing a central discrete oval mass of increased density (arrow).

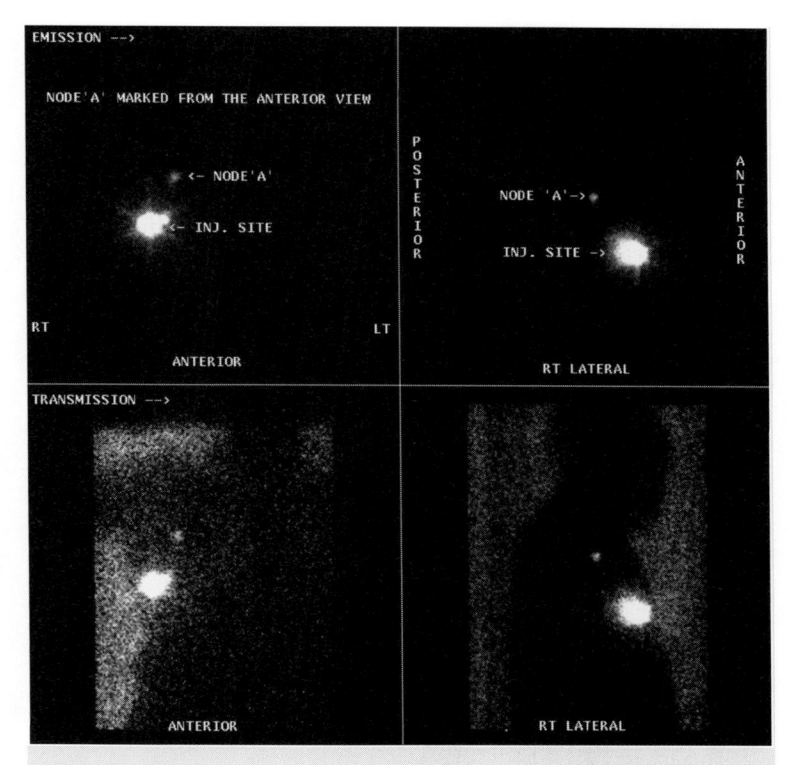

Radiolabelled sentinel node nuclear tracer confirming an involved axillary node (node A), which required clearance at the time of surgery.

Examination notes

What are the radiological signs of malignancy?

- Spiculated or irregular mass
- Distortion
- Skin tethering or thickening
- Nipple retraction
- Clustered micro-calcification
- Enlarged lymph nodes

What information can be deduced from the density of a breast mass?

- High-density lesion ('white'): malignancy, fibroadenoma, haematoma, cysts, post-surgical fibrosis, post-traumatic fat necrosis
- Low-density lesion ('dark'): lipoma, galactocoele, hamartoma

What information can be deduced from the microcalcification pattern in a breast?

- < 1 mm, ≥ 5 in cluster, fine, linear: more likely to be malignant
- > 1 mm, < 5 in cluster, round, lucent centre, solid rods: more likely to be benign

What is the role of breast imaging in screening for breast cancer?

- Imaging with mammography is the mainstay in the NHS Breast Screening Programme (NHSBSP) within the UK.
- Mammography is used to identify a mass, and for mass localisation, which allows further evaluation with focused ultrasound.
- Ultrasound-guided or stereotactic (x-ray-guided) core biopsy is used to obtain histological diagnosis and, if confirmed malignant, for preoperative localisation with wire placement.

Section 11 Surgical radiology

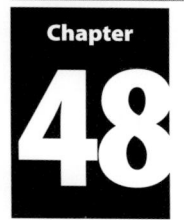

Chapter 48

Facial x-ray

Hardi Madani, John Curtis and Helen Marmery

Introduction
'This is an OM/OPG/PA view x-ray of the face/mandible.'

Views
- Occipitomental (OM) view at 0°: frontal sinuses, orbits, maxillary antra, nasal bones and ethmoid air cells
- Occipitomental (OM) view at 30°: additional features – zygoma, mandible, infraorbital foramina, odontoid peg
- Orthopantomogram (OPG): mandible, maxilla, teeth, TMJ and inferior alveolar canal
- PA mandible: mandibular fractures

Anatomy
Bones
- Frontal bones and sinuses
- Orbits and orbital floor
- Maxilla: medial and lateral walls of maxillary antra
- Zygomatic arch
- Mandible: symphysis, body, angle, ramus, condyle and coronoid process
- Teeth
- Temporomandibular joint (TMJ)

Physical Examination for Surgeons, ed. Petrut Gogalniceanu, James Pegrum and William Lynn. Published by Cambridge University Press. © Cambridge University Press 2015.

Circles: broken circle indicates a possible fracture
- Frontal sinuses
- Orbits
- Maxillary sinuses
- Nasal and ethmoid spaces

Lines: broken line indicates a possible fracture
- Lines of Dolan (OM30)
- McGrigor's lines
- Elephant trunks of Rogers (zygomatic arch fractures): formed from lines of Dolan

Pathology
Fractures
- Maxillary fractures: alveolar process; lateral and medial walls of maxillary antra.
- Zygomatic arch fracture: look at 'elephant trunks'.
- Tripod fractures: zygoma detachment (complex zygomaticomaxillary fracture). Suture lines involved are: 1. zygomaticofrontal suture; 2. orbital floor; 3. infraorbital rim; 4. lateral wall of maxillary sinus.
- Inferior orbital margin fracture.
- Orbital floor 'blow-out' fracture.
  - 'black eyebrow' sign: surgical emphysema in the upper orbital rim area
  - 'teardrop sign': herniation of orbital soft tissues in the maxillary antrum
  - fluid level in antrum of maxilla
- Mandibular fractures.

Tumours
- Bone: lytic lesions and cysts
- Soft tissues: contour changes

Infections
- Sinusitis (OPG and OM): opacity of maxillary and frontal sinuses
- Osteomyelitis (OPG and OM): opacity of mandible and maxilla

Dislocations
- TMJ (OPG).

Teeth
- Fractures and caries.

To complete the examination...
- If suspecting a complex fracture or inadequate views, ask for CT face/skull to determine.
- Facial trauma is associated with C-spine and head injuries, so consider CT head and C-spine imaging.

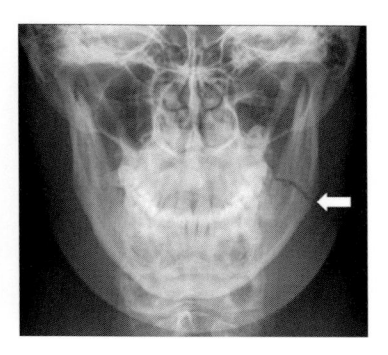

Mandible radiograph showing an oblique fracture of the left mandible at the angle (arrow).

Examination notes
What are the three McGrigor's lines?

Line 1   Upper lines: zygomaticofrontal sutures (laterally), upper orbits (centrally) and frontal sinuses

Line 2   Middle line: zygomatic arches (laterally), inferior orbits (medially) and bridge of nose (midline)

Line 3   Lower line: mandibular condyle and coronoid processes (laterally), lateral and medial walls of maxillary antra (medially) and floor of nose / upper teeth (midline)[33]

---

[33] Raby N, Berman L, de Lacey G. *Accident and Emergency Radiology*, 2nd edn. Edinburgh: Elsevier Saunders, 2006.

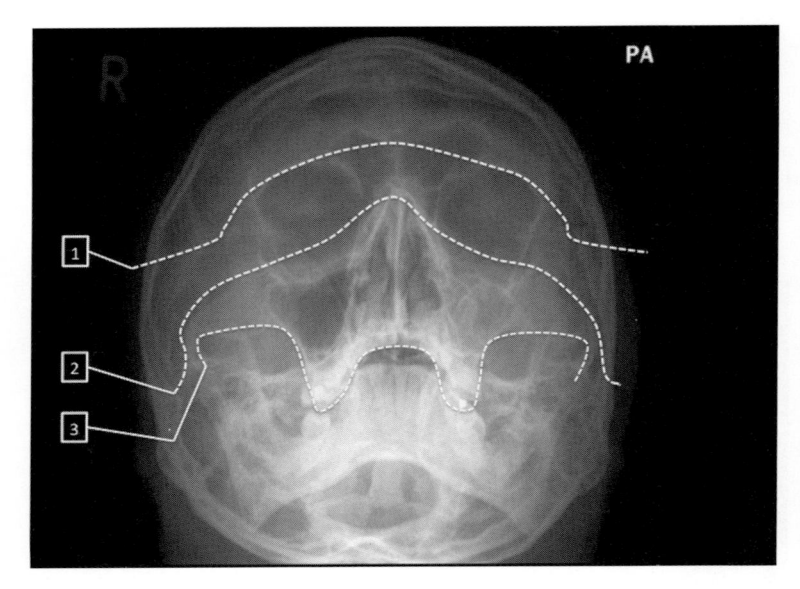

McGrigor's lines.

What vertical line should be checked?
Midline: nasal septum and mandibular symphysis.

What are the lines of Dolan?
A. Orbital line: medial aspect of lateral orbital rim and orbital floor
B. Zygomatic line: outer orbital rim and superior surface of zygomatic arch
C. Maxillary line: lateral wall of maxillary sinus and inferior surface of zygomatic arch

What are the elephant trunks of Rogers?

Two imaginary elephants' heads are formed from the lines of Dolan. The heads are seen in profile, placed on the edges of the skull with the trunks pointing outwards. The elephant's head is formed by the lateral orbital rim and lateral maxilla. The zygomatic arch forms the elephant's trunk, pointing laterally/outwards. In zygomatic arch fractures the 'elephant trunks' are distorted.

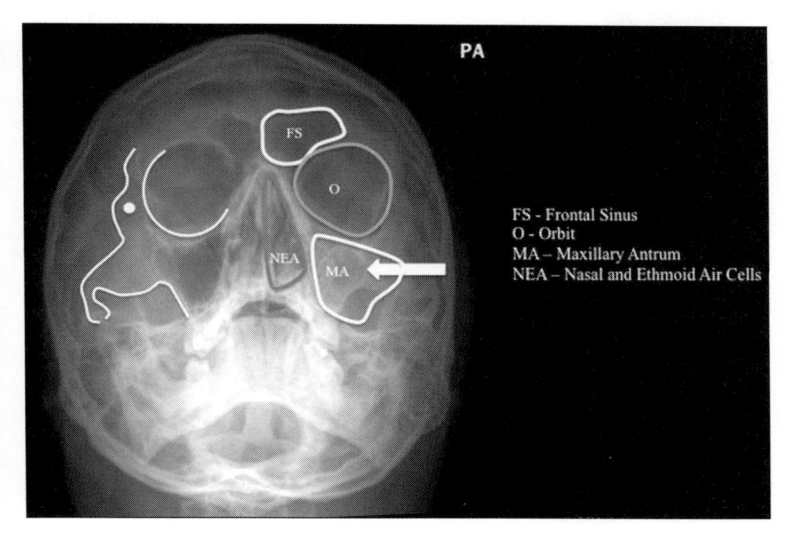

Facial x-ray showing increased density of the left maxillary antrum (arrow), suggestive of fluid and fracture, and the lines of Dolan forming an 'elephant's head' on the right.

Section 11 Surgical radiology

Chapter 49

Cervical spine x-ray

Hardi Madani, John Curtis and Helen Marmery

Introduction

'This is an x-ray of the cervical spine in AP/lateral/open-mouth view. It is (is not) an adequate film because C1 to C7/T1 junction have (have not) been included.'

Summary

- **A** Address
- **A** Adequate
- **A** Alignment
- **B** Bone
- **C** Cartilage
- **E** Everything else

Checklist

Address
- Name and date of birth

Adequate (views)
- Non-trauma : AP and lateral
- Trauma:
  1. AP
  2. lateral, C1 to C7/T1
  3. peg view/open mouth

Physical Examination for Surgeons, ed. Petrut Gogalniceanu, James Pegrum and William Lynn. Published by Cambridge University Press. © Cambridge University Press 2015.

Alignment

- Lateral view:
  - anterior longitudinal line
  - posterior longitudinal line
  - spinolaminar line
  - spinous process (interspinous) line

- AP view:
  - transverse spinous processes line up
  - posterior spinous processes align themselves when seen 'end on'

- Peg view:
  - equal spaces on either side of C1 peg to C2 body
  - lateral margins of C1–C2 align; if not aligned, suggestive of C1 blow-out (Jefferson) fracture

Bone

- Lateral view:
  - all vertebral body heights must be the same
  - anterior and posterior aspects of vertebral bodies should be concave

- AP view:
  - spinous processes lie in straight line and are equidistant from each other
  - the lateral edges of the vertebral bodies should all be equally aligned
  - all vertebral bodies have two pedicles (owl eyes) – if not this suggests lytic destruction of pedicle (spinal tumour – usually metastatic)
  - an increase in the interpedicular distance compared to the vertebral levels below is indicative of a burst type fracture

- Peg view:
  - C2 vertebra odontoid process (peg) intact
  - lateral margins of C1 and C2 align; failure of alignment suggests blow-out fracture of C1 (Jefferson's fracture)

Cartilage and ligaments

- Increased prevertebral soft tissue thickness is abnormal and can be a sign of a haematoma and occult fracture. Abnormal thickness is defined either in relation to the size of the adjacent vertebra or in millimetres. Normal soft tissue thickness is:

  C1–C4 = up to 7 mm
  C5–C7 = up to 22 mm
  or

≤ 30% of the vertebral width at the level of C1–C4
< 100% of the vertebral width at the level of C5–C7

- Intervertebral disk distances must be approximately the same.
- All inter-spinous process distances should be equal; an increased gap is suggestive of an occult fracture.

Everything else
- Soft tissue around spine: calcifications
- Lung apex: pneumothorax

Tip

In an exam situation, if presented with only one view, ask for a second view x-ray.

Examination notes

What injuries should not be missed?
- Spinal fracture
- Lower skull fracture: occiput
- Atlantoaxial subluxation
- Soft tissue widening
- Apex lung lesion

What is a hangman's fracture?
This is a C2 fracture through both pedicles or pars interarticularis. This is caused by hyperextension with/without distraction, most commonly in the setting of RTA. This is an unstable fracture.

What is a clay shoveler's fracture?
This is an avulsion fracture of a vertebral spinous process caused by a hyperflexion injury. This is a stable fracture usually affecting C6 and C7.

What are the common stable C-spine fractures?
- Avulsion injuries of spinous processes

What are the common unstable C-spine fractures?

- Tear-drop fracture of the vertebral body (associated with ligamentous disruption)
- Any fracture associated with subluxation or dislocation (associated with ligamentous disruption)
- Jefferson's fracture
- Hangman's fracture

Section 11: **Surgical radiology**

Chapter 50

Shoulder x-ray

Hardi Madani, John Curtis and Helen Marmery

Introduction

'This is an AP/Y/axial view radiograph of the right/left shoulder.'

Checklist

Views
- AP
- Axial or armpit view – golf ball (humeral head) lies on tee (glenoid fossa) and finger/thumb are acromion and coracoid processes
- Lateral or 'Y-shaped'

Anatomy
- Identify at shoulder/humerus: 'should look like a walking stick'.
- Identify clavicle and AC joint.
- Identify scapula and three bony eminences:
    - spine and acromion
    - coracoid process
    - glenoid

Pathology

Shoulder dislocation
- Anterior dislocation complications:
    - fracture of greater tuberosity of humerus: Hill–Sachs deformity (compression fracture of posterolateral margin of humeral head)
    - anteroinferior glenoid rim fracture: bony Bankart's lesion

Physical Examination for Surgeons, ed. Petrut Gogalniceanu, James Pegrum and William Lynn. Published by Cambridge University Press. © Cambridge University Press 2015.

- Posterior dislocation:
    - 'light bulb sign' on AP radiograph (NB: painful arm held with internal rotation will also look like 'light bulb sign')
    - incongruous relation of the glenoid rim and the humeral head (loss of parallelism)
    - 'trough sign': anterior fracture of humeral head as the anterior head is compressed against the posterior glenoid

Acromioclavicular joint injury (use AP view only)
- > 8 mm distance is abnormal
- Inferior cortices of acromion and clavicle should be aligned

Coracoclavicular ligament injury
- Distance between the coracoid and clavicle: < 1.3 cm is normal

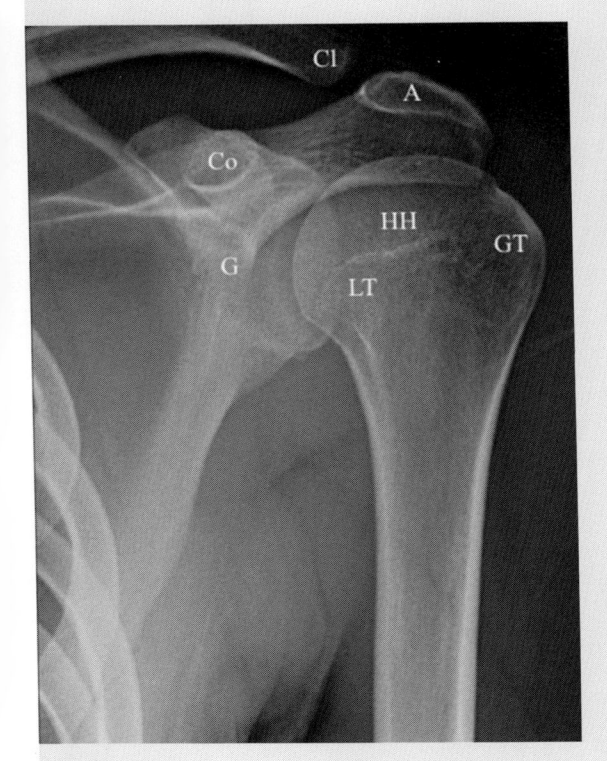

Normal shoulder: AP view, with key anatomy and review lines highlighted. A, acromion; Cl, clavicle; Co, coracoid process; G, glenoid; GT, greater tuberosity; HH, humeral head; LT, lesser tuberosity.

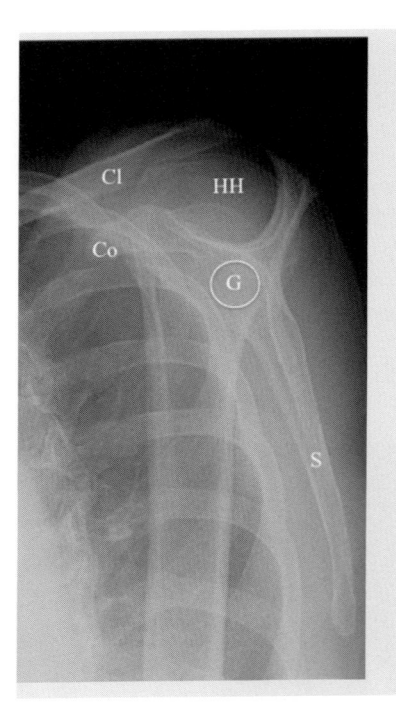

Normal shoulder: lateral (or Y) view. Cl, clavicle; Co, coracoid process; G, glenoid; HH, humeral head; S, scapula.

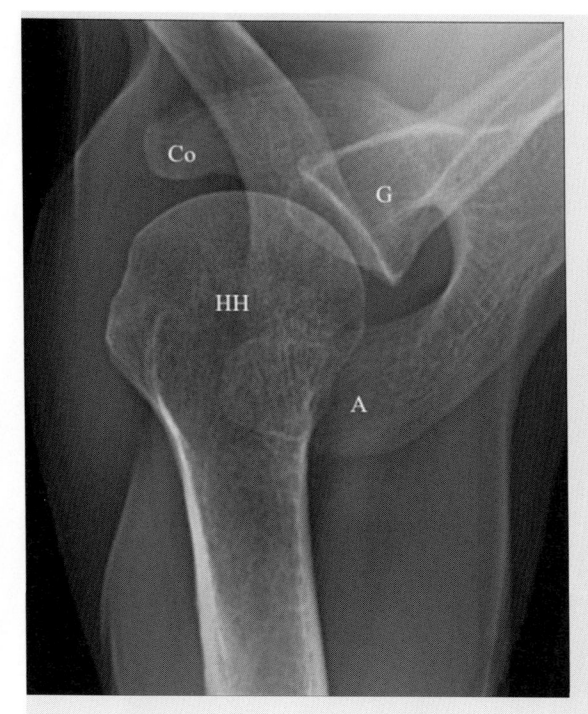

Chapter 50: Shoulder x-ray | 421

Normal shoulder: axial (or armpit) view. A, acromion; Co, coracoid process; G, glenoid; HH, humeral head.

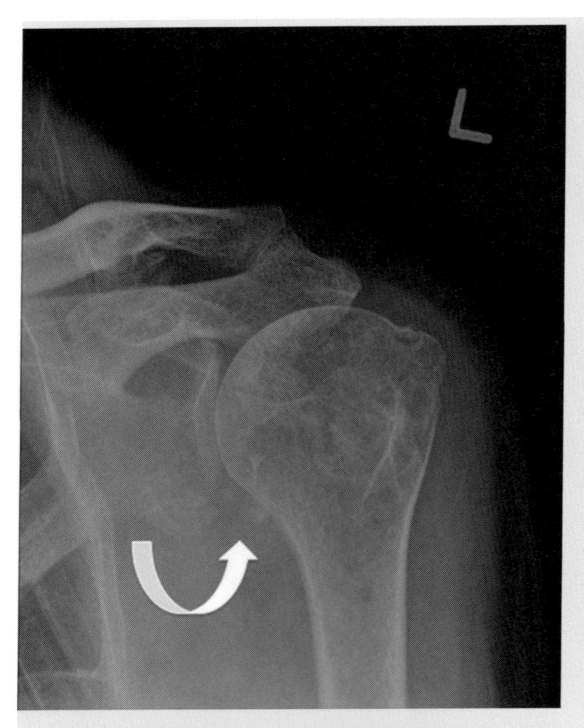

View of the left shoulder showing subtle anterior dislocation and multiple fractures of the anterior inferior glenoid labrum (Bankart's lesion) (curved arrow).

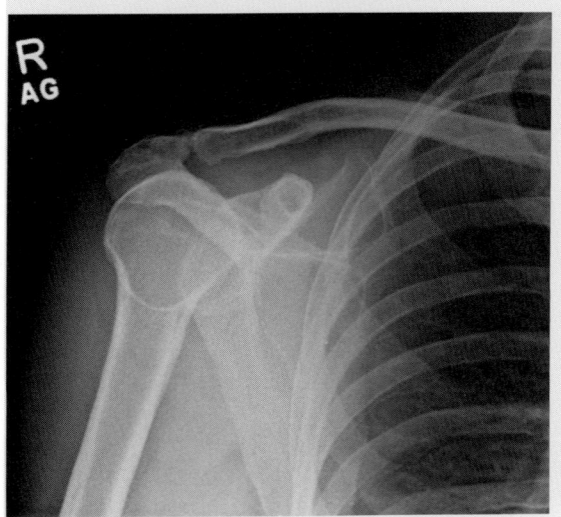

Light bulb sign indicates a posterior shoulder dislocation.

Examination notes
Which lesions should not be missed?
- Anterior dislocation.
- Posterior dislocation – may look like a light bulb and symmetrically shaped. This is due either to the shoulder being held in internal rotation or to a posterior dislocation. Look for an incongruous relation of the glenoid rim and the humeral head and the trough sign. If in doubt, request axial view.
- Greater tuberosity fracture.
- ACJ subluxation.
- Pneumothorax.

Section 11 Surgical radiology

Chapter 51

Elbow x-ray

Hardi Madani, John Curtis and Helen Marmery

Introduction
'This is an AP/lateral/oblique x-ray of the right/left elbow.'

Anatomy
Bones
- Humerus, radius, ulna

Lines
Lateral views:
- Anterior humeral line: includes anterior third of capitellum. Deviation suggests possible supracondylar fracture.
- Mid radial line (radiocapitellar line): should pass through middle of capitellum; failure to do so suggests possible dislocation.

Pathology
Fractures
- Check lines.
- Anterior fat is normal; displacement is seen with elbow effusion due to radial head fracture.
- Posterior fat pad is always abnormal – effusion inside the joint after trauma this indicates a haemoarthrosis and if present an occult fracture if no bony injuries are seen.

Physical Examination for Surgeons, ed. Petrut Gogalniceanu, James Pegrum and William Lynn. Published by Cambridge University Press. © Cambridge University Press 2015.

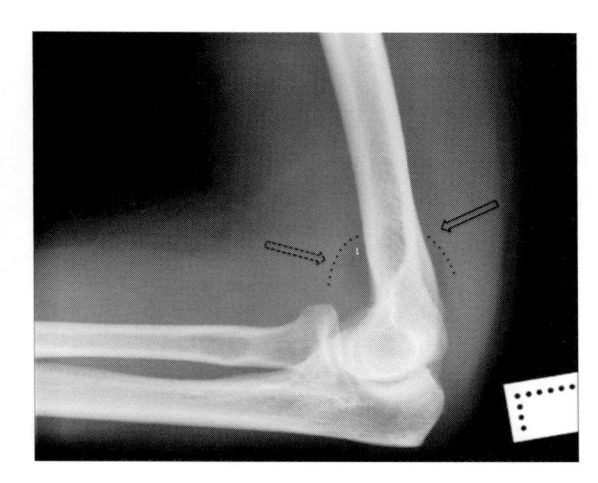

Lateral radiograph of the left elbow showing anterior (dotted arrow) and posterior (black arrow) effusions ('fat pads': dotted lines) consistent with an occult fracture. This was confirmed to be an undisplaced intra-articular fracture of the radial head.

Examination notes
What injuries should not be missed?
- Supracondylar fracture (associated with vascular injuries)
- Radial head/neck fracture
- Radial/ulnar dislocation
- Lateral epicondyle fracture
- Missed paediatric fracture – knowing CRITOL is critical (see below)

What is the order of appearance of bony ossification centres in the elbows of children?
Occurs from 1 to 11 years. Remember '**CRITOL**' for order. **The order of ossification is more important than the absolute dates.**

- **C** Capitellum (radial side of humerus) – 1 year
- **R** Radial head – 3 years
- **I** Internal epicondyle – 5 years
- **T** Trochlea (ulnar side of humerus) – 7 years
- **O** Olecranon (back piece of ulna) – 9 years
- **L** Lateral epicondyle – 11 years

Section 11: Surgical radiology

Chapter 52
Wrist and distal forearm x-ray
Hardi Madani, John Curtis and Helen Marmery

Introduction
'This is an AP/lateral/oblique radiograph of the right/left wrist, or scaphoid series.'

Views
- AP and lateral.

Anatomy
Bones
- Distal radius and ulna.
- Carpal bones: scaphoid, lunate, triquetral, pisiform, trapezium, trapezoid, capitate, hamate.
  - If the lunate is anteriorly displaced this is termed a lunate dislocation.
  - If the lunate (which is moon-shaped – with the concave side holding the rest of the carpus) – or cup of the lunate are empty then this is termed a perilunate dislocation – the capitate is displaced dorsally.
- Space > 2 mm between scaphoid and lunate is abnormal (scapholunate dissociation) (Terry Thomas sign).

Lines
- Normal radius has palmar/volar tilt (2–20°). If lost, suspect a fracture of the radius.
- Radial wrist normally more distal than ulna. If lost, this may suggest that the radius has impacted and is shortened.

Physical Examination for Surgeons, ed. Petrut Gogalniceanu, James Pegrum and William Lynn. Published by Cambridge University Press. © Cambridge University Press 2015.

- Dorsal angulation fracture of radius = Colles' fracture.
- Volar angulation fracture of radius = Smith's fracture.
- If there is an intra-articular fracture involving either the posterior cortex or more commonly the anterior cortex of the radius, the vertical fracture pattern causes subluxation of the carpal bones= Barton's fracture (unstable).

Pathology

Radius fractures

- Fractures involving the growth plate. Salter–Harris classification:

    I   S – Straight through
    II A – Above/metaphyseal
    III L – Lower/epiphyseal
    IV T – Through both metaphyisis and epiphysis
    V   S – Squashed

- Colles' and Smith's fractures: distal radial fracture with no joint involved.
- Barton-type fracture: distal radial fracture that is longitudinal and involves the joint space; it can have a volar or dorsal angulation and is associated with carpal displacement (unlike Colles' or Smith's).

Scaphoid

- Tenderness in anatomical snuffbox: ask for four-view scaphoid series.
- Normal radiographs but clinical suspicion: treat as fracture and repeat radiographs in 10–14 days.
- 80% waist: most common fracture (avascular necrosis likely).
- 10% proximal pole (avascular necrosis very likely).
- 10% distal pole (avascular necrosis unlikely).
- Scaphoid fractures may be associated with perilunate dislocation.

Subluxations and dislocations

- Galeazzi fracture: fractured shaft of radius with distal radioulnar joint dislocation
- Monteggia fracture: fractured ulna with dislocation of proximal radioulnar joint

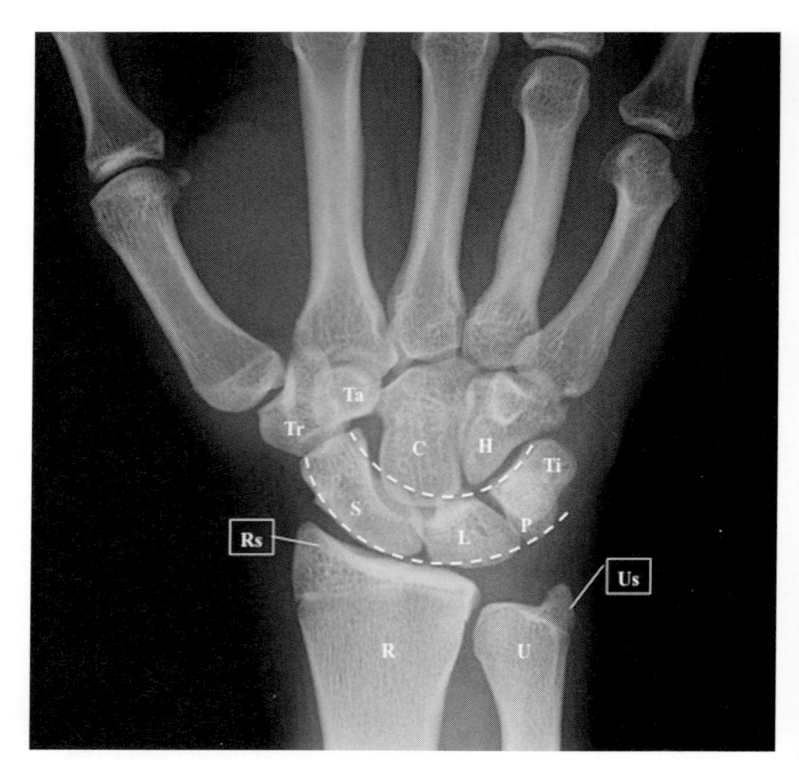

AP and lateral radiographs of the wrist, showing normal anatomy and radiocarpal and carpocarpal alignment review lines, applied when assessing for fracture and dislocation. In the lateral view, the capitate, lunate and radius (CLR) should be in alignment. Failure of alignment suggests a lunate or perilunate dislocation. Tr, trapezium; Ta, trapezoid; C, capitate; H, hamate; Ti, triquetrum; P, pisiform; L, lunate; S, scaphoid; Rs, Radial styloid; Us, ulnar styloid; R, radius; U, ulna.

Chapter 52: Wrist and distal forearm x-ray | 429

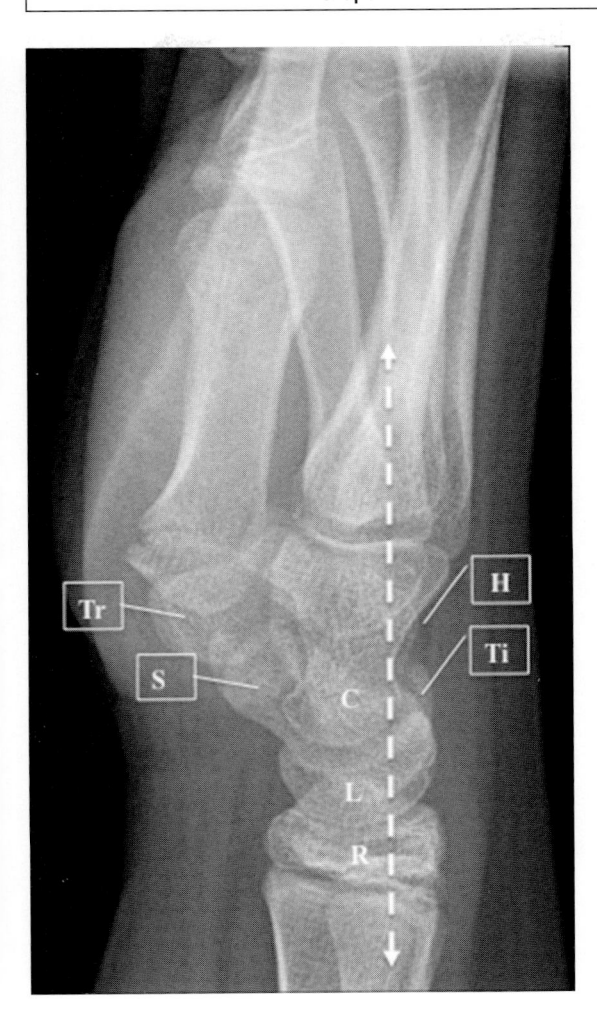

(cont.)

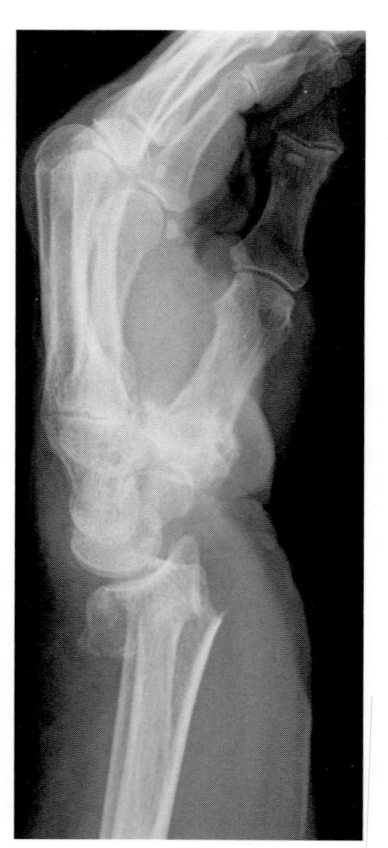

Radiograph of the wrist showing fracture of the distal radius with dorsal angulation (Colles' fracture). The reverse would constitute a Smith's fracture.

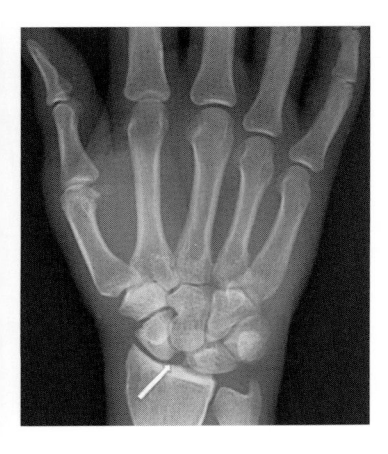

Radiograph of the right hand showing a widening of the scapholunate joint (Terry Thomas sign) (arrow).

Examination notes

What injuries should not be missed?

- Subtle distal radius fracture: look for normal volar tilt of radius, radius distal to ulnar (AP view) and smooth cortical outline (lateral view).
- Carpal fractures: normally waist of scaphoid intact.
- Lunate/perilunate dislocation – capitate normally sits in lunate (lateral view).
- Triquetral fracture: small fragment over dorsal wrist (lateral view).
- Radioulnar dislocation.
- Joint spaces > 2 mm (Terry Thomas sign) suggests ligament injury: scapholunate dissociation.
- 4th or 5th CMC joint dislocation.

What are the common eponymous names of different fractures?

- Colles' fracture:
  - low-energy extra-articular radius fracture in osteoporotic bone, resulting in radial shortening, dorsal translation and angulation
- Barton's fracture:
  - volar or dorsal fracture causing carpal dislocation

- Smith's fracture:
  - 'reverse Colles'
- Chauffeur's fracture: radial styloid fracture:
  - unstable (brachioradialis)
- Ulnar styloid fracture:
  - tip neutral plaster for 3–4 weeks
  - base suggests triangular fibrocartilage complex (TFCC) injury: ORIF
- Die punch:
  - distal radial pilon from scapholunate

How can you remember the normal anatomy of the radius?

11 + 12 = 23:

- Volar tilt = 11°
- Whole radial height = 12°
- Radial inclination = 23°
- Ulnar shortening compared to radius = 0–2 mm

Section 11 **Surgical radiology**

Chapter 53

Pelvis and hip x-ray

Hardi Madani, John Curtis and Helen Marmery

Introduction

'This is an AP/lateral/cross-table oblique radiograph of the pelvis or right/left hip.'

Views

- AP and lateral

Anatomy

Rings

- Inner and outer pelvic rings
- Obturator foramina

Lines

- Sacroiliac joint lines and symphysis pubis
- Sacral arcuate (foraminal) lines
- Iliopectineal and ilioischial lines
- Shenton's line: femoral neck fracture

Pathology

Pelvic fractures (3 × 3 rule)

- Three rings: pelvic brim and two obturator foramina
- Three bones: ilium, ischium and pubis
- Three joints: pubic symphysis and two sacroiliac joints

Physical Examination for Surgeons, ed. Petrut Gogalniceanu, James Pegrum and William Lynn. Published by Cambridge University Press. © Cambridge University Press 2015.

Femoral fractures (AP and cross-table horizontal lateral views)

- Femoral fractures: buckling, step, ridging and loss of normal trabecular pattern or transverse sclerotic line (suggesting impacted fracture of the subcapital femur)
- Extra- vs. intracapsular fracture of neck of femur

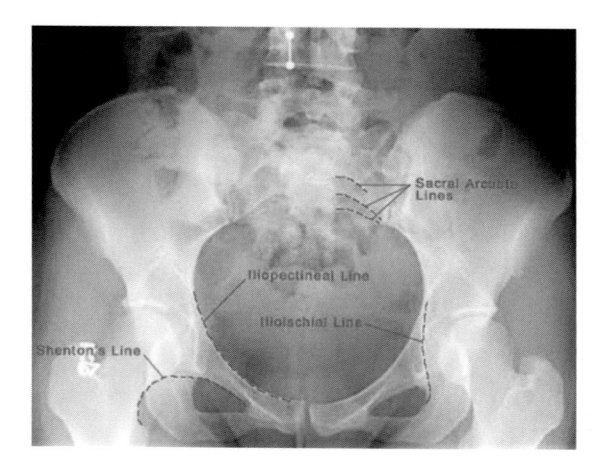

AP radiograph of the pelvis, summarising the lines to review when excluding subtle fractures: sacral arcuate lines, iliopectineal line (sciatic notch, along superior pubic ramus to symphysis pubis), ilioischial line (sciatic notch to medial border of the ischium) and Shenton's line (medial edge of the femoral neck and the inferior edge of the superior pubic ramus).

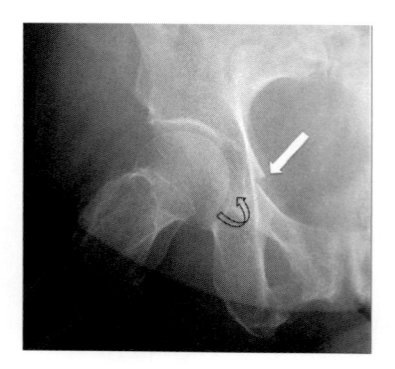

AP radiograph of pelvis and right hip showing fracture of the right superior ischial spine (arrow) and subtle fracture of the acetabulum (curved arrow). The patient presented with hip pain post fall.

Examination notes

What are the common fracture patterns in the pelvis?

- Acetabular and pubic rami (inferior or superior)
- Sacral and sacroiliac joint
- Apophysis avulsion fractures

> **Tips**
>
> A fracture at any site in the pelvic ring is associated with a second fracture (double fractures are inherently unstable).
>
> If no second fracture seen, look for apophysis avulsion fractures or disruption (widening or diastasis) of joints (e.g. symphysis pubis and sacroiliac joint).

What injuries should not be missed?

SAND:

- **S**uperior or inferior pubic fractures in patients with hip pain
- **S**ubtle sacral foraminal fractures
- **A**vulsions and avascular necrosis
- **N**on-accidental injuries
- **D**iastasis of pelvic ring: assess widening of pubic symphysis and symmetry or widening of sacroiliac joints

Why is it necessary to determine whether a femoral neck fracture is intra- or extracapsular?

This will influence further management, as intracapsular fractures carry a risk of avascular necrosis of the femoral head.

The capsule is attached to the base of the femoral neck and conveys arterial blood from a distal to proximal direction.

- Fractures proximal to the capsular attachment are intracapsular and are at risk of avascular necrosis due to impaired blood supply.
- Fractures lateral to the basicervical region are extracapsular, and thus the head and neck can generally be preserved with metal implants such as a dynamic hip screw.

How are intracapsular fractures of the femoral neck classified?

The Garden classification – and implications:

Garden stage 1	Partial fracture, undisplaced
Garden stage 2	Complete fracture, undisplaced
Garden stage 3	Complete fracture, partially displaced
Garden stage 4	Complete fracture, completely displaced

How are extracapsular femoral neck fractures classified?

- Intertrochanteric fractures are divided into number of pieces: 2, 3 or 4 (involves the two intertrochanteric pieces and the lesser and greater trochanters).
- Subtrochanteric: suggests a pathological fracture.

How can the hip joint be dislocated?

- Anterior or posterior dislocation

> **Tip**
>
> Posterior hip dislocations are the more common – e.g. 'dashboard injury'

Section 11: Surgical radiology

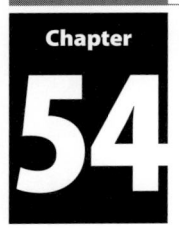

Chapter 54: Knee x-ray

Hardi Madani, John Curtis and Helen Marmery

Introduction
'This is an AP/lateral/skyline radiograph of the right (left) knee.'

Views
- AP and lateral/HBL (horizontal beam lateral) in trauma for effusion/lipohaemarthrosis
- Skyline view over patella (for patellofemoral joint pathology)

Anatomy

Bones
- Femur, tibia, fibula and patella

Lines
- Lateral view: distance from tibial tuberosity to inferior pole of patella should approximately equal length of patella:
  - if increased = patella alta (high-riding), and may indicate patella tendon rupture
  - if reduced = patella baja (low-lying), and may indicate quadriceps tendon rupture

Pathology

Intra-articular fractures
- Avulsion of the lateral aspect of the tibial plateau adjacent to Gerdy's tubercle: **Segond fracture** (suggests anterior cruciate ligament rupture)

Physical Examination for Surgeons, ed. Petrut Gogalniceanu, James Pegrum and William Lynn. Published by Cambridge University Press. © Cambridge University Press 2015.

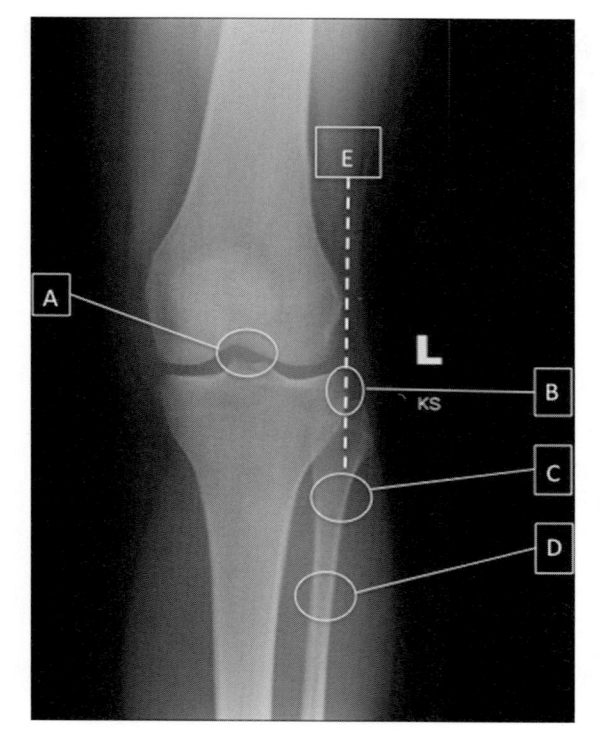

AP and lateral x-rays of the knee, illustrating the review lines and areas (circled) for subtle fractures.
(A) Fracture fragment in intercondylar notch indicative of cruciate ligament injury.
(B) Fracture fragment near the lateral border of the tibia (Segond fracture), indicating tear of the anterior cruciate ligament and medial meniscal injury.
(C) Fracture line of the neck of fibula indicating cruciate and collateral ligament tear.
(D) Fracture line of the proximal fibula (Maisonneuve fracture) associated with ankle fracture (ask for an ankle x-ray).
(E) Vertical line running through lateral femoral condyle. If the line contains more than 5 mm of tibial condyle a plateau fracture should be suspected.
(F) Line showing distance from tibial tubercle to inferior patella equals approximately (± 20%) the length of the patella. If increased, consider patella tendon rupture.

Chapter 54: Knee x-ray | 439

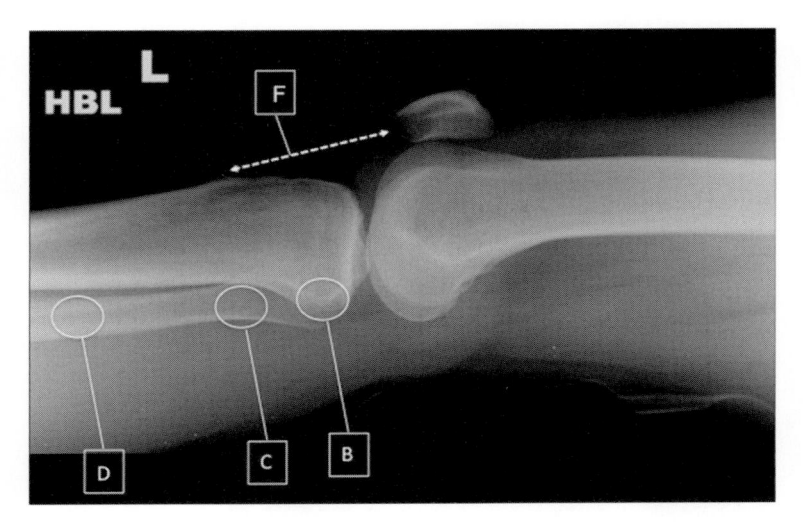

(cont.)

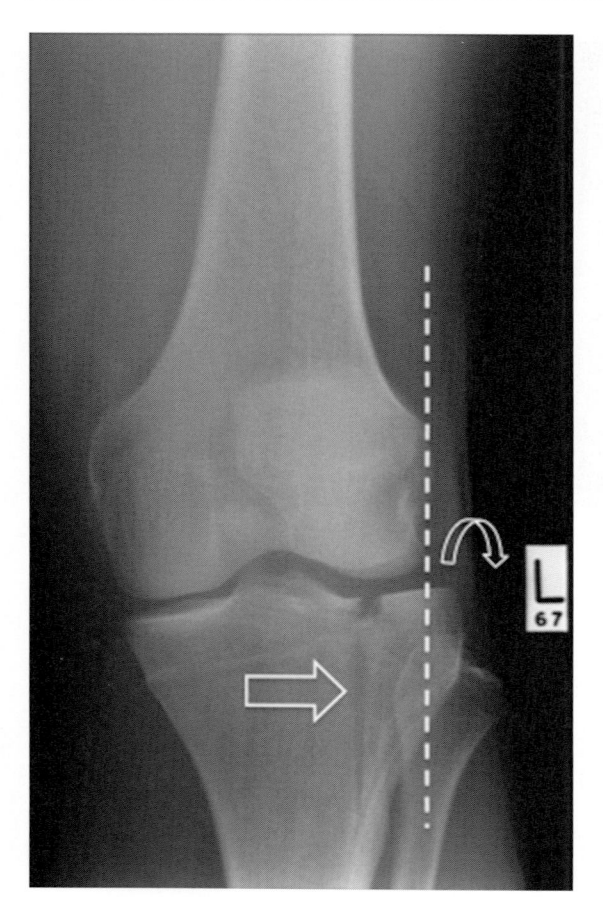

AP and HBL x-rays of the knee show a lipohaemarthrosis (arrow) due to displaced vertical lateral tibial plateau fracture (curved arrow).

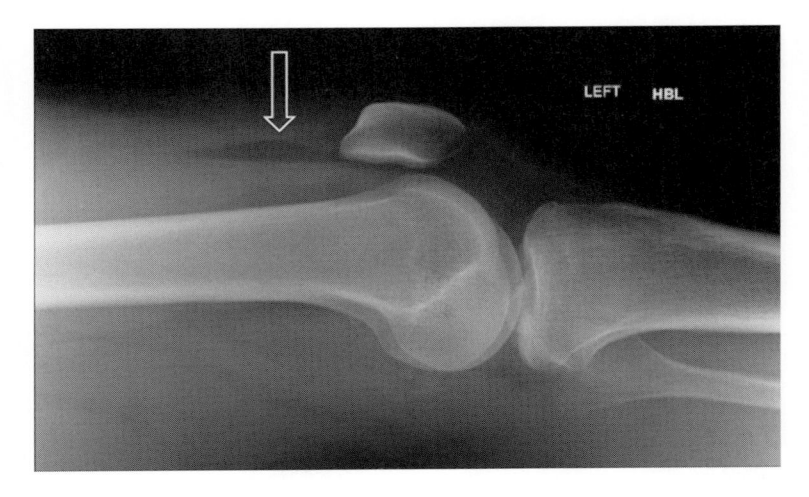

(*cont.*)

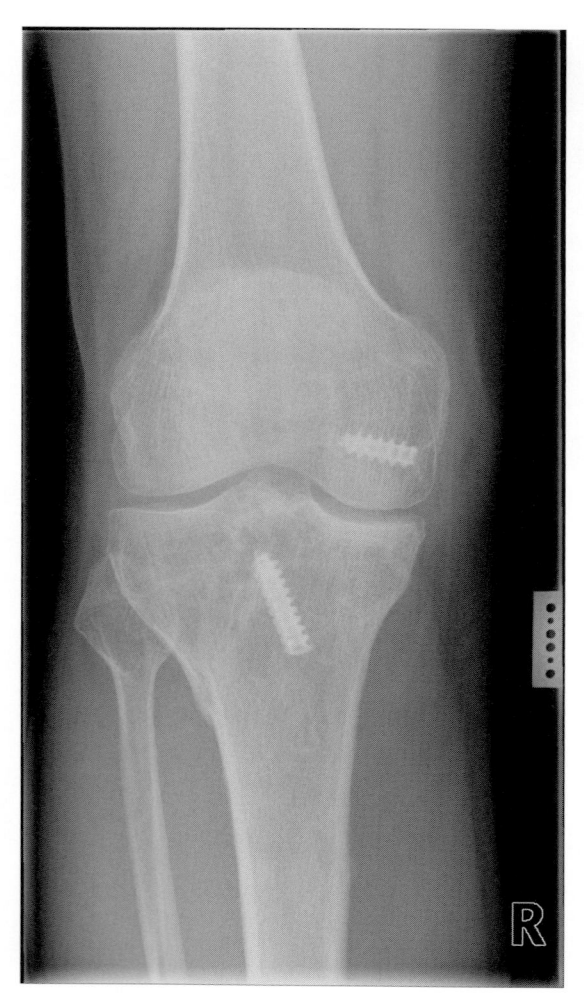

AP x-ray of the right knee shows anterior cruciate ligament (ACL) repair fixation screws in the tibia and femur.

- Fat fluid level (lipohaemarthrosis) on a horizontal beam lateral radiograph suggests intra-articular fracture with the release of marrow fat into the joint
- Intercondylar eminence fragment suggests ligament injury

Tibial plateau fractures
- 80% are lateral

Patella fractures
- Unfused ossification centres may mimic a fracture – typically lateral and/or superior (suggestive of a bipartite patella)

Fibula fractures
- Fracture involving proximal third of fibula is associated with **ankle fractures** (Maisonneuve fracture): ask for ankle x-ray

Examination notes

What are the indications for a knee x-ray in the context of trauma?
Indication for knee x-ray: **Ottawa rules** (any one factor present requires a knee radiograph):
- > 55 years old
- fibula head tenderness
- patella tenderness
- inability to flex to 90°
- inability to take 4 steps

What injuries should not be missed?
- Plateau fracture
- Segond fracture
- Osteochondral lesion

> **Tip**
>
> Isolated fractures of the fibula occur rarely.
> Fractures of the fibula are associated with lateral collateral or cruciate injury.

Section 11 Surgical radiology

Chapter 55

Foot and ankle x-ray

Hardi Madani, John Curtis and Helen Marmery

Introduction
'This is a radiograph of the right/left foot/ankle.'

Views
- Ankle – AP (shows medial clear space), lateral and mortice view (shows lateral clear space more clearly)
- Foot – DP (dorsoplantar: equivalent to AP) and oblique

Anatomy
Bones
- Malleoli, talus, calcaneus, tarsal bones, metatarsal bones, phalanges

Lines
- Foot DP – 2nd metatarsal medial border lines up with medial border middle cuneiform.
- Foot oblique – 3rd metatarsal medial border lines up with medial border of lateral cuneiform.
- Ankle AP – talar dome line is smooth throughout.
- Ankle lateral – Bohler's angle (normal 28–40°). The angle formed by the intersection of a line drawn from the highest point of the posterior tuberosity to the top of the posterior facet, and a line from the top of posterior facet to the tip of anterior process of calcaneum. If reduced can signify an occult calcaneal fracture.

Physical Examination for Surgeons, ed. Petrut Gogalniceanu, James Pegrum and William Lynn. Published by Cambridge University Press. © Cambridge University Press 2015.

Pathology

Fractures

- March fracture: 2nd or 3rd metatarsal stress fracture.
- Inversion injuries: base of 5th metatarsal.
- Lisfranc injury: disruption of Lisfranc ligament with or without fracture leads to lateral displacement of the 2nd metatarsal base with respect to the middle cuneiform. Weight-bearing views very useful in unmasking subtle injury.

Diabetic foot

- If no obvious fracture is seen, look for signs of osteomyelitis; bone destruction/osteolysis, usually involving calcaneum, 1st/5th metatarsal heads or distal phalanges; or bone changes and deformities suggestive of Charcot foot, typically involving the tarsometatarsal joints.

Foreign object

- Look for metallic objects, nails or glass in the soft tissues.

Examination notes

What injuries should not be missed?

- Lisfranc fracture – use weight-bearing views to demonstrate displaced metatarsals
- Stress fracture of 2nd and 3rd metatarsals (MT)
- Osteochondral lesion – 'blistering' to the cartilage surface and damage to the underlying bone, usually as a result of trauma, and commonly affects the talus
- Osteomyelitis
- Malignancy

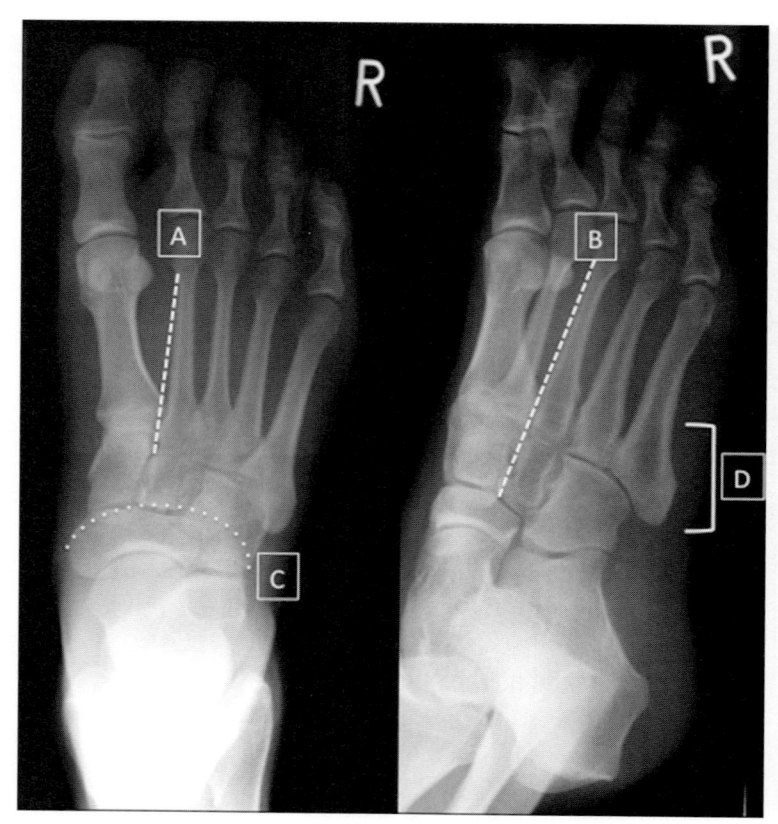

DP and oblique x-rays of a normal foot, with normal alignment lines and review areas. Line A shows the medial margin of the second MT lining up with the medial margin of intermediate cuneiform bone. Line B shows the medial margin of the third MT lining up with the medial margin of the lateral cuneiform. Disruption of these alignments suggests Lisfranc fracture dislocation. Line C highlights the normal mid-foot arc. Line D highlights typical site of 5th MT avulsion and Jones fractures.

Chapter 55: Foot and ankle x-ray | 447

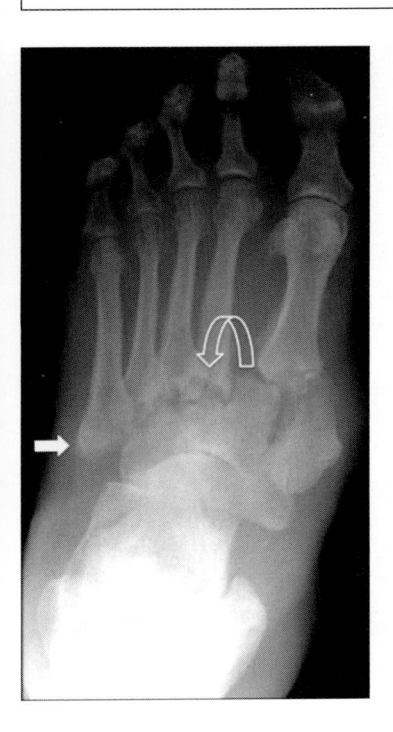

DP x-ray of the left foot showing displacement of the tarsometatarsal joints (arrows) due to Lisfranc fracture dislocation (note the misalignment of the normal review lines).

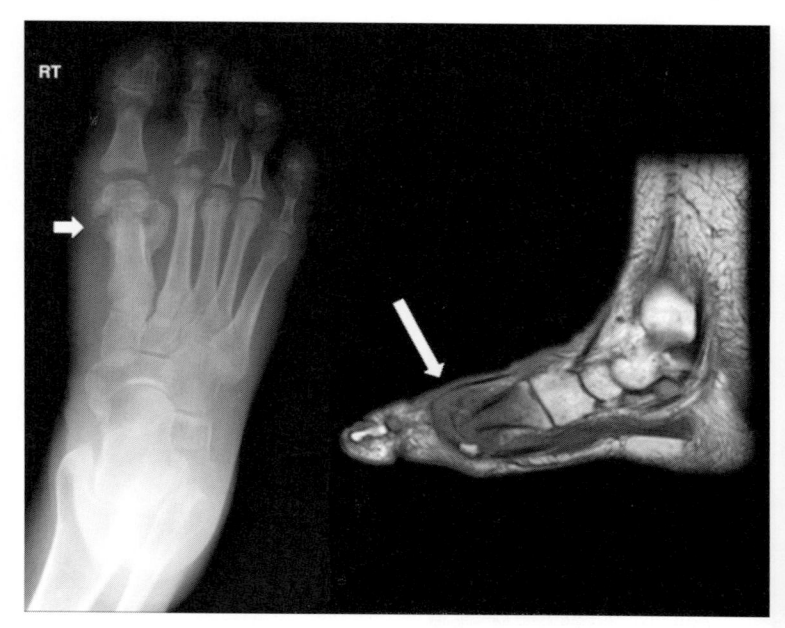

DP view of the right foot shows destructive process in the first MT head and metatarsophalangeal joint (short arrow) consistent with an infective or malignant process (osteosarcoma). Sagittal MRI of the foot confirmed osteomyelitis (long arrow).

Section 11 Surgical radiology

Chapter 56

Principles of CT

Hardi Madani, John Curtis and Helen Marmery

Basics

- X-rays are used to image thin transverse sections of the body (axial 1–10 mm thick slices).
- Slices are stacked on top of one another to produce series.
- Each tissue has a Hounsfield unit (HU) value, which represents the density of an object and ranges from −1000 to +1000.
- Objects can be described as low (black) or high (white) density:
  - Air is low density, with an HU value of −1000, and appears black.
  - Water is intermediate in density, with an HU value of 0, and appears grey.
  - Bone is high density, with an HU value of +1000, and appears white.
  - Soft tissues and organs have a range of values and are different shades of grey (see table).

Tissue types: densities and CT numbers (Hounsfield units)

Tissue	Density/colour	CT number (HU)
Bone	**White (high density)**	**+1000**
Stones	White	+100 to +900 or more
Fresh blood	Light grey/white	+60 to +80
Liver	Grey	+40 to +60
Water	**Grey (intermediate density)**	**0**
Fat	Murky grey/black	−50 to −100
Air	**Black (low density)**	**−1000**

Physical Examination for Surgeons, ed. Petrut Gogalniceanu, James Pegrum and William Lynn. Published by Cambridge University Press. © Cambridge University Press 2015.

Contrast
- Iodinated material is given intravenously, orally, rectally or into joints to help enhance and improve tissue differentiation between normal and abnormal tissues.
- Intravenous contrast is potentially nephrotoxic and can be fatal if aspirated.
- Oral contrast (water-soluble) can be used to visualise bowel or diagnose leaks.

Reconstruction and windowing
- Images can be viewed in different 'windowing' to help enhance tissue contrast and view different densities.
- CT can be used to reconstruct organs.

> **Example**
>
> CT virtual colonoscopy is now a well-accepted investigation for polyps and malignancy. Air is insufflated per rectum into a pre-prepared bowel and a CT is performed to visualise the dilated large bowel in various views including 3D reconstruction.

Section 11 **Surgical radiology**

Chapter 57

Head CT

Hardi Madani, John Curtis and Helen Marmery

Introduction

'This is an unenhanced (pre- and post-contrast) axial/coronal/sagittal view of the brain.'

Summary

'Concentric rings' model (external to internal):
- Skin and soft tissues
- Bones
- Circulation and perimeningeal spaces
- Brain parenchyma
- Cisterns and ventricles
- Everything else

Checklist

Skin and soft tissues
- Soft tissue haematoma
- Surgical emphysema
- Obvious lacerations

Bones
- Traumatic: skull, facial, mastoid, paranasal sinuses and paraorbital fractures (fluid, bleed and surgical emphysema with loss of normal bone contour)

Physical Examination for Surgeons, ed. Petrut Gogalniceanu, James Pegrum and William Lynn. Published by Cambridge University Press. © Cambridge University Press 2015.

- Neoplastic: bone lesions – primary, secondary metastases or erosion from intrinsic mass
- Infective/inflammatory: mastoid air cells and inner ear collection or paranasal sinusitis – air fluid level and localised abscess
- Iatrogenic: post-craniotomy or burr holes – smooth well-demarcated bone gap

Circulation and perimeningeal spaces

- Traumatic:
    - acute bleed: subarachnoid haemorrhage (SAH), subdural haematoma (SDH), extradural haematoma (EDH)
    - chronic hematoma or collection

- Arterial: aneurysm and AVMs (difficult to identify without contrast)
- Venous sinus thrombosis and occlusion: suspect in high-risk groups
- Infective: abscess
- Iatrogenic: surgical clips

Brain parenchyma

- Displacement and midline shift: mass effect from lesion, bleed, obstruction
- Herniation:
    - subfalcine
    - transtentorial (uncal)
    - tonsillar

- Vascular: infarction, small vessel change, intracerebral bleed
- Neoplastic:
    - 80% metastates and 20% primary lesions
    - primary: gliomas, meningioma, mixed glial/neuronal or pituitary

- Post-surgical: parenchymal loss or change, clips, shunts, craniotomy or screws

Cisterns and ventricles

- Infective: ventricular abscess collection
- Traumatic: acute haemorrhage secondary to trauma
- Obstructive: hydrocephalus

Everything else

- Orbits: periorbital masses or lens loss (dark ellipse in posterior orbit), post-trauma foreign body
- Pituitary: enlarged and hyperdense in haemorrhage

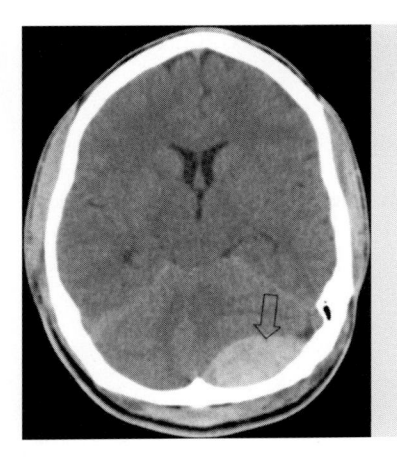

CT head showing a biconvex extradural (or epidural) haemorrhage in the left posterior cerebellum (arrow).

Examination notes

- Any suspicion of intracranial space-occupying lesion, e.g. AVM, aneurysm, venous thrombus or collection, requires a pre- and post-contrast CT scan.
- When describing any mass, start by attempting to localise to either parenchymal (intra-axial) or outside the brain, e.g. dural, bone, nasal (extra-axial).
- Look for high-density material – mass or haemorrhage:
  - SAH: blood in foramen magnum, ventricles, interpeduncular cisterns
  - SDH: crescent (concavo-convex)
  - EDH: biconvex (lens-shaped)
  - Contusion: small (2–3 mm) spots of blood, temporal lobes
  - Diffuse axonal injury: small spots of haemorrhage at the grey/white matter junction
  - Hemorrhagic or ischaemic infarct
- Look for abnormal low-density air (pneumocranium): fractures.
- Midline shift is always a clue to pathology.
- Ventricular dilatation or loss of normal cisterns and CSF spaces (especially around cord and central 3rd ventricle) are signs of impending herniation.

How can you differentiate between acute and chronic blood loss?

- Acute blood is generally of high density.
- Chronic blood is of low density.
- Subacute blood can be difficult to detect if it is isodense with brain (i.e. the same density).
- Clues should be sought such as displacement of sulci in the case of subacute subdural collections.

Section 11 Surgical radiology

Chapter 58

Chest CT

Hardi Madani, John Curtis and Helen Marmery

Introduction

'This is a post-contrast/non-contrast CT of the thorax in axial/coronal/sagittal view.'

Summary

A   Airway – trachea and main bronchi
B   Breathing – lungs and pleura
C   Circulation and mediastinum – great vessels, heart and oesophagus
D   Diaphragm
E   Everything else

Checklist

Airway (trachea)
- Tracheostomy
- ET tube: normally 2 cm from carina
- Foreign bodies
- Collapse
- Deviation
- Tracheobronchial laceration (lung cut off from hilum)

Physical Examination for Surgeons, ed. Petrut Gogalniceanu, James Pegrum and William Lynn. Published by Cambridge University Press. © Cambridge University Press 2015.

Breathing (lungs)
- Infections: unilateral or bilateral consolidation, collapse or pleural empyema
- Inflammation: ARDS, pleural effusion
- Vascular: PE +/– infarcted lung
- Tumour: primary lung, secondary metastases
- Trauma: lung contusions, laceration, haemothorax, pneumothorax, pnemomediastinum
- Iatrogenic: pneumonectomy or lobectomy, sternotomy wires, clips, chest drains

Circulation and mediastinum
- Infective/inflammation: acute mediastinitis, pericarditis
- Vascular:
  - aortic dissection or aneurysm
  - superior vena cava syndrome secondary to thoracic mass
- Traumatic: pericardial haematoma
- Mechanical: oesophageal perforation/dissection (e.g. post-endoscopy)

Diaphragm
- Mechanical: diaphragmatic hernias, phrenic nerve palsy and associated diaphragmatic elevation
- Tumour: primary mesothelioma

Everything else
- Bones: thoracic vertebra, clavicle, sternum, scapula, ribs: fractures, metastases, collections

Quick look
- Upper abdomen: air, fluid, blood, liver, spleen, adrenals, kidney and abdominal aorta

Section 11 Surgical radiology

Chapter 59

Abdomen CT

Hardi Madani, John Curtis and Helen Marmery

Introduction

'This is a post-contrast/non-contrast axial/coronal/sagittal CT of the abdomen and pelvis.'

Summary

- Life-threatening pathology
- Peritoneal cavity and abdominal wall
- Upper abdominal viscera
- Small and large bowel
- Pelvic viscera
- Retroperitoneum
- Extra-abdominal structures

Checklist: emergencies

First exclude life-threatening pathology: $A^3B^2C^1$:

- **3 As**
  - **A**bdominal aortic aneurysm
  - **A**cute pancreatitis
  - **A**ir (free air caused by perforation)

- **2 Bs**
  - **B**owel ischemia
  - **B**owel obstruction

Physical Examination for Surgeons, ed. Petrut Gogalniceanu, James Pegrum and William Lynn. Published by Cambridge University Press. © Cambridge University Press 2015.

- **1 C**
  - **C**ollections (free fluid, blood or abscesses).

Proceed to systematically review the abdomen and pelvis.

Checklist: systematic

Peritoneum and abdominal wall
- Free air
- Free fluid
- Collections: pelvic, subdiaphragmatic, paracolic gutters, inter-loop, lesser sac
- Abdominal wall: hernias, laparotomies, stomas, other tissue defects, surgical emphysema

Upper abdominal organs
- Liver
- Gallbladder and biliary tree
- Pancreas
- Spleen

Intestines
- Stomach and duodenum
- Small bowel
- Large bowel
- Appendix

Pelvic viscera
- Rectum and sigmoid colon
- Bladder and prostate
- Uterus and adnexae

Retroperitoneum
- Kidneys, ureters and bladder
- Aorta

Extra-abdominal checks
- Lung bases
- Bones
- Foreign objects and medical devices

Examination notes: general
What are the general principles of CT scanning?
- CT scans are normally performed with intravenous contrast, which appears white.
- Non-contrast CTs are performed in patients with renal impairment (e.g. eGFR < 45) or contrast allergies, or in CT scans that do not require contrast (e.g. CT KUB for renal calculi).
- A basic CT scan uses a *venous phase*, in which the veins (e.g. IVC) appear dense ('bright').
- Trauma or acute haemorrhage scans require an *arterial phase* (e.g. aorta appears dense/'bright') to identify contrast extravasation/active arterial bleeding.
- CT scans investigating bowel malignancy or strictures require IV and oral contrast (gastrografin). This makes the bowel look dense ('bright').
- CT virtual colonoscopy involves 3D reconstruction of the large bowel and is used to diagnose intraluminal lesions such as polyps or cancers, as an alternative to standard colonoscopy.

Examination notes: upper abdominal viscera
What are the features of portal hypertension?
- Dilated portal vein, varices, splenomegaly and ascites

What are the features of a liver abscess?
- Low-density (dark) mass with ring enhancement

What are the features of liver cirrhosis?
- Small, lobulated liver

How do liver metastases present?
- Low-density (dark) masses or nodules. These can be difficult to differentiate from benign cysts, and US confirmation may be required.

What are the features of acute cholecystitis?
- The gallbladder is thick-walled with surrounding fluid or 'fat stranding'.
- Gallstones may or may not be seen on a CT scan, so proceed to US scanning.

- Look for associated features such as intra- or extrahepatic bile duct dilatation, liver abscesses, a pancreatic head mass, cholangiocarcinoma or gall bladder adenocarcinoma.

What are the features of acute pancreatitis?

- The pancreas is diffusely enlarged with surrounding fluid and 'fat stranding'. By contrast, the pancreas is atrophied and calcified in chronic pancreatitis.
- Look for associated features such as pseudocyst formation, pancreatic necrosis, portal vein thrombosis or splenic artery pseudoaneurysm.

What pancreatic complications can be seen in blunt trauma?

- Identify pancreatic lacerations (linear/wedge low-density line) or surrounding fluid. If the pancreatic duct is involved, duct dilatation may be seen.

What spleen-related changes may be seen?

- Identify splenic rupture secondary to infectious mononucleosis or malaria.
- Splenic infarcts are wedge-shaped low-density (dark) areas which may be associated with a splenic artery thrombus.
- In the context of trauma, identify lacerations (linear/wedge dark line) with or without evidence of contrast extravasation (bleeding) or intraparenchymal pseudoaneurysms (high-density/bright foci), which are at risk of delayed rupture.

Examination notes: intestines

What are the features of small bowel obstruction?

- Normal diameter < 2.5 cm
- Look for air/fluid levels or dilated fluid-filled bowel
- Causes: adhesions, hernias, tumors, gallstone ileus

What are the features of large bowel obstruction?

- Dilated > 5.5 cm
- Causes: neoplastic or inflammatory masses, diverticulitis, volvulus, hernia, impaction
- Risk of perforation with diameters > 6–9 cm
- Toxic megacolon occurs in ulcerative colitis, Crohn's or infectious colitis (*Clostridium difficile*)

- Large bowel obstruction associated with a collapsed or non-dilated small bowel is suggestive of a patent ileocaecal valve. This prevents large bowel decompression into the small bowel and is associated with an increased risk of large bowel perforation.

What intestinal structures must not be missed?
- Appendix: acute appendicitis
- Meckel's diverticulum

How can visceral inflammation be identified?
- 'Fat stranding' or 'dirty fat' around organs and hollow viscera is a sign of inflammation – e.g. diverticulitis or infectious colitis.

What are the general features of intestinal ischaemia?
- Thrombus present in the mesenteric vessels (coeliac axis, SMA, IMA)
- Stenotic plaques involving the origins of the mesenteric arteries in the aorta
- Loss of normal haustral pattern
- Bowel wall thickening
- Bowel wall gas – pneumatosis, or portal venous gas

Examination notes: retroperitoneum

What are the obvious renal tract pathologies that must not be missed?
See Chapter 61, *Kidneys, ureter and bladder CT*.
- Renal masses
- Calculi anywhere in the kidneys, ureters or bladder
- Hydronephrosis or hydroureter
- Pyelonephritis and perinephric abscesses
- JJ stents (suggestive of previous obstruction)

What changes in vascular anatomy must be identified?
See Chapter 60, *Aorta CT*.
- Abdominal aortic aneurysms
- Standard findings in AAA: mural calcification and intraluminal thrombus

- Mycotic aneurysms: thick aneurysmal wall associated with a collection or evidence of wall inflammation
- Complications of AAA: rupture (contrast extravasation intra- or extraperitoneally), fistula formation (contrast seen in bowel or IVC) or haematoma formation (no contrast outside AAA)
- Aortic or iliac stenosis or occlusion
- Aortic dissection
- Mesenteric embolic occlusion or venous thrombosis

Examination notes: extra-abdominal changes

What medical devices must be identified?
- Aortic or iliac stents
- Surgical clips
- Staples/anastomosis clips

What bony features should be checked on an abdominal CT?
Check the lower ribs, spine, pelvis and femoral heads for fractures or metastatic lesions. Metastases can be lytic (dark) or sclerotic (bright) – e.g. prostatic metastases.

What changes in the lung bases must be identified?
- Effusions
- Consolidations
- Masses

Section 11: Surgical radiology

Chapter 60: Aorta CT

Hardi Madani, John Curtis and Helen Marmery

Introduction

'This is a CT aorta in arterial phase axial/coronal/sagittal view imaged at the thoracic/abdominal/bifurcation level.'

Summary

- A Aneurysm
- B Branches
- C Contrast extravasation/haematomas
- D Dissection
- E Endoprostheses/endovascular devices

Checklist: systematic check

Aneurysm

- Thoracic aortic aneurysm: dilatation ≥ 3.0 cm
- Abdominal aortic aneurysm: dilatation ≥ 2.5 cm (suprarenal, juxtarenal or infrarenal), ectatic
- Pseudoaneurysm (involving less than three layers of the wall): focal outpouching
- Dissection flap: pencil-thin curvilinear low-density line in a contrast-enhanced aorta separating true and false aneurysm
- Thrombus: low-density filling defect in contrast-enhanced lumen

---

Physical Examination for Surgeons, ed. Petrut Gogalniceanu, James Pegrum and William Lynn. Published by Cambridge University Press. © Cambridge University Press 2015.

Branches
- Thoracic aorta: extension of thrombus, aneurysm or dissection in the common carotid artery (CCA), left subclavian artery (LSA), brachiocephalic trunk (BCT), right subclavian artery (RSA)
- Abdominal aorta: occlusive disease affecting coeliac, SMA, IMA, renal artery, iliac artery

Contrast
- Rupture: periaortic fluid or active contrast leak
- Contained rupture: break in contour, haematoma in periaortic or retroperitoneal rupture
- Imminent sign of rupture (AAA): 'crescent sign' (high-density crescent within sac but outside perfused area)
- Aortoenteric fistula: high density in IVC or loop of bowel
- Inflammatory/mycotic aneurysm : 'dirty' periaortic fat and air

Dissection site
- Ascending thoracic aorta: above aortic root (Stanford type A)
- Descending thoracic aorta: distal to left subclavian artery (Stanford type B)
- Abdominal aortic dissection: double lumen

Endoprostheses
- Examine for endovascular grafts
- Look for evidence of upper limb revascularisation (carotid–carotid/carotid–subclavian bypass)
- Calibre and tortuosity of common femoral and iliac arteries

Quick look

Heart
- Pericardial recess and pericardial space: leak, rupture or trauma

Mediastinum
- Mass
- Subcutaneous air: surgical emphysema
- Higher-density fluid: leak (haematoma)

Bone
- Metastases, fractures (post road traffic accident)

Chapter 60: Aorta CT | 465

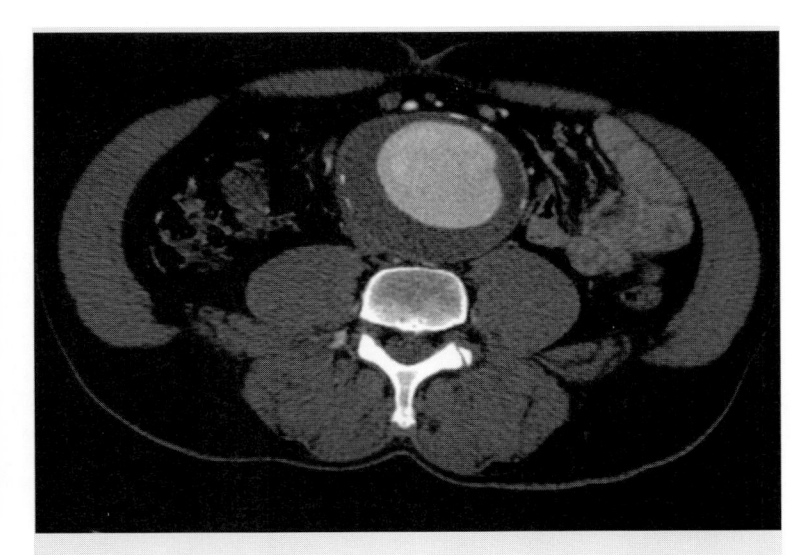

CT abdomen demonstrating abdominal aortic aneurysm.

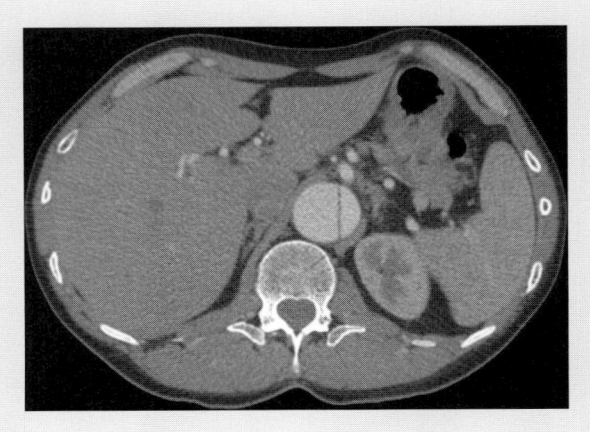

CT abdomen demonstrating abdominal aortic dissection.

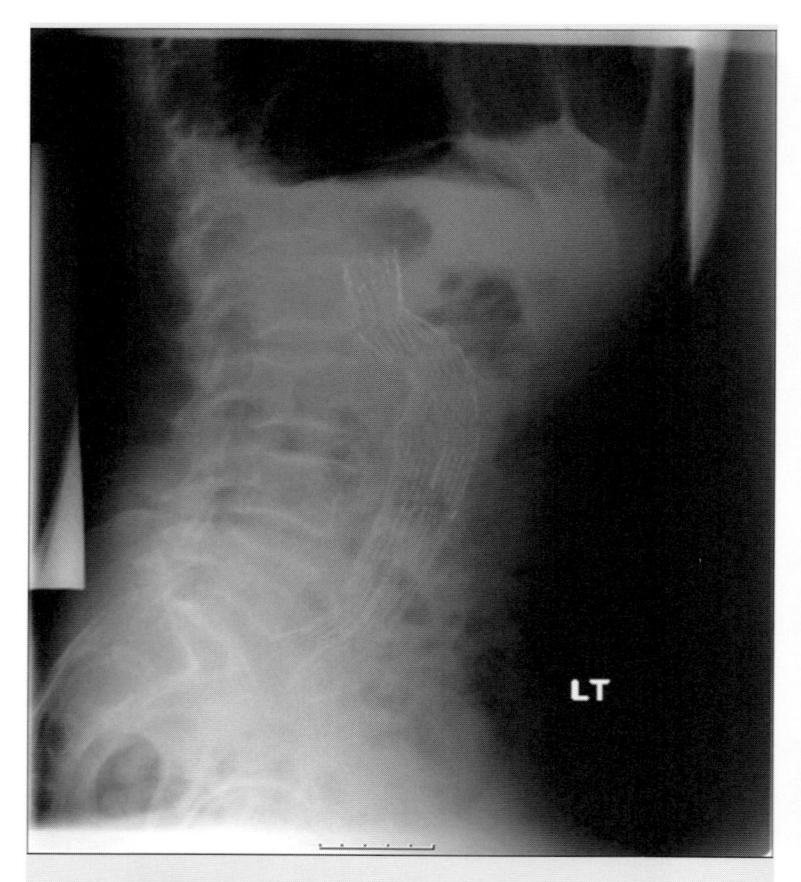

Lateral abdominal radiograph demonstrating an endovascular aortic prosthesis used to repair an abdominal aortic aneurysm using EVAR.

Tips

Common cases are a ruptured or leaking aneurysm and dissection.

Look for complications – end organ damage: infarcts and ischemia of kidney or bowel.

Examination notes

How is thoracic aortic dissection classified?

Stanford classification:
- Type A: includes ascending aorta (up to and including left subclavian artery)
- Type B: descending aorta only (distal to left subclavian artery)

e.g. a dissection involving the entire thoracic aorta (from root to diaphragm) is still a Stanford type A dissection, as it includes the ascending thoracic aorta).

> **Tip**
>
> Stanford **A** for **a**scending.
> Stanford **B** for **b**elow LSA.

DeBakey classification:
- Type I: ascending and descending aorta
- Type II: only ascending aorta
- Type III: only descending aorta

What are the features of an EVAR?

- Metallic mesh in aorta and iliac arteries.
- Normally there should not be contrast in the excluded aneurysmal sac.
- If contrast is present outside the graft this suggests the presence of an endoleak.
- If the distal part of an endovascular graft is seen only in one limb look for evidence of femoral–femoral crossover grafts in the suprapubic soft tissues.

How are endoleaks classified?

- Type I: leak at sites of graft attachment to aortic wall (inadequate seal at graft ends):
  - Type 1a: proximal endoleak
  - Type 1b: distal endoleak
- Type II: sac filling retrogradely via patent aneurysm side branches (e.g. lumbar or inferior mesenteric artery) – the most common type

- Type III: leak through a defect in graft fabric (mechanical failure of graft)
- Type IV: leaks through material of graft caused by graft porosity

Why should the common femoral and iliac arteries be assessed?

- If the patient is waiting for AAA repair, the calibre and tortuosity of the common femoral and iliac arteries (access vessels) needs to be assessed to determine if the endograft can be inserted safely.
- Presence of atheromatous changes may lead to distal ischaemia.

Section 11 **Surgical radiology**

Chapter 61

Kidneys, ureter and bladder CT

Hardi Madani, John Curtis and Helen Marmery

Introduction
'This is an unenhanced low-dose CT scan of the kidneys, ureter and bladder in axial/coronal/sagittal view.'

Summary

A **Air**: perforation from GI or urinary system

B **Blood**: high-density haemorrhage from tumour, trauma or obstruction

C **Calcifications**: renal, collecting system, ureteric, bladder calculi, prostate calcification

D **Dilatations**: renal or ureteric obstruction

Checklist: 'KUBE'

Kidney
- Site – horseshoe or ectopic kidney
- Size – masses, obstruction (calculi), reflux
- Content – stones, staghorn calculi

Ureter
- Site – on psoas: mass/lesion
- Size – obstruction:

Physical Examination for Surgeons, ed. Petrut Gogalniceanu, James Pegrum and William Lynn. Published by Cambridge University Press. © Cambridge University Press 2015.

- unilateral = calculi, ureteric or bladder tumour, stricture from previous surgery
- bilateral = bladder outflow obstruction

Bladder
- Air (dark): trauma, instrumentation or fistula to bowel (e.g. Crohn's disease) or infection
- Calcification of wall: schistosomiasis, TB infection, post radiation

Everything else
- Retroperitoneal and peritoneal spaces
- The 3 Fs – fat inflammation, fluid collection (e.g. urinoma) and "fast" (acute) haemorrhage
- Prostatic calcification may be detected on a KUB radiograph and is usually a sign of chronic inflammation

Quick look
- Bowel dilatation
- Free fluid, collection or air
- 'Dirty fat' around other organs, e.g. liver, gall bladder, pancreas

Tips

The scan is specifically an unenhanced 'grainy' low-dose scan looking for calculi.

CT KUB scans are good for artefacts – e.g. stents, calcifications and air – but lack of contrast limits diagnosis of solid organ pathology.

However, 'dirty'-looking fat or fluid around solid or hollow organs suggests inflammation, which requires a post-contrast scan.

If a ureteric cancer is suspected CT IVU should be requested (a delayed phase post-contrast scan). Contrast fills the renal pelvis, ureter and bladder, highlighting any mass or filling defects.

The commonest findings in exams are calcifications and secondary signs of obstruction (hydronephrosis or hydroureter).

Section 11 **Surgical radiology**

Chapter 62

Lower limb CT angiogram
Hardi Madani, John Curtis and Helen Marmery

Introduction
'This is a CT angiogram, in axial/coronal/sagittal view of lower limb arteries'

Summary
- A Arterial anatomy
- B Blockage
- C Contrast extravasation
- D Dissection
- E Extra-arterial – bone and soft tissue
- F Flow improvements: stents, bypasses

Checklist

Arterial anatomy
- Aorta:
  - divisions : single and bilateral

- Iliac:
  - internal
  - external

- Femoral:
  - common
  - profunda

Physical Examination for Surgeons, ed. Petrut Gogalniceanu, James Pegrum and William Lynn. Published by Cambridge University Press. © Cambridge University Press 2015.

- superficial
- popliteal
- Run-offs:
  - anterior tibial (AT)
  - posterior tibial (PT)
  - peroneal

Blockage
- Filling defect: stenosis or occlusion
- Collaterals
- Calcification

Contrast extravasation
- Intramural
- Extramural

Dissection

Extra-arterial
- Bone:
  - fractures, osteomyelitis secondary to amputation or vascular ulcers
- Soft tissue:
  - ulcers, cellulitis, collections

Flow improvements
- Bypasses: vein vs. prosthetic; patent vs. blocked
- Stents

Look for associated pathology
- Bony fracture and soft tissue haematomas, foreign body, gas (trauma or infection)
- Metallic mesh: arterial stents
- High concentration arterial calcification: arteriosclerosis

---

Tips

It is essential to know normal vascular limb anatomy.

Compare one limb to the other to identify pathology.

Section editor: Petrut Gogalniceanu
Senior author: Vijay M. Gadhvi

Section 12: Airway, trauma and critical care

Chapter 63: Examination of the trauma patient

Petrut Gogalniceanu and Vijay M. Gadhvi

Checklist

System
A-T-I (Assess, Treat, Investigate/Image)

Sequence
ATLS algorithm:[34]

- **A** Airway and C-spine control
- **B** Breathing and ventilation
- **C** Circulation and haemorrhage control
- **D** Disability and neurological deficit
- **E** Exposure and environment

---

[34] Practitioners should consult the ATLS manual for a definitive description of trauma care. Committee on Trauma, American College of Surgeons. *ATLS: Advanced Trauma Life Support Program for Doctors*, 8th edn. Chicago: American College of Surgeons, 2008.

Physical Examination for Surgeons, ed. Petrut Gogalniceanu, James Pegrum and William Lynn. Published by Cambridge University Press. © Cambridge University Press 2015.

Physiological parameters
- Respiratory rate and oxygen saturation
- Heart rate and blood pressure
- Temperature and blood glucose levels

Airway and C-spine control

Assess
- Cervical spine trauma is inferred from the mechanism of injury, the presence of neck pain or focal neurology in the arms or legs. Patients with polytrauma, unconsciousness or head injuries are presumed to have C-spine injuries unless otherwise proven.
- The airway is assessed by asking the patient to answer a simple question. The ability to phonate implies that the airway is patent.
- Inspect for evidence of a compromised or threatened airway by identifying stridor, hoarse voice, inhalation injuries, facial or laryngeal trauma and the presence of foreign objects in the mouth.

Treat
- The C-spine is controlled by immobilisation with a collar applied to the neck and blocks and tape which secure the neck and collar onto the bed.
- High-flow oxygen (15 L) is given via a non-rebreathe mask.
- The airway is opened by performing a basic manoeuvre (jaw thrust).
- Liquids in the oropharynx (blood, saliva or vomitus) are removed by suction with a Yankauer sucker.
- Solid foreign bodies or loose teeth are removed with Magill's forceps.
- An airway which cannot be spontaneously maintained should be supported with an airway adjunct such as an oropharyngeal or nasopharyngeal airway or laryngeal mask.
- A definitive airway may be established using a cuffed endotracheal tube or tracheostomy tube. In the emergency setting a needle crycothyroidotomy may be created by inserting a wide-bore cannula through the crycothyroid membrane.

Investigate
- Perform an arterial blood gas (ABG).
- Image the cervical spine with an AP and lateral plain film.
- If the C-spine x-rays are inconclusive, maintain cervical spine immobilisation until a CT scan can be performed.

Breathing and ventilation

Assess
- Look for evidence of cyanosis.
- Look for misting of the oxygen mask.
- Inspect the movement of the chest and use of accessory muscles.
- Palpate the position of the trachea, which may be deviated in a pneumothorax or haemothorax.
- Feel the chest wall for evidence of surgical emphysema.
- Assess chest expansion.
- Percuss the chest for dullness or hyper-resonance.
- Auscultate for air entry.

Identify
- Apnoea
- Flail chest
- Pneumothorax
- Haemothorax

Treat
- Deliver high-flow oxygen.
- If the patient is apnoeic use a bag-valve mask to ventilate.
- Needle decompression of tension pneumothoraces.
- Insert chest drains for definitive treatment of a pneumothorax or haemothorax.
- Cover any chest wall defects with an occlusive dressing.

Investigate
- Chest x-ray
- Perform an ABG if not already done

Circulation and haemorrhage control

Assess
- Assess cerebral perfusion by determining patient's level of consciousness or agitation secondary to cerebral hypoperfusion.
- Feel the radial and femoral pulses and assess rate and character.

- Look at the JVP to determine whether the patient has a reduced venous return (flat JVP, e.g. haemorrhagic shock) or evidence of cardiac-related shock (raised JVP, e.g. cardiac tamponade). In the trauma setting in the presence of neck immobilisation, JVP assessment is not always possible.
- Look for external sources of bleeding: floor, bed pan, in the bed.
- Identify sources of bleeding in the chest, abdomen, pelvis or fractured long bones:
    - Brief examination of the chest (haemothorax, cardiac tampoande, thoracic aortic injuries). Listen for muffled heart sounds in cardiac tamponade or absent breath sounds in a tension pneumothorax.
    - Examination of the abdomen: peritonism, masses, palpable AAA, RUQ (liver) or LUQ (spleen) tenderness.
    - Stability of pelvis.
    - Look for blood at the urethral meatus, perineal bruising or scrotal ecchymosis suggestive of pelvic fracture or urethral injuries.
    - Inspect and palpate upper and lower limbs for evidence of fractured long bones.
- Feel the peripheries and assess capillary refill time to determine the extent of peripheral hypoperfusion.

Identify shock

- Haemorrhage
- Fluid loss
- Cardiac tamponade
- Tension pneumothorax
- Sepsis
- Anaphylaxis
- Spinal trauma

Treat

- Stop bleeding by direct manual pressure or tourniquet.
- Stabilise pelvis with a sheet, towel or pelvic binder if there is a suspicion of bleeding secondary to a pelvic fracture.
- Splint any fractured limbs.
- Decompress cardiac tamponade using needle pericardiocentesis.
- Needle decompression of tension pneumothoraces, then proceed to inserting a chest drain.
- Gain bilateral wide-bore intravenous access.

- Resuscitate with intravenous fluids or blood products.
- Gain definitive control of haemorrhage either surgically or using endovascular techniques.
- Treat sepsis and anaphylaxis accordingly.

Investigate

- Check bloods for low haemoglobin and clotting abnormalities. Renal function is important in assessing the risk of cross-sectional imaging in the context of trauma.
- Group and save blood as well crossmatch.
- ECG.
- Urine dipstick (haematuria may be a sign of renal trauma).
- Pelvic x-ray (sacroiliac joint disruption with laceration of iliac vessels).
- Perform a FAST scan to identify free fluid in the chest, abdomen or pelvis.

Disability and neurological deficit

Assess

- Neurological deficit:
  - Consciousness is assessed using the Glasgow Coma Scale.
  - Pupil symmetry and reaction is used to determine evidence of central neurological deficits or raised intracranial pressure.
  - Lateralising signs are determined by assessing movement and sensation in the upper and lower limbs.

- Diabetes:
  - Blood sugar levels are measured to identify hypo- or hyperglycaemia.

- Pain:
  - Site and severity of pain.

Treat

- Hydration and blood pressure are controlled to allow good perfusion of the brain initially in the presence of any intracranial trauma, prior to definitive neurosurgical care. Anticonvulsants may be used to temporarily treat seizures. Uncontrolled seizures are treated by inducing general anaesthesia.
- Correct blood glucose abnormalities.
- IV or IM analgesia.

Investigate

- CT head.

Exposure and environment

Assess
- Fully expose the patient to assess any unidentified injuries.
- Perform a logroll to assess missed injuries to the posterior trunk. Identify spinal or paraspinal tenderness or deformities.
- Perform a digital rectal examination to assess for bleeding, high-riding prostate, rectal tone and perianal sensation.
- Core temperature is measured to rule out hypothermia.

Treat
- Warm the patient to treat hypothermia.
- Remove cold or wet clothing.
- Insert a Foley catheter and NG tubes if necessary.

Investigate
- Check bHCG for pregnancy, and amylase for blunt trauma to the pancreas.

Examination notes

How should inpatient trauma patients be treated?

All trauma patients need to be treated according to the American College of Surgeons Advanced Trauma Life Support (ATLS) principles.[35] This chapter does not teach ATLS principles, and only gives a simple system of assessing the trauma patient. All surgeons treating trauma patients should receive formal ATLS training in an accredited centre.

What system can be used in assessing the trauma patient?

A-T-I: assess – treat – investigate/image.

How is the care of trauma patients structured?

- Triage: prioritises the allocation of healthcare resources in order of clinical need.
- Primary survey: identification and treatment of life-threatening injuries; resuscitation of patient to a stable physiological state; basic investigations. e.g. haemorrhage from traumatic amputation of distal forearm.

---

[35] Committee on Trauma, American College of Surgeons. *ATLS: Advanced Trauma Life Support Program for Doctors*, 8th edn. Chicago: American College of Surgeons, 2008.

- Secondary survey: history, head-to-toe assessment of patient and specialist investigations to identify other serious injuries.
  e.g. fractured distal radius.
- Tertiary survey: repetition of primary and secondary survey; identification and review of all injuries after the patient has been resuscitated and stabilised. This includes all imaging and laboratory studies. Should be performed within 24 hours and on discharge.
  e.g. dislocation of left 5th finger.

How is trauma assessment different from other examination methods?

- Clinical assessment happens concomitantly with resuscitation and treatment of life-threatening injuries.
- Steps in the examination algorithm cannot be missed or selectively applied by the examining surgeon. All resuscitation steps need to be performed and completed sequentially.
- Specialist investigations are carried out after the initial stabilisation.

What is AMPLET?

AMPLET is a mnemonic for taking an essential rapid history in a severely injured patient who may deteriorate suddenly and become unable to give further vital information:

- **A** Allergies
- **M** Medications (drug history)
- **P** Past medical history and Pregnancy
- **L** Last ate (essential in deciding on safest method of anaesthesia)
- **E** Events that led to or followed the trauma; Environment in which trauma occurred
- **T** Tetanus prophylaxis status

What do you do after you complete the ABCDE algorithm?

3 **Rs**:

- Re-assess (repeat patient survey).
- Resuscitate.
- Refer to a trauma centre if local resources are unable to meet level of care needed.

What are the lethal injuries that should be identified and treated in the primary survey?

- **A** Airway obstruction and C-spine injuries
- **B** **T**ension pneumothorax, **L**arge haemothorax, **S**ucking chest wound (open pneumothorax), **F**lail chest, **C**ardiac tamponade
- **C** shock: cardiac, hypovolaemic, spinal, anaphylactic or septic
- **D** brain or spinal cord injury
- **E** hypothermia and hypoglycaemia

What is the mnemonic for life-threatening airway and breathing complications?

ATLS FC (see above)

What is a good basic method of assessing a patient's airway?

Speak to the patient and ask him or her a question. This tests consciousness, brain perfusion, airway patency, ability to phonate (and therefore ventilate).

How can the severity of trauma be determined?

ISS: Injury Severity Score

> **Trauma tips**
>
> Put out trauma call.
> Observe vital signs.
> Speak to patient.

Trauma summary

	Assess	Treat	Identify injuries	Investigate	Image	Question
Physiological parameters (vital signs)	Respiratory rate and oxygen saturation Heart rate and blood pressure Temperature and blood glucose levels			AMPLET history		Are the vital signs normal?
Airway and C-spine control	**C-spine control Airway patency:** – stridor – speech – foreign bodies – facial/laryngeal fractures	C-spine immobilisation Oxygen Chin lift or jaw thrust Suction or Magill's forceps Airway adjunct Definitive airway	Airway compromise: – not patent – not maintained – not protected	ABG	C-spine x-ray (AP & lateral)	Is the airway patent? Is the C-spine immobilised?

481

(cont.)

	Assess	Treat	Identify injuries	Investigate	Image	Question
Breathing and ventilation	**Inspect:** – cyanosis and accessory muscle use – chest movement – sucking chest wounds – misting of O_2 mask **Palpate:** – tracheal position – surgical emphysema – chest wall tenderness – chest expansion **Percussion:** dullness or hyper-resonance **Auscultate:** air entry	High-flow oxygen (15L) Bag-valve mask ventilation Needle decompression and/or chest drain insertion Cover chest wall defects with an occlusive dressing	Apnoea Impaired breathing – flail chest – pneumothorax – haemothorax	O_2 saturation Capnography	Chest x-ray	Is the patient ventilating? – lungs – chest wall – diaphragm – GCS

482

| Circulation and haemorrhage control | **External bleeding**: chest, abdomen, pelvis, long bones, floor
CNS: consciousness
Cardiovascular system:
– pulses
– JVP
– heart sounds
– skin temperature/colour/perfusion
– capillary refill time
Abdomen: peritonism, tenderness, masses
Pelvis: pelvic stability (AP/lateral)
Perineum: vaginal/meatal bleeding or bruising
Musculoskeletal: long bone fractures | Stop bleeding:
– direct manual pressure
– tourniquet
– stabilise pelvis
– splint fractures
– interventional radiology
– operating room
IV access and bloods
IV fluids and blood products | Shock:
Hypovolaemic
– haemorrhagic
– fluid loss
Non-hypovolaemic
– cardiac tamponade
– tension pneumothorax
– sepsis
– anaphylaxis
– neurogenic | ECG
Blood in urine | Pelvis x-ray
FAST scan
DPL | Is the patient in shock? What type of shock? |

(cont.)

	Assess	Treat	Identify injuries	Investigate	Image	Question
Disability and neurological deficit	GCS **Pupils:** symmetry and reaction to light **Lateralising sign:** power, sensation, tone, reflexes × 4 **Blood glucose** **Pain control**	Perfuse brain with fluid resuscitation Anticonvulsants Neurosurgical consultation	Intracranial bleed ↑ ICP	Blood sugar	CT head	Is there a neurological deficit?
Exposure and environment	Full exposure **Logroll:** back injuries, DRE	Warm patient NG tube Foley catheter Orthopaedic consultation	Hypothermia Hypoglycaemia Musculoskeletal injury	bHCG Amylase	Limb x-ray	Is there back injury? Is the patient cold?

AMPLET history: modified rapid history algorithm. **A**llergies, **M**edications, **P**ast medical history, **L**ast ate, **E**vents leading to trauma and trauma **E**nvironment, **T**etanus prophylaxis.

ABG, arterial blood gas; bHCG, beta human chorionic gonadotropin; CNS, central nervous system; DPL, diagnostic peritoneal lavage; DRE, digital rectal examination; FAST, focused assessment with sonography in trauma; GCS, Glasgow Coma Scale; ICP, intracranial pressure; JVP, jugular venous pressure; NG, nasogastric.

Section 12 Airway, trauma and critical care

Chapter 64
Examination of the critically ill surgical patient

Petrut Gogalniceanu, Julia Niewiarowski and Vijay M. Gadhvi

History
- Age/sex
- Background medical problems
- Operation and postoperative day number
- Cause of admission to ITU, and ITU day number
- Current problems
- Recent imaging
- Events in last 24 hours

Examination
A Airway
- Airway: maintaining own airway, respiratory adjuncts, intubated
- FiO_2
- C-spine status

B Breathing
- Respiratory rate (RR)
- O_2 saturation percentage (sats)
- Ventilation method: self-ventilating/non-invasive ventilation (CPAP or BiPAP)/invasive ventilation
- Trachea position
- Surgical emphysema
- Air entry in lungs

Physical Examination for Surgeons, ed. Petrut Gogalniceanu, James Pegrum and William Lynn. Published by Cambridge University Press. © Cambridge University Press 2015.

- Abnormal breathing sounds
- Chest wall: chest drains and rib/sternum fractures
- ABG:

pH	HCO$_3$	Hb
pCO$_2$	Lactate	Na$^+$
pO$_2$	Base excess	K$^+$

- Chest x-ray (CXR)

C Cardiovascular

Pump:

- Heart rate and rhythm (HR) and blood pressure (BP)
- Mean arterial blood pressure (MAP) and central venous pressure (CVP)
- Jugular venous pressure (JVP) and carotid pulse
- Heart sounds: I + II + other
- Inotropes
- Peripheral oedema
- ECG
- Troponin and BNP[36]

Circuit:

- Full examination of pulses:
  - neck: carotid
  - upper: supraclavicular, axillary, brachial, radial, ulnar
  - central: aorta
  - lower: femoral, popliteal, dorsalis pedis (anterior tibial artery), tibialis posterior (posterior tibial artery)
- Peripheral perfusion: warmth and capillary refill time

Fluid:

- Vascular access: central, peripheral, intraosseous
- Evidence of external bleeding: urinary catheter, drains, stoma bags, rectal, vaginal or oral
- Evidence of internal bleeding (chest, abdomen, pelvis and long bones)

---

[36] Troponin: marker of myocardial ischaemia; BNP, brain natriuretic peptide: marker of heart failure.

D Neurological Deficit
- GCS
- Pupils: size and reaction to light and accommodation
- Limb movement and sensation (all four limbs)
- Cerebral function
- Sedation status
- Rashes/meningism

D Diabetes
- Blood sugar levels
- Insulin requirements
- Method of blood sugar control

D DVT prophylaxis
- Calves: swelling or tenderness
- Heparin or low-molecular-weight heparin: treatment vs. prophylaxis
- Venous compression devices (antiembolic stockings)

E Everything else (abdomen)
(see Chapter 4, *Examination of the abdomen*)
- Wounds and scars
- Abdominal distension, tenderness, peritonitis, organomegaly
- Stomas
- Hernias and abdominal wall

F Fluid balance
- In: oral, intravenous
- Out:
    - urine output per hour over last 1, 2 and 3 hours
    - drains, stomas, fistula, vomit, nasogastric aspirate, diarrhoea
    - blood loss
- Total balance in 24 hours

G Gastrointestinal
- Oral intake/NG feed
- Vomiting

- Bowel motility
- Liver function tests, amylase, albumin

H Haemorrhage
- Haemoglobin
- Platelets
- Clotting: INR/APTT ratio
- Blood/blood product transfusions

K Kidneys/potassium (K$^+$)
- Haemofiltration or dialysis
- Urea, creatinine, sodium and potassium, magnesium
- pH, lactate, base excess, bicarbonate
- Urine dipstick

L Lines: date of insertion, site infection, output/function
- Intravenous lines
- Arterial lines
- Nasogastric tubes
- Drains
- Catheters

M Medications
- Allergies
- Drugs/doses/duration/routes

N Nutrition
- Nutrition method: enteral vs. parenteral
- Phosphate, magnesium, Ca^{2+}

I Infections
- Temperature
- Localised infections/abscesses
- Antibiotic therapy
- Microscopy, culture and sensitivity: blood, urine, sputum, cerebrospinal fluid, drain or wound discharges
- Urine analysis

List of current problems
A → I

Action plan
A → I

Examination notes
What should be assessed together with the airway?
Airway assessment always involves assessment of the cervical spine status in trauma patients: immobilised or cleared of fractures (clinically or radiologically)

What are the different ventilation options?
- Self-ventilation (SV)
- Non-invasive ventilation (CPAP and BiPAP masks)
- Invasive ventilation (pressure/volume support via endotracheal tube or tracheostomy)

When are CPAP and BiPAP used?
- CPAP: type I respiratory failure (low pO_2, normal pCO_2)
- BiPAP: type II respiratory failure (low pO_2, high pCO_2)

> **Tip**
>
> Type I respiratory failure: one abnormal parameter
> Type II respiratory failure: two abnormal parameters

How can oxygen be delivered?
Nasal speculum, facemask, laryngeal mask, endotracheal tube or tracheostomy

What is the minimal urine output?
- Adults: minimum 0.5 ml/kg/h
- Children: minimum 1 ml/kg/h
- Also examine the colour/concentration of urine

> **Tip**
>
> For adults, the minimum urine output per hour (in ml) equals half their body weight (in kg).

> **Example**
>
> A 70 kg man should produce a minimum of 35 ml urine/hour.

What are the different nutritional options?
- Nil by mouth
- Oral intake: sips of water, clear fluids, liquid diet, soft diet, fat-free diet, normal diet
- Enteral nutrition via nasogastric or nasojejunal tubes or via feeding gastrostomy or jejunostomy
- Parenteral nutrition via a central line or long-term line

What are the main blood products that can be transfused?
Red blood cells (RBC), fresh frozen plasma (FFP), platelets, human albumin solution (HAS)

How is the GCS assessed in the intubated patient?
GCS assessment is typically carried out in the neurological intensive care environment, whilst withholding sedation. In this scenario verbal response (intubated) is marked as presence or absence of voice (0 or 1), and the maximum verbal response with an intubated patient is 1

$E = n/4$

$V = n/1$

$M = n/6$

Maximum total $= n/11$

Section 12: Airway, trauma and critical care

Chapter 65: Assessment of the airway for intubation

Julia Niewiarowski, Rajeev Mathew and Vijay M. Gadhvi

Checklist

WIPER
- Patient sitting at examiner's eye level

Physiological parameters

Look
- **General**: obese, pregnant, beard present, posture
- **Jaw**: receding mandible, mouth opening
- **Oral cavity**: swelling, vomit, tumour, infection, burns
- **Teeth**: prominent, loose
- **Face**: syndromes, acromegaly
- **Neck**: cervical spine immobility, scarring, masses

Feel
- **Neck**: masses

Move
- **Neck**: flexion/extension
- **Jaw**: opening

Physical Examination for Surgeons, ed. Petrut Gogalniceanu, James Pegrum and William Lynn. Published by Cambridge University Press. © Cambridge University Press 2015.

Special tests
- Mallampati score
- Wilson's score
- Interdental distance
- Thyromental distance
- Atlanto-occipital movement
- Mandibular protrusion

Examination notes

What is the OBESE mnemonic for predicting a difficult airway?

- **O** Obese
- **B** Bearded
- **E** Elderly (> 55 years old)
- **S** Snorers (suggesting sleep apnoea; syndromes pose additional difficulties)
- **E** Edentulous (no teeth)

What syndromes pose airway difficulties?

- Down's syndrome can indicate cervical instability and potential contraindication to neck hyperextension during intubation.
- Pierre–Robin and Treacher–Collins syndromes are associated with micrognathia, making direct laryngoscopy difficult.

What specific features do you look for in the examination of the airway?

- Asking the patient to open the mouth as wide as possible assesses the degree of mouth opening and also allows inspection of the mouth.
- Loose or prominent teeth should be assessed; these can obscure the view at laryngoscopy or even be dislodged and cause airway obstruction during intubation.
- Patients with acromegaly will have a large tongue and jaw. Large tongues are difficult to depress out of view and impair the visualisation of the glottis in direct laryngoscopy.
- Scarring of the neck can indicate previous trauma or radiotherapy. Both of these can mean tethering of internal airway structures and rigidity leading to poor views at laryngoscopy.

How is movement of the neck assessed?

Ask the patient to maximally extend the neck, and estimate the angle that the upper teeth have moved through from the neutral to the maximally extended position. Movement of less than 20° is associated with difficult intubation.

How can a difficult intubation be predicted?

1. **Mallampati test**: The patient sits with his or her head in the neutral position; the examiner's eye is level with the patient's mouth. The patient is asked to 'open your mouth as wide as you can, now stick out your tongue as much as you can.' There is no need for the patient to say 'aah'. Mouth opening is a predictor of difficult intubation if the patient has a Mallampati score of III or IV.
2. Wilson's score > 3.
3. **Interdental distance < 3 cm** (or < 2 finger breadths).
4. **Thyromental distance < 6.5 cm** – this is the measurement from the chin to the upper edge of the thyroid cartilage with the neck fully extended.
5. **Atlanto-occipital movement < 35°** of neck extension from neutral.
6. **Poor mandibular protrusion** – the lower incisors cannot be protruded to oppose the anterior surface of the upper incisors.

Section 12: Airway, trauma and critical care

Chapter 66: Assessment of the compromised airway

Julia Niewiarowski, Rajeev Mathew and Vijay M. Gadhvi

Checklist

WIPER
- C-spine immobilisation if indicated

Physiological parameters

Look
- Level of consciousness
- Cyanosis
- Abnormal respiratory movements
- Burns/injuries involving head and neck
- Foreign bodies/blood in the oral cavity

Listen
- Stridor
- Voice change
- Gurgling

Feel
- Air movement through nose/mouth
- Chest movement
- Airway reflexes

Physical Examination for Surgeons, ed. Petrut Gogalniceanu, James Pegrum and William Lynn. Published by Cambridge University Press. © Cambridge University Press 2015.

Examination notes

How do you prepare for an examination of the compromised airway?

- In trauma scenarios use ATLS principles with cervical spine control, using either triple immobilisation or in-line manual stabilisation.
- Ensure there is working suction and oxygen at the bedside.

What are the general observations to be made in the examination?

- Check the patency of the airway. Is there any sign of chest movement and air movement? If there is no air movement, you need to state that you will use simple airway manoeuvres to open the airway – i.e. chin lift/head tilt (avoided in the trauma patient) or a jaw thrust.
- Use an airway adjunct such as a Guedel or nasopharyngeal airway. Once you are satisfied that there is both air movement and chest movement, you can then observe the general appearance of the patient.
- Look for cyanosis, decreased level of consciousness and any obvious signs of trauma or foreign body in or around the airway. If a patient insists on sitting forwards and/or is drooling, this can be a sign of impending airway obstruction: the patient should not be laid flat, and there should be minimal manipulation of the airway.

What may be heard during the examination of a patient with a compromised airway?

- Stridor – a high-pitched sound caused by obstruction of the larynx or lower airway. Changes in the tone of voice may be a sign of airway swelling or vocal cord abnormality.
- Stertor – a low-pitched snoring sound caused by obstruction above the larynx.

How do you check the airway reflexes?

The two main reflexes which protect the lungs from being soiled are:

1. **Cough reflex**: can be severely impaired in comatosed states.
2. **Gag reflex**: can be tested by using a tongue depressor and gently stimulating the oropharynx.

In general, a patient with a head injury recording a GCS < 8 will not be able to maintain the reflexes needed to protect his or her own airway, and will need definitive airway protection with a cuffed endotracheal tube.

What are the causes of a compromised airway?

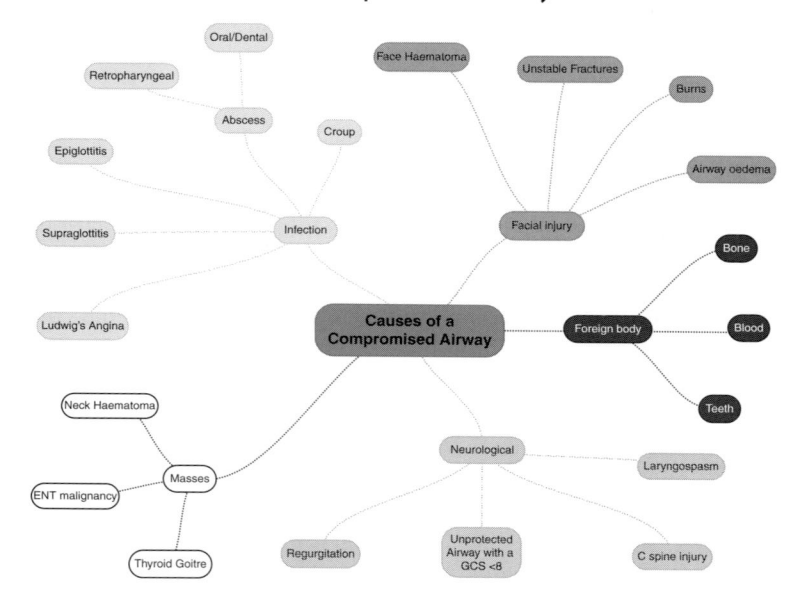

- **Causes of a Compromised Airway**
  - **Infection**
    - Oral/Dental
    - Retropharyngeal
    - Abscess
    - Croup
    - Epiglottitis
    - Supraglottitis
    - Ludwig's Angina
  - **Facial injury**
    - Face Haematoma
    - Unstable Fractures
    - Burns
    - Airway oedema
  - **Foreign body**
    - Bone
    - Blood
    - Teeth
  - **Masses**
    - Neck Haematoma
    - ENT malignancy
    - Thyroid Goitre
  - **Neurological**
    - Laryngospasm
    - Regurgitation
    - Unprotected Airway with a GCS <8
    - C spine injury

Section 12: Airway, trauma and critical care

Chapter 67: Examination of a tracheostomy

Julia Niewiarowski, Rajeev Mathew and Vijay M. Gadhvi

Checklist

WIPER
- Gloves/eye protection if handling the airway

Physiological parameters

Look
- Agitation
- Cyanosis/desaturation
- Respiratory rate
- Tube position
- Chest movement

Listen
- Air entry into chest
- Air leak around cuff

Feel
- Surgical emphysema
- Suction catheter passage

Examination notes

What do you look for in the initial observation of a tracheostomy?

- See-sawing chest movements are a sign of airway obstruction.
- Agitation, hypertension and tachycardia may be the first indicators that there could be a problem with the tracheostomy.
- Cyanosis and desaturation are late signs, and should not be relied on as the sole means of indicating a problem.
- Examine the tracheostomy tubing more carefully: most of the tube should be within the trachea via the stoma.

What are the various types of tracheostomy?

There are two ways of performing a tracheostomy:

1. **Percutaneous** – performed in ITU by intensivists/anaesthetists using the Seldinger technique with progressive dilatation over a guidewire.
2. **Surgical** – performed in the operating theatre under direct vision.

How do you assess whether a tracheostomy has become misplaced?

Observe the patient and auscultate the chest to hear any signs of air entry. If there is a leak around the tracheostomy cuff or stoma then this would normally be heard as a 'gurgling' sound or slow release of air when applying positive-pressure ventilation. If there is no air entry into the chest you should suspect that the tracheostomy has become displaced.

Index

Abbreviated Mental Test Score (AMTS), 326
abdomen
  anatomical divisions, 35
  bruits, 50–2
  distension, 42
  emergency checklist, 457
  hernia location, 39–41
  imaging, 47–8 *See also* abdominal x-ray
    CT, 48, 457–62
    MRI, 48
    transabdominal ultrasound, 47
  inspection, 34–60
  palpation, 34–7, 41–2
  percussion, 35
  skin changes, 38
    ecchymosis causes, 50
abdominal aortic aneurysm (AAA), 208–11, 227, 461, 463
  history, 209
  imaging, 211
  sign of imminent rupture, 464
abdominal incisions, 61–8
  classification, 68
abdominal pain
  anatomical origins, 43
  gynaecological causes, 53
  inflammation, 44
  non-surgical causes, 55
  surgical causes, 52
  urine tests, 46
  visceral pain, 43
abdominal scars, 61–8
  easily missed scars, 68
abdominal x-ray, 47, 396–8
  artefacts, 397
  bowel gas pattern, 397
  calcifications, 398
  extraluminal gas, 397
  soft tissues, 398
abducens nerve testing, 332
accessory nerve testing, 333
acellular dermal matrix (ADM), 94
Achilles tendon
  rupture assessment, 200
acromioclavicular joint (ACJ), 142
  injury, 419
  test, 147
adenocarcinoma, parotid gland, 313
adnexal fullness, 106
Adson's test, 218
airway assessment, 474, 480, 491–3
  for intubation, 491–3
airway management, 474
Allen's test, 215
AMPLET, 479
anaesthetic risk assessment, 21
anal examination, 99–100
  Goodsall's rule, 101
angiogram, lower limb, 471–2
ankle examination, 190–202
  causes of pain, 201
  movement assessment, 191, 195
  Ottawa rule, 194
  palpation, 191, 193–4
  skin changes, 192
  special tests, 191
ankle joint, 195, *See also* ankle examination
  fractures, 443
  range of movement, 196
ankle x-ray, 444–8
  anatomy, 444
ankle–brachial pressure index (ABPI), 234
  diabetic ulcers, 254
ankylosing spondylitis, 131

499

anosmia, 334
anterior cruciate ligament (ACL) injury, 184, 186
anterior drawer test
  ankle examination, 197
  knee examination, 148, 183
anterior tibial pulse, 227
anus examination, 99–101
aorta
  aneurysm. *See* abdominal aortic aneurysm (AAA); thoracic aortic aneurysm
  branches, 464
  CT examination, 463–8
  dissection, 464, 467
  endoleaks, 467
  endoprostheses, 464
  palpation, 45
aphasia, 327
apnoea test, 322
apprehension test, 148
arterial examination. *See also* abdominal aortic aneurysm (AAA); carotid artery examination
  lower limbs, 223–36
    arterial anatomy, 226
    bruits, 233
    Buerger's angle and test, 232
    bypass grafts, 228
    causes of ischaemia, 236
    causes of pain, 235
    investigations, 234
    neurological examination, 234
    skin changes, 223
    soft tissue changes, 224
    symptoms of disease, 225
    tests, 224
  upper limbs, 212–13
    Allen's test, 215
arteriovenous fistula, 86, 88, 246
  complications, 88
  steal syndrome, 88
ascites
  causes, 57
  shifting dullness, 58

auscultation, 11
  abdomen, 35
  cardiac examination, 265–6
  groin, 70
  thorax, 259
axilla, 91
axillobifemoral bypass, 211
axillounifemoral bypass, 211

Bartholin's gland, 106
Barton's fracture, 427, 431
basal cell carcinoma (BCC), 357
Battle's incision, 64
bedside observations, 6
Bell's phenomenon, 337
benign paroxysmal positional vertigo (BPPV), 278
Berry's sign, 312
biceps muscle test, 148
bicipital groove, 143
bladder, CT examination, 470
bleeding risk assessment, 21
Boas' sign, 49
bowel ischaemia, 397
bowel obstruction, 397
  causes, 56
  large bowel, 399, 460
  small bowel, 399, 460
brain CT, 451–4
brain death, 319–20
branchial cyst, 314
breast. *See also* mammography
  causes of lumps, 96
  chest x-ray and, 388
  focused systemic examination, 91
  implants, 93
  inspection, 90
  lump assessment, 90
  Paget's disease, 93
  palpation, 90
  post-mastectomy reconstruction, 94
  scars, 91
breast cancer screening, 408
Brudzinski's neck sign, 325

bruits, 50–2, 233
　carotid, 204, 206
Buerger's angle, 232
Buerger's test, 232
burns, 367–70
　acute, 368
　burn centre transfer criteria, 370
　depth estimation, 369
　life-threatening emergencies, 370
　management guidelines, 369
　size estimation, 370

callosities, 192
candidiasis, vaginal, 105
cardiac examination, 264–9
　cardiac scars, 267
　cardiac symptoms, 265
　differentiation of murmurs, 267
　preparation for, 265
carotid artery endarterectomy (CAE) scars, 204–5
carotid artery examination, 203–4
　bruits, 204
　　causes of, 206
　neurological deficit, 205
　　causes of, 206
　palpation, 203
　　carotid bifurcation, 204
　pulsatile neck mass causes, 207
　stenosis, 205
carotid–carotid bypass, 267
carotid–subclavian bypass, 216, 267
carpal fractures, 431
carpal tunnel compression, 380
　examination for, 380
cauda equina syndrome (CES) assessment, 346
CEAP classification, 239
cerebral perfusion assessment, 475
cervical lymphadenopathy, 259
cervical spine examination, 130–1, *See also* spine injury assessment
　bony contours, 132
　causes of cervical pain, 137
　initial observations, 131
　movement assessment, 132–3
　scars, 341
　Spurling's test, 133–4
　trauma patients, 474
cervical spine immobilisation, 474
cervical spine injuries, 138–9, 416
　common fractures, 416
　unstable fractures, 417
cervical spine x-ray, 416
　AP view, 415
　bone, 415
cervix examination, 106
chauffeur's fracture, 432
chest CT, 455–6
　airway, 455
　circulation and mediastinum, 456
　diaphragm, 456
　lungs, 456
chest drain, 258, 475
chest examination. *See* thorax examination
chest x-ray, 386–95
　abdominal pain and, 47
　airway, 387
　bones, 388
　breast, 388
　circulation, 388
　danger areas, 388
　diaphragm, 388
　foreign objects, 389
Chevrier's test, 242
chevron incision, 65
Chilaiditi's sign, 388
chondrodermatitis helicis nodularis, 274
chronic liver disease, signs of, 29
chronic venous disease, 239, *See also* venous system examination
chronic venous hypertension, 237
claudication, 18
　arterial versus neurogenic, 225
clay shoveler's fracture, 416
clonus, 345
closed kinetic chains, 128
cognitive function assessment, 326–7
Coleman block test, 196

Colles' fracture, 427, 431
colostomy, 80
common femoral artery assessment, 468
computed tomography (CT), 449–50
   abdomen, 48, 457–62
      extra-abdominal changes, 462
      intestines, 458, 460–1
      pelvic viscera, 458
      peritoneum, 458
      retroperitoneum, 458, 461–2
      upper abdominal organs, 458–60
   aorta, 463–8
   brain, 451–4
   chest, 451–4
   general principles, 459
   head, 456–9
   KUB (kidneys, ureter, bladder), 469–70
   lower limb angiogram, 471–2
   reconstruction, 450
   virtual colonoscopy, 450, 459
conductive hearing loss, 337
consciousness level assessment, 322–4, 477
consent form, 24–5
coracoclavicular ligament injury, 419
corns, 192
cortical localising features, 328
Cottle's manoeuvre, 283
cough reflex, 495
cough sign, 43–4
cranial nerve deficits, trauma patients, 303
cranial nerve examination, 333
critically ill patients, 11, 485–90
   abdomen examination, 487
   airway assessment, 485, 489
   blood transfusion, 490
   breathing and ventilation, 485, 489
   cardiovascular assessment, 486
   diabetes, 487
   DVT prophylaxis, 487
   fluid balance, 487
   gastrointestinal assessment, 487
   haemorrhage, 488
   history, 485
   infections, 488
   kidney function, 488
   lines, tubes and drains, 488
   nutrition, 488, 490
Crohn's disease, 27
crural vessels, 233
cubital tunnel compression, 380
Cullen's sign, 50
Cusco's speculum, 104
cyanotic limb causes, 221

DeBakey classification of aortic dissection, 467
deep venous thrombosis, 245
   prophylaxis in critically ill patients, 487
dental examination, 305, *See also* intra-oral examination
   dental occlusion, 305
   relevance to nose and sinus examination, 285
   tooth notation, 304
dermatome testing, 342, 345
desmoid tumours, 40
diabetes
   arterial investigations, 234
   critically ill patients, 487
dial test, 185
diaphragm, 388, 456
DIEP (deep inferior epigastric artery perforator) flap, 95
digital rectal examination, 76, 100
   cauda equina syndrome assessment, 346
diplopia, 336
Dix–Hallpike manoeuvre, 278
Dolan's lines, 412
dorsalis pedis pulse, 227
drug history (DH), 17
Dunphy's sign, 43
Dupuytren's contracture, 375
   scars, 376
dysphasia assessment, 327

ear examination, 271–80, 297
   flexible nasendoscopy, 277
   hearing tests, 272, 276

otoscopy, 271, 274
patient positioning, 272
pinna abnormalities, 273
Ehlers–Danlos syndrome, 361
elbow examination, 152–3
special tests, 153
elbow x-ray, 424–5
anatomy, 424
bony ossification centres in children, 425
fractures, 424–5
elephant trunks of Rogers, 413
Elevated Arm Stress Test (EAST), 220
endovascular aneurysm repair (EVAR), 211, 467
end-stage renal failure, 85
epididymis, 114
palpation, 114–15
epididymo-orchitis, 114
epigastric mass causes, 59
Eustachian tube, 285
extradural haematoma (EDH), 452–3
eyes
examination, 296
movement tests, 336
peripheral stigmata of disease, 28
reflex testing, 334
thyroid status examination, 309–10

FABER test, 157, 170
facial examination, 292–4
bones, 298
midface fractures, 302
facial nerve testing, 333
upper versus lower motor neuron pathology, 336
facial x-ray, 409–13
family history, 17
femoral canal, 74
femoral cut down, 76
incisions, 76, 211
femoral fractures, 434
neck fractures, 435
femoral nerve tension test, 158
femoral pulses, 211, 226

fever, differential diagnosis, 331
fibula fractures, 443
finger assessment, 373
deformities, 375
finger clubbing, 256
causes, 32
fitness for surgery, 21–2
Fitzpatrick classification of skin colour, 357
flaps, 362–6
classification, 363–4
free flaps, 365
common cutaneous donor sites, 365
common muscle donor sites, 365
reasons for, 365
types of, 364
flexible nasolaryngopharyngoscopy, 288
fluoroscopy, 384, 398
foot x-ray, 444–8
forearm x-ray. *See* wrist and forearm x-ray
fracture management, 12
Froment's sign, 379
full-thickness skin grafts (FTSG), 363

gag reflex, 337, 495
gait, 121, 123, 128–9
abnormalities, 345
ankle examination, 190
cervical spine examination, 131
gait cycle, 128
hip examination, 162, 164
knee examination, 175
lumbar spine examination, 154–5
thoracic spine examination, 131
typical patterns, 123
vestibular function assessment, 337
Galeazzi fracture, 427
Garden classification, 436
Gardner's syndrome, 40
gastrointestinal disease, peripheral stigmata, 27
Gerber's lift-off test, 146
Glasgow Coma Scale (GCS), 323, 477
intubated patients, 490
glossopharyngeal nerve testing, 333

golfer's elbow, 153
Goodsall's rule, 101
grafts, 364–8
Grey Turner's sign, 50
groin
   anatomy, 74
   causes of lumps, 77
   causes of pain, 116
   inspection, 69–79
   preparation for examination, 70
   scars, 76
gynaecological examination, 105–6
   digital bimanual examination, 103
   history, 103
   pudendum inspection, 102–3
   speculum examination, 103–4
gynaecomastia causes, 96

haematuria causes, 111
haemodialysis access. *See* renal access
haemoptysis causes, 260
haemothorax, 475
   causes, 261
hands, 371–82
   clawing, 381
   deformities, 375
   motor nerves, 372
   peripheral nerve examination, 377
   peripheral stigmata of disease, 27
   scars, 374
   sensory nerves, 372
   skin changes, 371
   special tests, 373
   thyroid status examination, 309
hangman's fracture, 416
Hawkins–Kennedy test, 147
head CT, 456–9
head trauma, 297, *See also* brain CT
   complications, 330
   CT indications, 324
   hospital discharge criteria, 325
headache
   differential diagnosis, 331
   ophthalmoscopy role, 335

hearing loss
   conductive, 280
   sensorineural, 280
hearing tests, 272, 276
heart examination. *See* cardiac examination
heart failure causes, 269
hepatomegaly causes, 56
hernias, 74
   classification, 79
   cough sign, 44
   direct, 75
   femoral, 74
   indirect, 75
   inguinal, 74–5
      scrotal, 75
   strangulated, 75
Hesselbach's triangle, 75
Hill–Sachs deformity, 418
hip examination, 162–74
   bone, 163
   causes of pain, 173
   movement assessment, 163, 166
      abduction, 168
      adduction, 168
      causes of reduced movement, 174
      extension, 168
      hip rotation, 167
      range of movement, 166
      resisted movements, 168
   skin, 162
   soft tissues, 163
   special tests, 163
hip x-ray, 433–6
history, 16–17
hoarseness, 304
hockey stick incision, 66
Hoffmann's sign, 343
Holmes–Adie pupil, 334
Homans' sign, 246
Horner's syndrome, 256
Howship–Romberg sign, 49
hydrocoele, 75, 114
hypertrophic scarring, 361
hypoglossal nerve testing, 333

ileostomy, 80–1
iliac fossa mass, 85
    causes, 59
impingement sign, 170
infective colitis, 18
information provision, 25–6
    explanation of procedure, 26
infrainguinal pulses, 225
infraspinatus muscle test, 145
inguinal canal, 71–4
inguinal hernia, 74–5
    repair scars, 76
    scrotal, 75
intestinal ischaemia, 461
intra-oral examination, 295–6, *See also dental examination*
    bimanual examination, 297
    investigations, 306
    maxilla tests, 302
    symptoms sought, 296
intubation
    airway assessment, 491–2
    difficult airway prediction, 492–3
investigations, 8
ischaemia severity, 235

jaundice causes, 33
Jefferson's fracture, 415
joint examination, 121–7, *See also specific joints*
    bones, 124–5
    limb measurements, 124
    movement assessment, 125–6
    skin, 124–5
    soft tissues, 124–5
    special tests, 126
jugulovenous pressure (JVP), 265, 476

Kehr's sign, 49
keloid scarring, 361
Kernig's sign, 325
kidney, CT examination, 469
Klippel–Trenaunay–Weber syndrome, 246
knee examination, 175–89
    bone, 175–6
    causes of pain, 187
    effusions, 178
        causes, 178, 189
    ligaments and menisci, 178, 181–5
        collateral ligaments, 181
        cruciate ligaments, 183–5
        meniscal tests, 182
    movement assessment, 176, 178
        causes of reduced movement, 188
    patella, 177
    patellar tracking assessment, 180
    skin, 175
    soft tissues, 175–6
    special tests, 176
knee x-ray, 437–43
    anatomy, 437
    easily missed injuries, 443
    fibula fractures, 443
    indications, 443
    intra-articular fractures, 437
    patella fractures, 443
    tibial plateau fractures, 443
Kocher's incision, 65

Lachman's test, 184
Lanz incision, 65
laparoscopic port scars, 67
large bowel obstruction, 399, 460
laryngopharyngoscopy, 288
lateral thoracolumbar incision, 66
LD (latissimus dorsi) flap, 95
Le Fort facial fracture classification, 302
Ledderhose's disease, 375
leg length measurement, 124
    discrepancy assessment, 165
leukoplakia, genital, 105
limb weakness causes, 351
line position, 394
lingual sulci, 304
Lisfranc injury, 445
liver
    abscess, 459
    cirrhosis, 459
    metastases, 459

lower limb biomechanical assessment, 128
lower limb CT angiogram, 471–2
lower limb neurology, 136
lower limb pulses, 225, 227, *See also* arterial examination
　anatomical landmarks, 226
lucid interval, 325
lumbar spine examination, 154–61
　cafe au lait patch relevance, 156
　causes of pain, 161
　flexion assessment, 156
　hairy patch relevance, 156
　initial observations, 155
　movement assessment, 155–6
　　causes of reduced movement, 160
　neurological assessments, 157–9
　special tests, 155
lumbosacral tension assessment, 158
lunate dislocation, 426
lunate–perilunate dislocation, 431
lung examination. *See* thorax examination
lymph node palpation, thyroid status examination, 310
lymphadenopathy causes, 315

magnetic resonance imaging (MRI), abdomen, 48
Maisonneuve fracture, 195, 443
malignant melanoma (MM), 356
Mallampati test, 493
mammography, 404–8
　breast cancer screening, 408
　breast mass density, 408
　breast tissue, 405
　calcification, 405, 408
　radiological signs of malignancy, 407
　skin changes, 405
mandibular fractures, 410
March fracture, 445
Marcus Gunn pupil, 334
Marjolin's ulcer, 357
maxillary fractures, 302, 410
McBurney's incision, 65
McMurray's test, 182

median nerve compression, 380
median nerve injury, 381
meningism assessment, 325–6
　causes of meningeal irritation, 326
Mercedes Benz incision, 65
metastatic cancer signs, 28–9
microtia, 273
midline laparotomy, 64
Monteggia fracture, 427
Morton's neuroma, 199
Murphy's sign, 49
muscle power grading, 342
myotome testing, 342, 345

nasal septal haematoma, 301
neck examination, 28, 307–17
　anterior triangle of the neck, 312
　causes of lumps, 316
　levels of the neck, 314
　neck lump, 310
　posterior triangle of the neck, 313
neck trauma, 297
Neer's test, 148
nerve root lesions, 382
nerve tension tests, 158
neurological examination
　focal, 332–52
　global, 319–31
neurological screen, 155
nipple discharge, 97
nose examination, 281–7, 297
　alar collapse, 283
　external examination, 281
　internal examination, 282, 284
　　nasal endoscopy, 284
　nasal mass causes, 287
　septal perforation causes, 286
nystagmus, 278

obturator sign, 49
oculocephalic reflex, 322
oculomotor nerve testing, 332
oedematous limb causes, 222
olfactory nerve function, 334
onycholysis, 312

open kinetic chains, 128
ophthalmoscopy, 335
optic nerve testing, 332
oral examination. *See* intra-oral examination
orbital blow-out fracture, 302, 410
orthopantomogram (OPG), 305
osteoarthritis, 376
  radiological features, 385
osteomyelitis, 410
otitis media with effusion, 277
otoscopy, 271, 274
Ottawa rules, 194, 443
ovarian cysts, 106

Paget's disease of the breast, 93
Paget–Schroetter disease, 220
palpation, 10–11
  abdomen, 34–7, 41–2
  aorta, 45
  arterial
    abdominal aortic aneurysm, 208–9
    carotid artery, 203–4
    femoral pulses, 211
    lower limbs, 224
    popliteal arteries, 211
    upper limbs, 212
  breast, 90
  face, 293
    facial bones, 301
  groin, 69–76
  gynaecological examination, 106
  hands, 371
  hip, 166
  lymph nodes, 310
  neck, 294, 303, 308
  nose, 282–3
  oral examination, 296–7
  pelvis, 45
  penis, 109–10
  scrotum, 112, 114
  shoulder, 142
  spine, 132, 156
  spleen, 45
  stoma, 81
  thorax, 259
  throat examination, 288
  venous examination, 238
Pancoast's tumour, 256
pancreatitis, 460
papilloedema, 335
Parkes–Weber syndrome, 246
parotid gland
  masses, 304
past medical history (PMH), 16
past surgical history (PSH), 16
patella
  apprehension test, 180
  bulge test, 178
  fractures, 443
  tap test, 178
  tracking assessment, 180
peau d'orange, 93
pelvic compression test, 159
pelvic distraction test, 159
pelvis
  easily missed injuries, 435
  fractures, 433, 435
  x-ray, 433–6
Pemberton's test, 312
penis examination 109–11
  causes of lesions, 111
  history, 110
perforator veins, 240
pericardial rub causes, 269
perilunate dislocation, 426
perioperative checks, 13
peripheral arterial disease, 254, *See also* arterial examination
  symptoms, 225
peripheral nervous system examination
  lower limbs, 344–5
  upper limbs, 341
    hands, 377, 379
peripheral stigmata of disease, 7, 27–33, *See also specific diseases*
peritonitis, 44
  classification, 44
  cough sign, 43
PermCath, 88

peroneal pulse, 227
Perthe's test, 245
pes anserinus palpation, 177
pes cavus, 192
  causes, 192
pes planus, 192, 195
  causes, 192
Peyronie's disease, 110, 375
Pfannenstiel incision, 66
Phalen's manoeuvre, 380
pharyngeal pouch, 314
phlegmasia caerulea dolens, 240
Pierre–Robin syndrome, intubation and, 492
pinna abnormalities, 273
pivot shift test, 185
pleomorphic adenoma, parotid gland, 313
pneumobilia, 397
pneumoperitoneum, 397
pneumothorax, 475
  causes, 262
popliteal fossa masses, 177
popliteal pulse, 227
portal hypertension, 459
portal vein gas, 397
posterior cruciate ligament injury assessment, 183
posterior drawer test, 183
posterior tibial nerve compression, 199
posterior tibial pulse, 227
postoperative assessment, 13–15
preauricular sinuses, 273
pregnancy test, 46
presenting complaint, 18
  assessment, 19
  history, 16
  orthopaedic, 18
pronator drift, 342
prostatic signs, 101
proximal fibula palpation, 195
pseudopneumoperitoneum, 397
psoas sign, 49
pudendum
  causes of masses, 107
  inspection, 102–3

pulmonary symptoms, 256
pulses. See lower limb pulses; *specific pulses*
pulse volume recording (PVR), 234
pupil abnormality causes, 340
pupillary light reflex, 334

quadriceps muscle assessment, 158

radiculopathies, 382
radioulnar dislocation, 431
radius anatomy, 432
radius fractures, 427
radius fractures, 427, 431
rectal bleeding, 48
renal access 86–7
renal angle tenderness, 50
renal mass
  causes, 60
  versus splenomegaly, 46
renal tract pathologies, 461
renal transplant, 86
  features of transplanted kidney, 87
retroperitoneum, 461–2
  vascular anatomy changes, 461
rheumatoid arthritis, 376
right iliac fossa pain, 44
Rigler's sign, 397
Rinne's test, 276, 337
Romberg's test, 337, 346
roof top incision, 65
Roos' test, 219
rotator cuff, 144
  muscle tests, 144
Rovsing's sign, 49
Rutherford Morison inicison, 65

sacroiliac joint examination, 154–61
  palpation, 156
salpingitis, 106
saphenofemoral junction (SFJ), 241
scaphoid fractures, 427
scapholunate dissociation, 426, 431
scapular winging, 142
scarf test, 147
scars, 359–61

abdominal, 61, 68
breast, 91
cardiac surgery, 267
carotid artery endarterectomy, 204–5
cervical spine, 341
classification, 361
groin, 76
hand, 374, 376
hernia repair, 76
hypertrophic scarring, 361
Schober's test, 156
sciatic nerve stretch test, 171
sciatic nerve tension test, 158
scrotum
  causes of pain, 120
  inspection, 112–14
  mass, 113–14
  palpation, 112, 114
Segond fracture, 437
seizures, causes of, 329
Semon's law, 290
sensorineural hearing loss, 337
sentinel lymph node biopsy (SLNB), 93
serratus anterior muscle assessment, 144
shock, 476
shoulder examination, 140–51
  bone, 140–1
  causes of pain, 151
  impingement tests, 147
  individual muscle tests, 144
  initial observations, 142
  instability assessment, 148
  movement assessment, 141, 143
  skin, 140
  soft tissues, 140
shoulder joint, 142, *See also* shoulder examination
  abduction failure causes, 144
  range of movement, 143
    causes of reduced movement, 150
  rotator cuff, 144
    muscle tests, 144
shoulder x-ray, 418–23
  acromioclavicular joint injury, 419
  anatomy, 418

coracoclavicular ligament injury, 419
dislocation, 418, 423
views, 418
sialography, 306
Sims' speculum, 104
Simmonds–Thompson test, 200
sinusitis, 410
Sister Mary Joseph nodule, 48
skin
  abdomen, 34
    pathological changes, 38
  colour changes, 10
  examination, 355–60
  face, 292
  hands, 371
  inspection, 9
  joints, 124–5
  lower limb arterial examination, 223
  lumps and lesions, 353–4
    benign lesions, 356
    description of, 356
    malignant lesions, 355
skin grafts. *See* grafts
small bowel obstruction, 399, 460
Smith's fracture, 427, 432
social history, 17
Speed's test, 148
spinal cord
  compression causes, 351
  injury management, 348
spine injury assessment, 138
  clinical clearance, 138–9
  radiographic clearance, 139
spleen
  palpation, 45
splenomegaly
  causes, 57
  versus left renal mass, 46
split-thickness skin grafts (STSG), 363
Spurling's test, 133–4
squamous cell carcinoma (SCC), 357
Stanford classification of aortic dissection, 467
steal syndrome, 88

Stensen's duct, 304
stoma, 80–3
   complications, 80, 82
   definition and types, 81
   palpation, 81
   scars, 80
stork test, 157
straight leg test, 157
stridor, 495
subacromial impingement, 144
subarachnoid haemorrhage (SAH), 452–3
subdural haematoma (SDH), 452–3
subscapularis muscle test, 146
superior labrum anterior to posterior (SLAP) tears, 149
superior vena cava (SVC) obstruction, 257
   causes, 261
   differential diagnosis, 261
supra-aortic pulses, 225
supraspinatus muscle
   tear, 144
   test, 145
surgical consent, 24–5
surgical consultation, written communication of, 22–3
   example, 23–4
surgical emphysema causes, 263
surgical management, 11
   operation structure, 12
surgical risk assessment, 21
surgical signs, 49

talar tilt test, 198
teeth. *See* dental examination
telangiectasia, 283, 357
tennis elbow, 153
teres minor muscle test, 145
Terry Thomas sign, 426, 431
Terson's syndrome, 335
testicular atrophy causes, 119
testicular cancer, 114–15
testicular torsion, 115
testis, 114
   palpation, 114–15

Thessaly test, 182
thigh thrust test, 159
Thomas's test, 169
thoracic aortic aneurysm, 216, 463
thoracic aortic arch aneurysms, 216
thoracic outlet syndrome (TOS), 216
   areas of compression, 217
   causes, 217
   imaging, 220
   provocation tests, 213, 218–20
thoracic spine examination, 130–1
   initial observations, 131
   movement assessment, 132–3
thorax examination, 255–63
   thoracic scars, 257, 260
throat examination, 288–91
   asymmetrical tonsil causes, 291
   laryngopharyngoscopy, 288
   vocal cord immobility causes, 291
Thudicum's speculum, 284
thumb assessment, 373
thunderclap headache, 330
thyroid mass investigation, 313
thyroid status examination, 308–9
   history, 312
   lymph node palpation, 310
   specific examination points, 310
tibial plateau fractures, 443
Tinel's sign, 380
Tinel's tap test, 199
tinnitus, 277
toe–brachial pressure index (TBPI), 234
tongue, 28, 304
tooth notation, 304
tourniquet test, 243
toxic megacolon, 460
trachea, 387, 455
tracheal deviation causes, 263
tracheostomy examination, 497–8
   types of tracheostomy, 498
TRAM (transverse rectus abdominis myocutaneous) flap, 94–5
transverse abdominal incision, 65
trapezius muscle assessment, 144
trauma patients, 11, 297, 483–94

airway, 473–5, 480
AMPLET, 479
breathing and ventilation, 475
cervical spine, 473–5
circulation and haemorrhagic control, 475–7
cranial nerve deficits, 303
disability assessment, 477–8
exposure and environment, 478
neurological deficit, 477
physiological parameters, 474
trauma severity assessment, 480
treatment principles, 478
Treacher–Collins syndrome, intubation and, 492
treatment principles, 11–13
Trendelenburg's test (orthopaedic), 164
Trendelenburg's test (vascular), 242
trigeminal nerve testing, 333
  nerve divisions, 336
tripod fractures, 410
triquetral fracture, 431
trochlear nerve testing, 332
Troisier's sign, 48
tympanic membrane, 274
  perforations, 275
  retraction pockets, 275

ulcers, 247–54
  aetiology elucidation, 248, 250
  arterial, 254
  causes of, 249
  diabetic, 253–4
  foot, 192
  genital, 105, 108
  Marjolin's ulcer, 357
  toes, 18
  venous, 254
ulnar nerve compression, 380–1
ulnar nerve injury, 381
ulnar styloid fracture, 432
ultrasound, transabdominal, 47
undescended testis, 75
Unterberger's test, 279

urine tests, 46
urostomy, 80–1
uterus
  palpation, 106
  prolapse, 106

vagina
  causes of masses, 107
  digital manual examination, 104–5
  prolapse, 106
  speculum examination, 103–4
vagus nerve testing, 333, 337
Vancouver Scar Scale (VSS), 361
varicocoele, 115
varicose veins, 237, 253, 265, *See also* venous system examination
  arterial system assessment, 240
VasCath, 88
vas deferens, 114
venous system examination. *See also* varicose veins
  CEAP classification, 239
  lower limbs, 237–46
    arteriovenous fistula, 246
    disease processes, 240
    skin complications, 237
    superficial vein anatomy, 239
    tests, 238, 241–6
venous thromboembolism (VTE) risk assessment, 21
vertebral artery insufficiency, 134
vertigo, 277
vestibular function assessment, 337
vestibulocochlear nerve testing, 333
vestibulo-ocular reflex, 322
Virchow's node, 48
visual field assessment, 334
  deficit causes, 338
vital signs, 5

Waddell's signs, 134
Warthin's tumour, 313
Weber's test, 276, 337
Wharton's duct, 304

wrist and forearm x-ray, 425
  easily missed injuries, 431
  lines, 426
  radius fractures, 427
  scaphoid injuries, 427
  subluxations/dislocations, 427
wrist movement assessment, 373
wrist x-ray, 426–8
written communication of surgical consultation, 22–3

x-ray
  abdominal, 47, 396–403
  ankle, 444–8
  cervical spine, 414–17
  chest, 47, 386–95
  different densities, 383
  elbow, 424–5
  facial, 409–13
  fluoroscopy, 384, 398
  foot, 444–8
  hip, 433–6
  joints, 122
  knee, 437–43
  orthopaedic radiograph description rules, 384
  pelvis, 433–4
  plain film radiology, 383–5
    basic checks, 383
    osteoarthritis, 385
  shoulder, 418–19
  wrist and distal forearm, 426–32

zygomatic arch fracture, 302, 410